SEMINARS IN DYSPHAGIA

Edited by **Renée Speyer and Hans Bogaardt**

Seminars in Dysphagia
http://dx.doi.org/10.5772/58665
Edited by Renée Speyer and Hans Bogaardt

Contributors

Alfredo M.B. De Paula, Carlos Henrique F Camargo, Helio Teive, Edna Márcia Abdulmassih, Rosane Sampaio Santos, Pedro Melo, Catiuscia Greco, Livia Scelza, Agnaldo Lopes, Vishal Shelat, Garvi Pandya, Elizabeth Ward, Rebecca Louise Nund, Nerina Scarinci, Bena Cartmill, Hisao Hiraba, Hadeer Akram AbdulRazzaq, Syed Azhar Syed Sulaiman, Takashi Sawai, Akihisa Kamataki, Miwa Uzuki, Eddy Dejaeger, Hiroshi Makino, Daniele Farneti, Elisabetta Genovese, Nicoll Kenny

Published by InTech

Janeza Trdine 9, 51000 Rijeka, Croatia

Publishing Process Manager Ana Pantar

Technical Editor InTech DTP team

Cover InTech Design team

First published August, 2015

Printed in Croatia

Additional hard copies can be obtained from orders@intechopen.com

Seminars in Dysphagia, Edited by Renée Speyer and Hans Bogaardt

p. cm.

ISBN 978-953-51-2151-0

For EU product safety concerns :
IN TECH d.o.o., Prolaz Marije Krucifikse Kozulić 3, 51000 Rijeka, Croatia,
info@intechopen.com or visit our website at intechopen.com.

Meet the editors

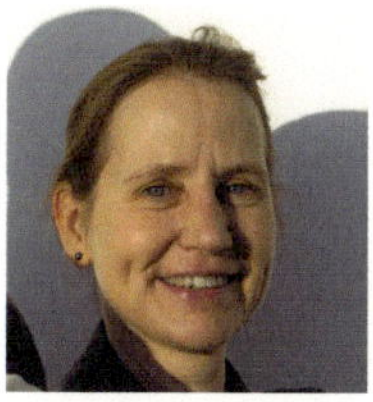

Dr Renée Speyer is currently employed as Associate Professor at James Cook University in Australia where she is the Head of Speech Pathology. After graduating as a speech pathologist in the Netherlands, she earned master degrees in Speech and Language Pathology, Epidemiology and Health Professions Education and completed a PhD in 2004. Dr Speyer's career included working as a speech pathologist in different health care settings and in academia. Over the last two decades Dr Speyer has developed an international research track record in the field of oropharyngeal dysphagia. She is currently undertaking research projects both nationally and internationally involving clinimetrics, instrument development, and developing evidenced based interventions in allied health for different disability population groups. She published over 50 internationally peer-reviewed research articles, mainly in the field of oropharyngeal dysphagia.

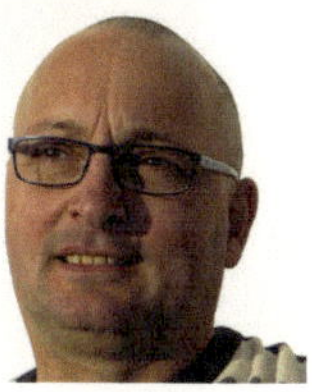

Hans Bogaardt is a Speech Pathologist and Clinical Epidemiologist, who is specialized in assessment and treatment of dysphagia. Currently Hans works as Lecturer in Speech Pathology at The University of Sydney, Australia. Hans completed his undergraduate degree in Speech Pathology at the Leidse Hogeschool in Leiden, the Netherlands and worked for several years in Germany and the Netherlands in different hospitals and rehabilitation centers. In 2004 he obtained his master's degree in Evidence Based Practise / Clinicial Epidemiology at the University of Amsterdam. In the following years Hans worked as a clinician and researcher at the Department of Otolaryngology of the Academic Medical Center in Amsterdam. In 2009 he finished his PhD with a thesis titled 'Current Aspects of Assessment and Treatment of Dysphagia'. Next to his teaching, Hans is involved in several research projects looking into assessment and treatment of swallowing disorders in a range of different patient populations.

Contents

Preface

In the last decades, the assessment and treatment of dysphagia has become an increasingly important part of the work of speech pathologists in clinical setting. As the general population ages, this population is confronted with an increase in disease and consequent the sequalae of these diseases. Also, changes in lifestyle have contributed largely to an increase in medical conditions and the incidence of certain diseases.

These ever changing situations in the general population, and subsequent in health care, has without a doubt led to a shift of practice for speech pathologists. In most countries in the 1990s, the care for dysphagic patients was only a part of the daily activities of a speech pathologist working in a clinical setting. Whereas nowadays, worldwide speech pathologists have a full-time job in managing swallowing disorders in a range of different settings, ranging from ICUs to rehabilitation centers to even private practices.

Since the 1990s, the quality of care has increased for dysphagic patients as researchers have gained more insight in factors that lead to swallowing problems and therapy has become more targeted, improving the outcomes. Although the quality of treatment and the research have increased, there is still a lot unknown about dysphagia and outcomes can still be improved. Fortunately as the world becomes more and more a global community, clinicians and researchers are now able to attend conferences on dysphagia in every corner of the world and share their ideas and thoughts. Nowadays there are several international organizations that focus solely on swallowing and swallowing disorders and in the last decades the dysphagia community has grown into a global family of researchers and clinicians.

This book reflects the current international status of dysphagia research, with contributions by esteemed colleagues from (in alphabetical order) Australia, Belgium, Brazil, Italy, Japan, Malaysia, Singapore and South-Africa. The book focuses on anatomy, assessment of dysphagia and the management of dysphagia in specific populations. Contributions are written in such a way, that they might help clinicians in their clinical decision making, by providing detailed background information or present novel approaches to assessment and treatment.

It was a pleasure to work with each of the authors and we are thankful that they participated with their original work. We hope this book will contribute to the knowledge of clinicians about swallowing disorders and will help them further to improve treatment outcomes and patients' quality of life.

August 2015,

Renée Speyer
Department of Otorhinolaryngology and Head and Neck Surgery
Leiden University Medical Center
Leiden, The Netherlands;
College of Healthcare Sciences,
James Cook University
Townsville, Queensland, Australia

Hans Bogaardt
Faculty of Health Sciences,
The University of Sydney,
Sydney, Australia

Section 1

Anatomy and (Patho-)Physiology

Chapter 1

Anatomical and Physiopathological Aspects of Oral Cavity and Oropharynx Components Related to Oropharyngeal Dysphagia

Ludmilla R. Souza, Marcos V. M. Oliveira,
John R. Basile, Leandro N. Souza, Ana C. R. Souza,
Desiree S. Haikal and Alfredo M. B. De-Paula

Additional information is available at the end of the chapter

http://dx.doi.org/10.5772/60766

1. Introduction

Dysphagia (from the Greek words *dys,* difficulty, and *phagein,* to eat) is a congenital or acquired swallowing disorder that has structural and functional causes that promote a delay or difficult in the passage of food and liquids from the oral cavity to stomach. Remarkably, dysphagia is an underestimated neuromuscular disorder, although its consequences frequently are associated with high rates of morbidity and mortality. Estimates of oropharyngeal dysphagia prevalence vary broadly (ranging from 10% to 80%) according to screening methods used and especially the type of study population [1-3]. Dysphagia exhibits a multifactorial etiology, with partipation of exogenous and endogenous factors. The most common causes of dysphagia are divided into the categories of iatrogenic (such as patients with previous history of intubation, tracheostomy, or nasogastric feeding tubes, or a history of infection or metaboic disorders), medications (such as polypharmacy, depressors of the central nervous system, anticholinergics, sympathomimetics, and diuretic drugs) neurological diseases (such as stroke, dementia, amyotrophic lateral sclerosis, Parkinson's disease, Alzheimer's disease, extrapyramidal disorders), neuromuscular (such as myasthenia gravis and inflammatory myopathies), or structural obstruction (such as Zenker's diverticulum, oropharyngeal tumors, and factors that causes extrinsic compression of the upper aerodigestive tract), as well as other causes [4-7]. Clinically, dysphagia might be classified into three major types: oropharyngeal dysphagia, esophageal dysphagia, and functional dysphagia. Oropharyngeal dysphagia is the inability to initiate the act of swallowing, whereas esophageal dysphagia is the perception of difficulty of passing solids or liquids from the throat to the stomach. Functional dysphagia refers to a condition in which some patients complain of dysphagia but do not have an organic cause for a swallowing disorder. The most common symptoms of oropharyngeal dysphagia include difficulty in manipulating food, problems with saliva production, and difficulty in chewing the food and swallowing the bolus (a soft mass of chewed food mixed with saliva at the point of swallowing), and an associated impaired quality of life. Frequently, patients with oropharyngeal dysphagia exhibit a series of complications such as nasal regurgitation, coughing, suffocating, gurgle or wet voice after swallowing, unexplained weight loss, anxiety, depression, low-tract respiratory infections and, it's most serious complication, aspiration pneumonia. Problems with social isolation and poor quality of life are a common feature of individuals with dysphagia. Notably, the occurrence of dysphagia is associated with high mortality rate [8].

The different parts of the oral cavity and oropharynx are made up of several cell types and tissues (nerves, fibrovascular, cartilaginous, lining and salivary glandular epithelia, and smooth and striated muscles) along with mineralized tissues (enamel and dentin of the teeth and bones) [8, 9]. Notably, there is an intimate relationship between dysphagia and anatomical, functional, and regulation disturbances of oral cavity and oropharynx components related to physiological salivation, chewing, and swallowing. Salivation depends of the anatomical and functional integrities of the minor and major salivary glands. The saliva lubricates the oral cavity and oropharynx, and an adequate salivary flow assists the initial digestive process by reducing the bolus size of food, begins the enzymatic digestion of some types of carbohydrates, and provides moisture and lubrication of the food particles in order to facilitate the swallowing mechanism, i.e., the movement of the bolus from oropharynx to esophagus [10]. Chewing and swallowing are likely complex and well-coordinated motor programs, combined together as a sequence. During chewing, the food particles are reduced in size and consistency. Chewing is highly dependent of an efficient participation of the teeth, a mineralized tissue whose occlusal surfaces are frequently used for cut off, rip, knead, and grind food during feeding. Moreover, the masticatory muscles have a pivotal role in establishing the muscle strength necessary for the implementation of chewing activity in order to manipulate and grind the food [11-13]. During swallowing two essential and vital functions must be executed: bolus transport and airway protection. After adequate bolus preparation, it needs to be swallowed through an involuntary transport process from the oral cavity and pharynx to the esophagus without allowing the entry of food particles or liquid in the respiratory trac [14, 15]. Together, salivation, chewing, and swallowing, therefore, plays a critical role in alimentary events, allowing food to be initially processed, formed into a bolus, and subsequently transported in the digestive system. Individuals with health problems related to these mechanisms often present with complaints of oropharyngeal dysphagia.

In this present chapter, we will highlight a series of morphological and physiological aspects related to the oral cavity and oropharynx. Moreover, we will discuss the physiopathological aspectos of the salivation, chewing, and swallowing mechanisms in order to allow to health professionals to obtain essential knowledge for management of oropharyngeal dysphagia.

2. Anatomical and functional aspects of the oral cavity and oropharynx

2.1. The oral cavity and the oropharynx

Anatomically, the oral cavity or mouth is an organ of the digestive system that is anteriorly delimited by the lips, posteriorly by the oropharynx, superiorly by the hard and soft palates, and inferiorly by the tongue (anterior 2/3) and floor of the mouth, and surrounded by a buccal mucosa that lines the cheeks, along with the upper and lower teeth and periodontum. The upper teeth are embedded in the maxilla and the lower teeth are embedded in the mandible, which articulates with the temporal bones of the skull. The oropharynx is the part of the throat just behind the mouth. It includes the base of the tongue, the soft palate, the tonsils, and the side and back wall of the throat. The oropharynx is the middle part of the pharynx (between the nasopharynx and hypopharynx/laryngopharynx) that is located behind the oral cavity (the palatoglossal arch) extending from the uvula to the level of the hyoid bone. It opens anteriorly into the mouth through the isthmus faucium. In this site, the oropharynx is delimited by the base of the tongue (posterior 1/3) and the upper border of the epiglottic vallecula. Laterally, it is formed by the palatine tonsils, tonsillar fossa, and tonsillar pillars located between the palatoglossal and palatopharyngeal archs. Superiorly, its wall consists of the inferior surface of the soft palate and the uvula [8, 16] [Figure 1].

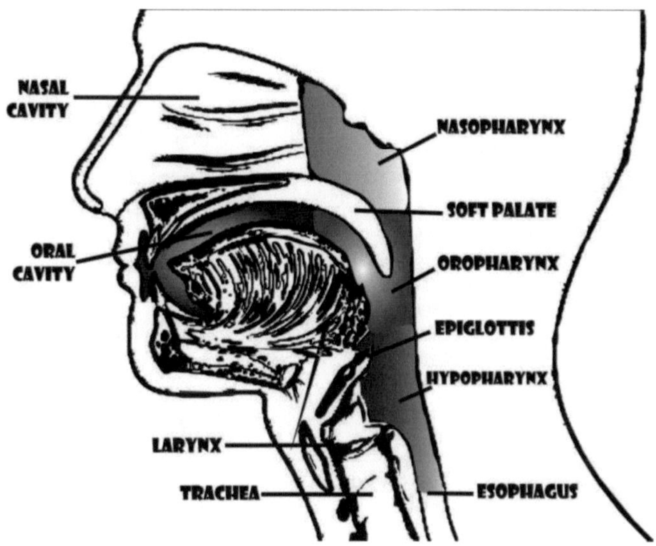

Figure 1. Anatomical aspects of the oral cavity and oropharynx.

2.2. The teeth

The tooth is an organ that consists of a mineralized, inert, and acellular superficial tissue (enamel, an exclusive hard tissue produced by epithelial cells of ectodermal origin known as ameloblasts) but supported by a less mineralized, more resilient, and vital hard tissue (dentin, which is secreted by a cells of neural crest origin known as odontoblasts) which is formed from and supported by a rich innervated and vascular connective tissue (the dental pulp, which is rich in fibroblast-like cells, blood vessels and nerves). Mammalian tooth development is regulated by means of sequential and reciprocal interactions between the cranial neural crest-derived mesenchymal cells and the ectoderm-derived dental epithelium. The teeth are found in the entrance of the oral cavity and constitute about 20% of the structural area of mouth. Anatomically, the tooth consists of a crown and a root, and the junction of the two regions is known as cervical margin (Figure 2A). The teeth have an important role in food processing due to different actions performed by their occlusal surfaces during chewing (Figure 2B). However, the teeth also exhibit other functions, such as defense, proper phonetic articulation, and esthetics in humans. Due to a specialized supporting biological apparatus that consist of the cementum (a mineralized and avascular tissue composed of apatite and organic matrix rich in collagen whose function is to anchor the fiber bundles of the periodontal ligament to the tooth root), periodontal ligament (a highly specialized connective tissue composed for collagen fibers bundles that connect the cementum that cover the tooth root to the alveolar bone whose roles are related to teeth flexibility and sensorial receptor functions), and the alveolar bone (mineralized tissue that support the teeth), the teeth are found firmly attached to the jaws. The hardness of teeth, which is determined by a rich hydrated biologic apatite crystal amid an organic matrix, the number of teeth, the total superficial area formed by the occlusal surfaces, and the supporting tissues allow the teeth to withstand to the forces of the chewing [17, 18].

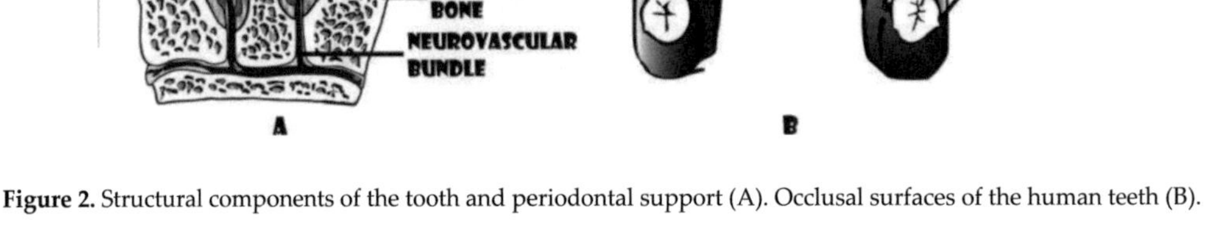

Figure 2. Structural components of the tooth and periodontal support (A). Occlusal surfaces of the human teeth (B).

2.3. The oral mucosa

The oral mucosa is lined by a mucous membrane that consists of a lining epithelial tissue and an underlying connective tissue. The oral mucosa can be classified as follows: lining, masticatory, and specialized. Among its functions, the oral mucosa has been related to protection, taste sensation, and chewing. The lining of oral mucosa must be as flexible as possible in order to be protective. Related to chewing, the oral masticatory mucosa permits a free movement of the lips, tongue, and cheek muscles. It exhibits a covering of keratinized epithelium and its connective tissues is strongly attached to the bone to withstand the constant mastication of food. The lips exhibit cutaneous (external face, skin), semi-mucosa (transition between external and internal surfaces), and mucosa (inner surface in contact with the anterior teeth) lining. The specialized mucosa that is found in the dorsal surface of the tongue exhibits papillae and taste buds responsible for taste sensation. In the case of the oropharynx mucosa, it is lined by non-keratinized squamous stratified epithelium [9].

2.4. The salivary glands

Three paired sets of major salivary glands (parotid, submandibular, and sublingual) and about 600 to 1,000 minor salivary glands scattered throughout the oral cavity and oropharynx make saliva that keeps the mouth moist and play a pivotal role for chewing, swallowing, and digestion. Histologically, the salivary glands exhibit a secretory unit known as an acinus that is composed by numerous secretory glandular epithelial cells (acinar cells) that surround a central space where the secretion is released. From this space, occurs the formation of the ductal structure, a closed channel lined by epithelial (ductal) cells that run through the gland and end as an opening on the oral mucosa surface. The ductal system contains specialized segments with distinct functions characterized as intercalated, striated/granular (middle portion), convoluted tubule, and excretory ducts (located next to the opening on oral mucosa). Beyond its transport role, the ductal cells alter the salivary electrolytic composition. Other important cell types found between the acinar/intercalated ductal epithelial cells and basal lamina are the myoepithelial cells. These cells show contractile capacity that helps to expel the salivary secretion from the acinus through the ductal system [19, 20]. The parotid glands are located inferior and anterior to the external acoustic meatus, lying posteriorly to the mandibular ramus and anteriorly to the mastoid process of the temporal bone. It drains its secretions (rich in proteins due to presence of acini with serous glandular epithelial cells) into the superior vestibule of oral cavity through Stensen's duct or the parotid duct. The parotid gland is responsible for providing about 25% of the total salivary volume. The submandibular glands are located superiorly to the digastric muscles and it is divided into superficial and deep lobes by the mylohyoid muscle. It drains its secretions (rich in glycoproteins due to presence of predominantly mucous acini, alonmg with some serous acini) into the submandibular duct in the sublingual caruncles, a small papilla near the midline of the floor of the mouth on each side of the lingual frenum. The submandibular gland is responsible for producing about 65% of the total salivary volume. The sublingual salivary glands are anteriorly located to the submandibular gland and inferiorly to the tongue and closest to the oral mucosa lining in the floor of the mouth. It drains its secretions (predominantly mucous, but it also contains some serous epithelial glandular cells) through 8-20 minor excretory ducts (the ducts of Rivinus) and one largest ducts, the sublingual duct or duct of Bartholin. These ductal structures join the submandibular duct to drain through the sublingual caruncle. The sublingual salivary gland is responsible for the production of 3-5% of the total salivary volumen. The minor salivary glands are mainly located in the lips, tongue, buccal mucosa, and palate, although they can also be found along the tonsils, supraglottis, and paranasal sinuses. Each minor salivary gland has a single duct which secretes serous, mucous, or mixed saliva directly into the oral cavity [21, 22] (Figure 3).

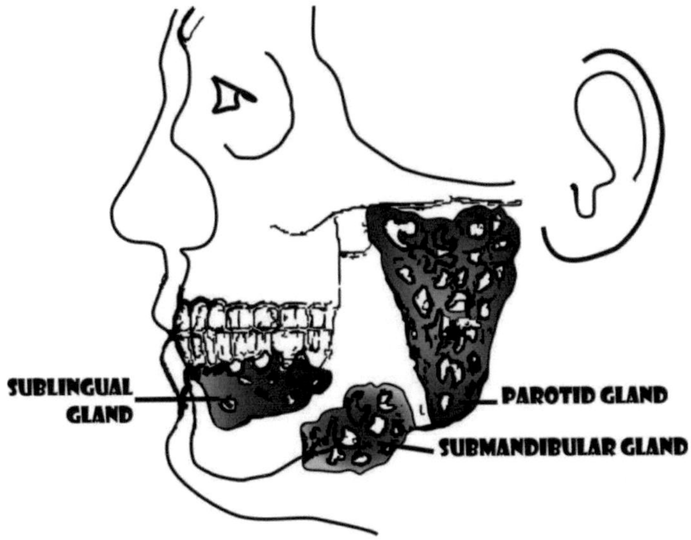

Figure 3. Anatomical localizations of major salivary glands.

2.5. The masticatory muscles

The masticatory muscles are voluntary striated muscles that are responsible for chewing actions, grinding the teeth, moving the mandible from side to side, opening the mouth, and also assisting in speech. During embryogenesis they develop from the mesoderm of the first brachial arch, also known as mandibular arch. In humans, the mandible is connected to the temporal bone of the skull via the temporomandibular joint, an extremely complex joint which permits movement in all planes. The masticatory muscles originate on the skull and insert into the mandible, thereby allowing for jaw movements during contraction. That group of muscles is represented by the masseter, temporalis, medial pterygoid, and lateral pterygoid muscles. The masseter muscle represents the most important masticatory muscle. The masseter is made up of outer and inner parts. The origin point of the outer masseter muscle is along the zygomatic arch, the bony arch of the cheek formed by the connection of the zygomatic and temporal bones. The insertion point of the outer masseter is on the surface of the ramus of the mandible. The origin point of the inner masseter muscle is from the rear of the zygomatic arch and it's insertion point is on the upper surface of the ramus of the mandible. The temporalis muscle is the muscle which assists in closing the mouth, grinding the teeth and moving the mouth from side to side when chewing. Its origin point is along the entire rim of the temporal fossa of the skull and its insertion point is the coronoid process of the mandible and temporal crest. The pterygoid muscle, made up of lateral and medial parts, is located on the inside of the ramus of the mandible. The lateral pterygoid muscle is located higher to the medial pterygoid muscle. These muscles work in tandem with the masseter muscles to assist in chewing, jaw rotation, side to side movement of the mouth, and the projection of the lower jaw. The lower head of lateral pterygoid muscle also assists in opening the mouth. Both lateral and medial parts of the pterygoid muscle have two heads and exhibit two origin points. The upper head of the lateral pterygoid muscle's origin point is from the lateral plate of the sphenoid bone and the origin point of the lower head is in the lateral pterygoid plate. Both heads merge to share the same insertion point which is the pterygoid fovea, but the upper head's insertion reaches the capsula and articular disc. The deep head of the medial pterygoid muscle has an origin point from the lateral pterygoid plate and the superficial head has an origin point from the palatine bone and maxillary tuberosity. Both heads merge to form a broad insertion point on the inner surface of the ramus of the mandible. Other muscles associated with the hyoid bone (such as sternohyoid, middle pharyngeal constrictor, hyoglossus, digastric, stylohyoid, geniohyoid, and mylohyoid muscles), also cooperate for opening the jaw in addition to the lateral pterygoid. The hyoid bone provides attachment for the muscles of the floor of the mouth and the tongue above, the larynx below, and the epiglottis and pharynx behind [13, 23] (Figure 4).

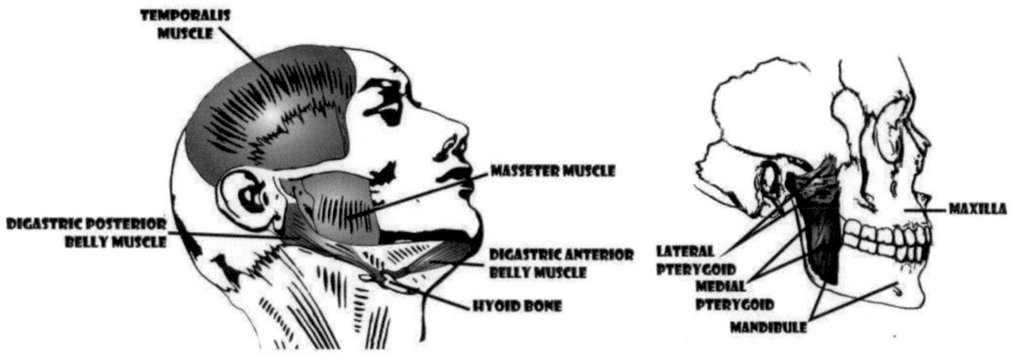

Figure 4. The muscles of mastication

2.6. The tongue

The tongue is an organ lined by an oral epithelium that contains numerous specialized structures related to taste sensation (receptor cells that can sense particular classes of tastes located in the taste buds, including filiform papillae, fungiform papillae, vallate papillae, and foliate papillae) (Figure 5A). Internally, however, the tongue exhibits its most remarkable characteristic in that it is predominantly composed of striated muscle. According to its embryological origin, the tongue might be classified by anterior and posterior regions. The anterior region, that represents about 2/3 of the length tongue, is visible, highly mobile, and directed forward against the lingual surfaces of the lower incisor teeth. The posterior region, which represents 1/3 of the length of the tongue, has its base on the floor of the mouth, connected with the hyoid bone, epiglottis, and soft palate, styloid process, and approximates the oropharynx. Both regions of the tongue exhibit a distinct nerve supply and are delimited by the terminal sulcus anteroposteriorly and by the lingual septum mediolaterally. The striated muscle tissues of the human tongue are classified as intrinsic (i.e. they originate and insert within the tongue, running along its length, and are responsible for changing the shape of the tongue, lengthening and shortening it, curling and uncurling its apex and edges, and flattening and rounding its surface in order to execute eating, swallowing, and speech) (Figure 5B) and extrinsic (i.e. they originate from bone and extend to the tongue, and are responsible for change the tongue position, allowing for protrusion, retraction, elevation and side-to-side movement) (Figure 5C). The intrinsic muscles of the tongue are: 1) the superior longitudinal muscle, that runs along the superior surface of the tongue under the mucous membrane, and elevates, assists in retraction of, or deviates the tip of the tongue. It originates near the epiglottis, the hyoid bone, and from the median fibrous septum, 2) the inferior longitudinal muscle, that lines the sides of the tongue and is joined to the styloglossus muscle, 3) the verticalis muscle, which is located in the middle of the tongue and joins the superior and inferior longitudinal muscles, and 4) the transversus muscle, which divides the tongue at the middle and is attached to the mucous membranes that run along the sides. On the other hand, the extrinsic tongue muscles are represented by: 1) the genioglossus, which arises from the mandible and depresses and protrudes the tongue, 2) the hyoglossus, which arises from the hyoid bone and retracts and depresses the tongue, 3) the styloglossus, which arises from the styloid process and elevates and retracts the tongue, and 4) the palatoglossus, which arises from the palatine aponeurosis and depresses the soft palate, moves the palatoglossal fold towards the midline, and elevates the back of the tongue [24-26] (Figure 5).

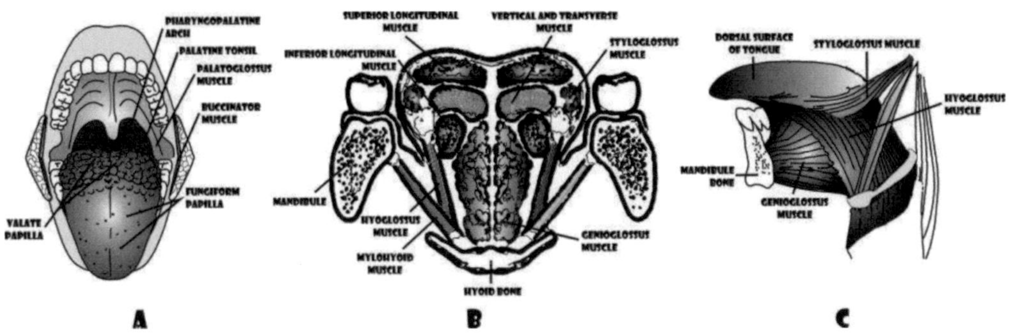

Figure 5. Anatomical aspects of dorsal (A), transversal (B), and lateral (C) views of the tongue.

2.7. The vascular and nervous network of the components of the oral cavity and oropharynx related to salivation, chewing, and swallowing

Almost all of the soft and hard components of the oral cavity and oropharynx exhibit rich vascular and motor-sensitive innervation networks [8, 27-32].

The maxillary teeth are supplied by the maxillary artery (a branch of the external carotid artery) and its branches: the middle and posterior superior alveolar arteries. The mandibular teeth are supplied by the inferior alveolar artery (a branch of the maxillary artery) and its branches: the mental artery and the incisive artery. The venous drainage of the maxillary and mandibular teeth occurs via the anterior, middle, posterior, and inferior alveolar veins. Like enamel, dentin is avascular. The odontoblasts located within the dentin receive nutrition through dentinal tubules from tissue fluid that originates from the blood vessels located in the dental pulp, the vital tissue of the tooth, characterized as a connective tissue with many cells (odontoblasts, fibroblasts, immune cells, and undifferentiated mesenchymal cells) and an extensive nerve and vascular supply. In the pulp chamber, there is the plexus of Raschkow that monitors painful sensations and participates of inflammatory events. In this plexus, there are two types of nerve fibers (A and C fibers) that mediate the sensation of pain. A-fibers conduct rapid and sharp pain sensations and belong to the myelinated group, whereas C-fibers are involved in dull aching pain and are thinner and unmyelinated. Within each dentinal tubule may contain an odontoblastic process and possibly an afferent axon characterized as an A-delta type sensitive fiber.

In the oral cavity, the palate is supplied by the maxillary and, sphenopalatine arteries (a branch of the maxillary artery) and its branches: the lesser and greater palatine, facial (a branch of external carotid artery) and its branches: the ascending palatine, tonsilar, submentual, upper and lower labial and angular arteries. The floor of the oral cavity is supplied by arteries: facial, ascending palatine, submental (a branch of the facial artery), and lingual (a branch of the external carotid artery). The masticatory muscles receive a blood supply from branches (the pterygoid portion) of the maxillary artery (masseteric, superficial temporal, anterior and posterior deep temporal, pterygoid branches, and buccal arteries). The tongue receives its blood supply primarily from the lingual artery but a secondary blood supply is supported by the tonsillar branch of the facial artery and the ascending pharyngeal artery. The tissues of the cheeks receive a blood supply from the facial artery. The tissues of the superior and inferior lips receive blood from the superior and inferior labial arteries, respectively, that are branches of the facial artery. The venous drainage of the palate and the floor of the mouth occur via thelesser and greater palatine veins, the sphenopalatine vein, the lingual vein, the submental vein and the pterygoid plexus. Veins of the tongue drain into the sublingual vein and the internal jugular vein. There is also a secondary blood supply to the tongue from the tonsillar branch of the facial artery and the ascending pharyngeal artery.

The salivary glands also receive a rich vascular network. When the oral mucosal surface is stimulated, afferent nerve signals travel to the salivatory nuclei in the medulla. The medullary signal may also be affected by cortical inputs resulting from stimuli such as taste and smell. Efferent nerve signals, mediated by acetylcholine, also stimulate salivary gland epithelial cells and increase salivary secretions. The parotid gland is mainly irrigated by the external carotid artery via its branches, the posterior auricular and transverse facial arteries. However it also receives a blood supply from the superficial temporal artery (a branch of the external carotid artery when it bifurcates into the superficial temporal artery and maxillary artery). The venous drainage of parotid glands is supported by the retromandibular vein (formed by the union of the superficial temporal and maxillary veins) while its lymphatic drainage is supported by the preauricular or parotid lymph nodes which ultimately drain to the deep cervical chain. The submandibular gland receives its blood supply from the facial and lingual arteries. Its venous drainage occurs through the anterior facial vein. The sublingual gland receives its blood supply from the sublingual and submental arteries.

The oropharynx receives vascular irrigation from the ascending pharyngeal artery, a branch of the external carotid. Iti s a long, slender vessel, deeply seated in the neck, beneath the other branches of the external carotid. Palatine tonsils are vascularized by the tonsillar branches of the facial, descending palatine and ascending pharyngeal arteries. The oropharynx venous drainage occurs through the parapharyngeal spaces to the region of the midportion of the peritonsillar plexus, which drain into the lingual and pharyngeal veins, which in turn drain into the internal jugular vein, particularly the jugulodigastric nodes.

Regarding innervation, the motor innervation of the oral cavity is supported by some branches of the mandibular division of the trigeminal cranial nerve (CN V) and the sensitive innervation is supported by branches of maxillary and some branches of the mandibular nerve. The maxillary teeth and their associated periodontal ligament are innervated by the branches of the maxillary division of the trigeminal nerve, the posterior, middle, and anterior superior alveolar nerves. The mandibular teeth and their associated periodontal ligament are innervated by the inferior alveolar nerve, a branch of the mandibular division. This nerve runs inside the mandible, within the inferior alveolar canal below the mandibular teeth, giving off branches to all the lower teeth.

The oral mucosa of the anterior region of maxilla (maxillary incisors, canines and premolar teeth) is innervated by the superior labial branches of the infraorbital nerve. The pterygopalatine nerve (nasopalatine nerve) is responsible for innervation of the anterior mucosa of maxilla (emerging from beneath the incisive papillae). The lingual nerve, a branch of the mandibular division of the trigeminal nerve, is responsible for innervation of the gingiva of the lingual aspect of the mandibular teeth. The mental nerve, a branch of the inferior alveolar nerve, is responsible for innervation of the facial aspect of the mandibular incisors and canines. The buccal nerve is responsible for innervation of the gingiva of the buccal region of the mandibular molars. The palate is innervated via the maxillary nerve, the nasopalatine nerve, the greater palatine nerve, the lesser palatine nerve and the glossopharyngeal nerve. The floor of the oral cavity is innervated through the lingual, mylohioid, hypoglossal, glossopharyngeal, internal laryngeal, and chorda tympani nerves. Unlike most of the other facial muscles, which are innervated by the facial cranial nerve (CN VII), the muscles of mastication are all innervated by the trigeminal nerve (CN V), more specifically they are innervated by its mandibular branch. The motor function of the trigeminal nerve activates the muscles of mastication and other accessory muscles (the tensor tympani, tensor veli palatini, mylohyoid, and anterior belly of the digastric). All intrinsic and extrinsic muscles of the tongue are supplied by the hypoglossal nerve (CN XII), with the exception of the palatoglossus muscle that is innervated by the vagus nerve (CN X). Regarding sensory nerves, the sensation of taste in the anterior region of the tongue is passed along the chorda tympani, a branch of the facial nerve. Sensation is passed along the lingual nerve, a branch of the trigeminal nerve. Posteriorly, both taste and sensation are passed along the glossopharyngeal nerve (CN IX).

Innervation of salivary glands is entirely autonomic. They are innervated by parasympathetic fibers (via cranial nerves V, VII, and IX) and sympathetic fibers (via preganglionic nerves in the thoracic segments T1-T3 and via postganglionic sympathetic fibers C2-C3) of the autonomic nervous system (Figure 6). The parotid salivary gland is innervated by the facial nerve and anterior branch of the great auricular nerve (composed of branches of spinal nerves C2 and C3 from the cervical plexus). Postganglionic sympathetic fibers from the superior cervical sympathetic ganglion reach the parotid gland as the periarterial nerve plexuses around the external carotid artery and their function is mainly vasoconstriction. Preganglionic parasympathetic fibers leave the brain stem from the inferior salivatory nucleus in the glossopharyngeal nerve (CN IX) and then through its tympanic and then the lesser petrosal branch pass into the otic ganglion where they synapse with postganglionic fibers that reach the parotid gland via the auriculotemporal nerve. The sympathetic nervous system also affects salivary gland secretions indirectly by innervating the blood vessels that supply the glands. Both sympathetic and parasympathetic stimuli result in an increase in salivary gland secretions. The submandibular and sublingual glands receive their parasympathetic input from the facial nerve (CN VII) via the submandibular ganglion. Their secretions are also regulated directly by the parasympathetic nervous system and indirectly by the sympathetic nervous system. The sympathetic nervous system regulates submandibular secretions through vasoconstriction of the arteries that supply it. Parasympathetic innervation of both submandibular and sublingual glands is provided by the superior salivatory nucleus via the chorda tympani nerve. Parasympathetic activity increases salivary flow, makingsaliva watery. On the other hand, increased sympathetic activity reduces glandular blood flow, making the saliva thicker, rich in glycoproteins and glycosaminoglycans. The lingual nerve is responsible by the postganglionic parasympathetic innervation of minor salivary glands. However, the minor salivary glands located on the superior jaw are innervated by fibers of the palatine nerve.

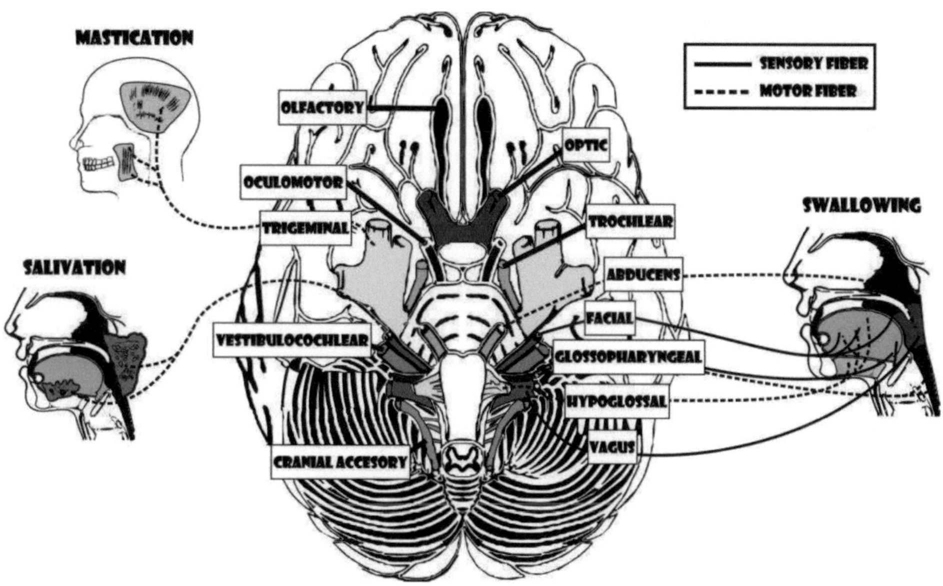

Figure 6. Cranial nerves and their relationship with salivation, chewing, and swallowing mechanisms.

The muscles of the oropharynx receive innervation from the pharyngeal plexus of the vagus nerve (CN X). This network of nerve fibers provides sensory and motor innervation from the pharyngeal branches of the glossopharyngeal nerve (CN IX), the pharyngeal branch of the vagus nerve (CN X), and superior cervical ganglion sympathetic fibers (a component of the autonomic sympathetic nervous system responsible for maintaining homeostasis of the body). However, the motor innervation of the oropharynx also receives nerve fibers from the cranial part of accessory cranial nerve (CN XI). The palatine tonsils receive afferent innervation via the tonsillar plexus, which has contributions from the general somatic afferent fibers of the maxillary division of the trigeminal nerve (CN V) via the lesser palatine nerves, and general visceral afferent fibers from the tonsillar branches of the glossopharyngeal nerve (CN IX) (Figure 6).

3. Physiological aspects of salivation, chewing, and swalloing

3.1. Salivation

Minor and major salivary glands are responsible for saliva production. These exocrine glands consist of a few fundamental cell types: i) acinar cells, which are responsible for secretion of salivary components; ii) myoepithelial cells, which usually form a thin layer above the basement membrane that support acinar and ductal cells and have contractile functions that help to expel the salivary secretions from the lumen to the duct; iii) ductal cells, which are distributed in specialized segments for transportation and modulation of salivary composition. Moreover, there are putative stem cells that reside in the ductal compartment and are related to repair and regeneration of salivary glandular tissue [19, 20].

Saliva is an exocrine secretion made by minor and major (parotid, submandibular, and sublingual) salivary glands that is expressed into the oral cavity. Saliva consists of approximately 99% water, containing a variety of electrolytes (sodium, potassium, calcium, chloride, magnesium, bicarbonate, phosphate), carbohydrates (glucose, glycosaminoglycans), proteins (represented by enzymes, immunoglobulins and other antimicrobial factors, mucosal glycoproteins, traces of albumin, and some polypeptides and oligopeptides), and traces of other biological products (urea, ammonia). Saliva exhibits pH is from 6 to 7 and varies in accordance with the salivary flow. Saliva is critical for preserving and maintaining the health of the oral tissues, allowing them to adequately perform a number of pivotal functions for taste sensation, mastication, digestion, deglutition, and speech. Also aided by the effects of saliva are tissue protection and repair, dilution of toxic substances and cleaning of microorganisms and residues. Saliva can be a useful auxiliary means of diagnosis, an indicator of risk, anda way to monitor local and systemic diseases [10, 33-37] (Table 1).

Saliva can be categorized as *whole saliva* and *specific glandular-derived saliva*. Whole saliva is representative of the typical status of the oral cavity, as it is a complex mixture of fluids from the salivary glands, the gingival crevicular fluid, mucous secretions from the oral cavity, nasal cavity, and pharynx, non-adherent oral bacterial, food remainders, desquamated epithelial

http://dx.doi.org/10.5772/60766

Function	Main chracteristics
Taste sensation	· The low levels of glucose, sodium, chloride, and urea hypotonicity in the saliva provides the ionic environment capable to dissolve substances and maintain taste cells; · Secretions from lingual salivary glands of von Ebner may modulate taste; · A salivary protein (gustin) seems to play a role in the growth and maturation of gustatory buds.
Hydration and lubrication of soft oral tissues	· Presence of mucin glycoprotein that forms seromucosal coverage on the soft oral tissues, hydrating and lubricating the soft oral tissues.
Chewing, swallowing, and digestion of carbohydrates and fats	· Saliva is fundamental for adequate crushing and lubrication of food particles and bolus formation ; · The presence of the digestive enzyme α-amylase (ptyalin) and lingual lipase (produced by minor salivary glands of tongue; the enzyme is only activate in the stomach) in saliva are responsible for the initial digestion of carbohydrates and triglycerides, respectively.
Protection of soft and hard oral tissues	· The coverage of mucin protects the oral tissues against the adhesion and colonization of pathogenic agents. · Prevent the colonization by potentially pathogenic microorganisms once saliva selectively modulates the adhesion of microorganisms to the oral tissue surfaces. · Saliva contains a spectrum of immunologic (immunoglobulins = IgA, more frequent, and IgM and IgG – less frequent, complement system) and non-immunologic (enzymes = lysozyme, lactoferrin, and peroxidase and non-enzymatic proteins = mucin glycoproteins, agglutinins, histatins, proline-rich proteins, statherins, and cystatins) which present antibacterial and antiviral properties. · Protection for tooth enamel through the formation of a biofilm, presence of antibodies, buffer capacity (sialin, urea, and carbonic acid-bicarbonate and phosphate buffer systems), and concentration of calcium, phosphate, and fluoride, which are decisive for the stability of teeth and enamel minerals. Moreover, its buffer capacity neutralizes gastric juices to protect the oral cavity and esophagus · Maintain the structural integrity of tooth enamel by modulating the remineralization and demineralization processes.
Tissue repair	· Saliva can stimulates blood coagulation, shortening bleeding time. · Components of saliva (such as EGF = epidermal growth factor) can increase wound contraction and stimulate rapid tissue repair.
Dilution and cleaning of toxic substances and residues	· Elimination of desquamated oral mucosa epithelial cells, non-adherent microorganisms, toxins, and food waste. · The salivary flux tends to eliminate excess nutrients (such as carbohydrates) that could favor the growth and colonization of microorganisms.
Auxiliary means of diagnosis, indicator of risk, and monitoring of diseases	· Saliva offers a highly potential non-invasive means for monitoring health status, disease onset and progression, treatment outcome, and decision making for patient care for both local and systemic diseases.

Table 1. Functions of saliva and main characteristics.

and blood cells, as well as traces of medications or chemical products. On the other hand, specific glandular-derived saliva is characterized as salivary production collected directly and exclusively from the output of the salivary ducts in the oral cavity. Another way to categorize the saliva flow rate is as *unstimulated* (resting) or *stimulated.* Unstimulated salivary flow rate has a continuous and low salivary flow (basal unstimulated secretion). With regard to the stimulated salivary flow, it is responsible for most of the daily production of saliva and it is usually stimulated by several mechanical, pharmacological, gustatory, and olfactory factors. In healthy subjects, the mean whole saliva production ranges from 1 to 1.5L daily. The clinical evaluation regularly monitored of the stimulated and unstimulated *salivary flow index* (SFI) can be used to categorize the individuals as exhibiting normal, high, low, or very low salivary flow. Adults with normal stimulated salivation exhibit SFI variations between 1 and 3 mL/min, low SFI ranges from 0.7 to 1.0 mL/min, and very low SFI (hyposalivation) is characterized as less than 0.7 mL/min. On the other hand, adults with normal unstimulated salivation exhibit SFI variations between 0.25 to 0.35 mL/min, low SFI ranges from 0.1 to 0.25 mL/min, and very low SFI is less of 0.1 mL/min. The sensation of oral dryness in healthy individuals usually occurs when the whole (both unstimulated and stimulated) SFI is reduced by more than 50% of the daily production [34, 38-40].

Salivary flow and composition varies between individuals and also in the same individual once it is affected by several exogenous and endogenous factors such as age, gender, anatomic and functional aspects of salivary glands, sensory stimuli to food, posture, weight, circadian and circannual cycles, type of nutritional characteristics of the diet, frequency of chewing and bite force, physical exercises, tobacco and alcohol drinking, use of medication, fasting and nausea, and presence of systemic diseases. Decreased salivary flow and alterations in salivary composition cause a clinically significant oral imbalance manifested by increased susceptibility to oral infections (dental caries, periodontal disease, oral candidosis); burning mouth; sore tongue (glossodynia); difficulties with speech, mastication, and swallowing; altered taste sensation (dysgeusia); and halitosis [35, 36, 41-44] (Table 2).

Factors	Main characteristics
Age	· Although with increasing age the salivary gland tissue undergoes atrophy and gradually is replaced by a fibro-adipose tissue, increasing age *per se* seems to not interfere significantly in production and salivary composition; · Unstimulated salivary flow seems to be more affected by advanced age (it is lower in elderly) compared to stimulated salivary flow.
Gender	· Although the findings are conflicting, it appears that women exhibit low unstimulated and stimulated salivary flow compared to males as a result of a smaller size of the salivary glands and the influence of female sex hormones.
Anatomic and functional aspects of salivary glands	· Salivary flow and its composition depend on the individual contribution of each major salivary gland (parotid, submandibular and sublingual) and minor salivary glands. In unstimulated salivary flow, the parotid, submandibular, sublingual, and minor glands contribute 20%, 65%-70%, 7%-8%, and <10%, respectively. When the salivary flow is stimulated, the parotid gland contributes with over 50% of the total salivary secretion;

Factors	Main characteristics
	· Salivary secretions may be serous, mucous, or mixed. The parotid gland contributes a rich serous secretion while the submandibular, sublingual and minor salivary glands contribute a mucous or mixed secretions rich in mucin.
Sensory stimuli for food	· A series of mechanical, chemical, memory, visual, and olfative stimuli may promote alteration in salivary production; Mechanical stimulus (such as chewing) is related to increased salivary secretion; · Food containing acid substances promote intense salivary flow; Greater stimulus to saliva production can occur when humans see or imagine favorite foods.
Posture, lightning, circadian and circannual cycles	· Higher saliva production is verified in individuals kept standing up; · Lower saliva production is observed in individuals in the dark or blindfolded;
Type of nutrition, consumption of water, and characteristics of diet	· Nutritional deficiencies promote lower salivary function and composition; · Higher the body hydration results in greater salivary flow; · The consumption of food with greater consistency promotes an increased salivary flow rate.
Frequency of chewing and bite forcé	· Decreases in the frequency of chewing or a reduced bite force are related to lower salivary flow.
Physical exercises	· Physical activities can affect both production as well as composition of saliva. During exercise, there is less production of saliva and changes in the concentration of salivary proteins and electrolytes levels.
Tobacco and alcohol drinking use	· Tobacco components affect the production of saliva from the salivary glands. Smokers have increased production of saliva; · In contrast, the ingestion of alcoholic beverages promotes a decrease of salivary components (enzymes and electrolytes) as well as salivary flow.
Use of medication	· A comprehensive class of drugs may direct or indirectly influence salivary production and composition, especially those with anticholinergic effects (antidepressants, anxiolytics, antipsychotics, antihistaminics, and antihypertensives).
Presence of systemic diseases	· A series of physical and emotional systemic diseases may directly or indirectly affect the production of saliva and its composition, such as Sjögren syndrome, celiac disease, diabetes mellitus, chronic renal insufficiency, anorexia, bulimia, mood disorders (anxiety and depression), obesity, paraneoplastic syndrome, nausea, vomiting, and others

Table 2. Factors associated with production and composition of saliva.

3.2. Chewing

Chewing is a complex integrative physiological mechanism involved in the early stages of digestion and absorption of nutrients. During chewing, the food particles are reduced in size and consistency due to manipulation of food by oral soft tissues and crushing of food by the occlusal surfaces of teeth. The saliva facilitates the chewing mechanism by moistening and coalescing the food particles. The chewed food is kept trapped laterally by the tongue and buccal mucosa and becomes soft and slippery to ensure an adequate swallowing and further processing in the gastrointestinal tract. Chewing involves the participation of diverse anatomical structures such as teeth, bone (mandible and maxilla), accessory and masticatory muscles, and sensory-motor activities. Biomechanically, the chewing in humans occurs in a stereotypical way: after ingestion of food it is transported from the front of the mouth to the occlusal surfaces of the post-canine teeth. Following this, the food is subjected to a series of masticatory cycles needed to process the food, making it softer and disintegrated until the food becomes more difficult to chew. At this stage, when food is ready to be swallowed, it is propelled posteriorly into the oropharynx where the food accumulates until it is finally swallowed [11, 13].

The muscles of mastication exhibit an adductor action (i.e., a motion that pulls a structure or part towards the midline of the midsaggital plane of the body) of mandible, while the lateral pterygoid muscle abducts (i.e., a motion that pulls a structure or part away from the midline of the midsaggital plane of the body). All four move the mandible laterally. Another accessory muscle, the sternohyomastoid is responsible for opening the mandible in addition to the lateral pterygoid. Anteriorly, the muscles of the lips (orbicularis oris) ensure the closing of the mouth in order to avoid escaping of the food. Posteriorly, at the moment of swallowing, the simultaneous contraction of perioral and jaw muscles, together with opening of the pharyngeal ring, causes a squeeze of the food toward the fauces. The coordinated activity of the trigeminal (CN V) and facial (CN VII) nerves during chewing may be controlled by the direct projections from the parvocellular reticular nucleus to the trigeminal and facial nuclei. Muscle activity during chewing requires complex neuromuscular control with a central pattern generator and peripheral feedback regulatory mechanisms. A distinctive population of brainstem neurons located on the corticobulbar projections play a role at the onset of rhythmicity of the chewing movements and swallowing mechanisms while peripheral afferent nerves modulate the activity of the brainstem central pattern generators. The rhythmicity of chewing movements may also be affected by basal ganglia dysfunctions. Only a small part of the muscle activity observed during chewing is needed for the basic rhythmic movements of the jaw. The peripheral feedback mechanisms that control masticatory muscle activity are supported by periodontal mechanoreceptors (rapidly conducting trigeminal sensory afferent neurons that innervate specialized receptors in the periodontal ligament of the teeth, located closest to collagen fibers) and muscle spindles (afferent sensory proprioceptors located within the belly of a muscle that primarily detect changes in the length of this muscle). Notably, muscle activity seems to start just when the intake food promotes resistance during chewing. The information provided by these mechanoreceptors is important for the specification of the forces used when food is manipulated and positioned between the teeth and prepared for chewing. Moreover, information about mechanical properties of food as well as the spatial contact patterns with the dentition is also provided by these mechanoreceptors. In this way, during cortical stimulation, the central pattern generator produces stereotyped open-close cycles that are mainly dependent on peripheral information about the position and velocity of the mandible, the forces acting on the mandible and on the teeth, and the length and contraction velocity of the muscles involved [45-47].

There are several factors that determine the performance of the masticatory system and, so, of chewing. Among them: the quantity and the total occlusal area of teeth, bite force, neuromuscular control of jaw movement, performance of food manipulation by the tongue, cheeks, and teeth, breakage behavior, taste and texture of food, number of chewing cycles until swallowing of food, and salivary flow [11, 48-50] (Table 3). Experimentally, the masticatory function of individuals might be evaluated and measured by using subjective and objective strategies. The subjective masticatory function (chewing ability) might be evaluated by interviewing subjects as to their own assessment of that function. In turn, the objective masticatory function (chewing performance) has often been measured by determining an individual's capacity to fragment a test food. The chewing performance can be determined by quantifying the degree of fragmentation of an artificial test food (Optosil, a silicon rubber commonly used as a dental impression material, 8 cubes of edge size of 5-8 mm) after a fixed number of chewing cycles (range from 10 to 160 cycles). The degree of fragmentation considers the size of food fragments forced through a stack of sieves. The distribution of particle sizes of the comminuted food can be adequately described by a Rosin-Rammler distribution function which is characterized by two variables only. In each sieve, the amount of test food is weighed and the median particle size of the particles is calculated from the weight distribution of particle sizes [51, 52].

Factors	Main characteristics
Teeth	· Form the occlusal area where the food particles are fragmented; · The fragmentation of food is directly dependent on the number of teeth and thus of its total occlusal area.
Bite forcé	· Depends on jaw muscle volume, activity, and the coordination between the chewing muscles; · Important for reduction of food particle size.
Neuromuscular control	· The brain stem has been shown to be an essential part of the central nervous system that is necessary for basic rhythmic activity of the jaw-opening and jaw-closing muscles. This type of control (central pattern generator) may be switched on by activity of higher centers or by intra-oral stimuli. Moreover, peripheral feedback mechanisms provide information (position and velocity of the mandible, forces acting on the mandible and on the teeth, length and contraction velocity of the masticatory muscles involved) to the central nervous system to improve the performance of mastication; · Responsible for the neurologic control of masticatory muscles and movement of the mandible, playing an important role in the fragmentation of the food; · Act to exert muscle forces that close, and abduct-adduct the mandible allowing the teeth cut and crush food; · A small part of the muscle activity observed during chewing is needed just for the basic rhythmic movements of the jaw, and additional muscle activity is required to overcome the resistance of the food; · The texture of food might simulate different breakage behavior. Crispy food decelerates (induces a decrease of the chewing muscle electrical activity after food breaks) and accelerates (induces an increase of the chewing muscle electrical activity with intact food) the mandible as result of resistance and breakage of food particles.

Factors	Main characteristics
Performance of food manipulation and trituration	· Depends on how well the tongue and cheeks manipulate the food while the teeth crushe the food and turn it in small particles; · Individuals with a high masticatory performance will, on average, swallow finer food particles (median particle size of about 1mm) than subjects with a less high performance (median particle size of about 3mm).
Characteristics of the food	· Depends of factors such as percent water content, fat percentage, taste, texture, volume, and consistency; · Consistency of food can make the jaw decelerate and accelerate as a result of resistance and breakage of food particles; · These characteristics also affect masticatory force, jaw muscle activity, and mandibular jaw movements.
Number of chewing cycles until swallowing of food	· During chewing cycles, the food particles are reduced in size and consistency. Together, the saliva, due to the presence of water and mucin glycoprotein, facilitates chewing by moistening the food particles for swallowing; · The number of chewing cycles needed to prepare the food for swallowing is importantly influenced by food characteristics; · The number of chewing cycles needed to prepare food before swallowing is rather constant within an individual for certain foods but varies among different individuals.
Salivary flow	· Responsible for mixing of food particles into a bolus that can be swallowed; · Salivary flow rate is weakly correlated to variation in the swallowing threshold, i.e., individuals with a relatively high salivary flow rate do not necessarily swallow the food after fewer chewing cycles compared to a subject with less saliva; · Saliva might modify food properties, which may lead to changes in chewing force, mandibular jaw movements, number of chewing cycles to prepare the food for swallowing, and, perhaps, the visual and sound perception of the food.

Table 3. Factors related to chewing and mains characteristics.

3.3. Swallowing

The process of swallowing includes the voluntary effort to ingest food and an involuntary effort of bolus preparation and transport. During early stages of swallowing, the bolus, which represents food particles bound together under viscous forces determined by components of saliva, is transported from the oral cavity and pharynx to the esophagus [14, 15, 53-55].

Briefly, swallowing mechanisms might be summarized as follows: in the oral cavity, where the initial preparation of swallowing occurs, the food is chewed, moistened, and coalesced. During chewing, the food particles are continuously moved towards the occlusal surface of the teeth through the actions of the tongue and masticatory muscles. A premature spillage of the bolus into the pharynx is avoided by the approach of the soft palate to the tongue that creates a glossopalatal seal, while various movements of the mandible are important for the adequate grinding of the bolus. When the bolus is ready for swallowing, the tongue forms a slit containing the bolus with the lateral edges curved upwards. The soft palate closes the nasopharynx, the larynx is elevated and closed, the pharyngeal constrictor muscles (superior, middle, and inferior) contract and the cricopharynx muscles relaxes. The tongue then contracts from anterior to posterior pushing the bolus back into the pharynx, the whole process taking about one second. The true cords, the false cords, the epiglottis and the aryepiglottic folds constrict to form a barrier of several layers to protect the airway and prevent aspiration. Elevation of the larynx occurs by the contraction of the suprahyoid musculature and relaxation of the cricopharyngeus musculatures. With this relaxation, negative pressure is created in the upper oesophagus, which helps in the movement of the bolus towards to stomach. The oropharyngeal stage has a short duration (less than a second), although it may vary depending on size of the bolus. Moments before the bolus enters the oropharynx, the soft palate elevates to close the nasopharynx, avoiding the regurgitation of the bolus through the nose, while the hyoid bone elevates and draws the larynx upwards and epiglottic folds down to protect its entrance. The tongue base moves in contact with the posterior pharyngeal wall, accompanied by an anterior movement of the hyoid. The cricopharyngeus muscle begins its relaxation resulting in the opening of the upper esophageal sphincter. The rhythm and pattern of the swallowing mechanism is involuntary controlled by a central pattern generator located in the medulla. Moreover, during the oropharyngeal stage of swallowing, it the participation of the voluntary cranial nerves trigeminal (CN V), abducens (CN VI), and hypoglossal (CN XII) is fundamental for muscle voluntary control. The involuntary control (sensitive) of the oropharyngeal stage of swallowing involves the pivotal participation of the glossopharyngeal (CN IX) and vagus (CN X) cranial nerves. The esophageal phase starts after bolus passage through the upper esophageal sphincter and is characterized by a single primary peristaltic wave movement travelling at 3-4 cm/sec. After opening of the lower esophageal sphincter, the bolus is directed towards the stomach. Several secondary peristaltic waves occur spontaneously in an hour helping to clear residue and any gastric reflux. The oesophageal transit time varies with age [15, 53, 54, 56, 57].

4. Local and systemic physiopathological conditions associated to oropharyngeal dysphagia

A plethora of endogenous and exogenous etiologic factors might disrupt the physiology and anatomical integrity of oral cavity and oropharynx components and, therefore, have an negative affect on salivation, chewing, and swallowing mechanisms. The occurrence of disturbances in these mechanisms play pivotal roles in the occurrence of oropharyngeal dysphagia [1, 5] (Figure 7).

4.1. Age

The aging process is currently viewed as the result of an accumulation of insults to orofacial structures and function. Dental caries on root surfaces uncovered by gingival tissue, periodontal disease, tooth loss, oral cancer, infectious diseases (such as oral candidosis), traumatic

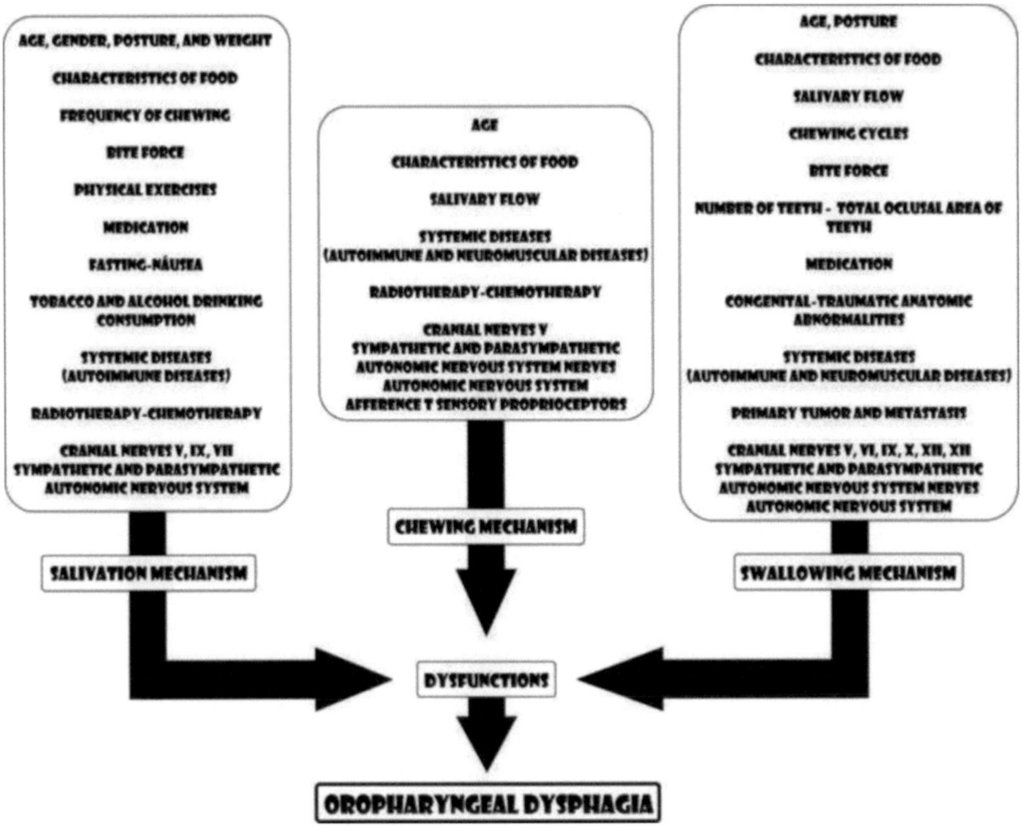

Figure 7. Schematic representation of the main etiological factors associated with dysfunction in salivation, chewing, and swallowing mechanisms, with promotion of oropharyngeal dysphagia.

lesions (hyperplastic and ulcerations caused by removable prosthodontic appliances), vesiculobullous autoimmune diseases (such as pemphigus vulgaris and cicatricial pemphigoid), and others remain as a constant threat to the maintenance of oral health in older individuals. Although many of these diseases might be promptly prevented, diagnosed and treated, a majority of older persons have encountered significant oral and pharyngeal problems that can ultimately have a profound impact on the quality of their lives. Many of these changes are directly connected to problems with genetic and epigenetic susceptibilities, socioeconomic inequalities, health behavior, access to oral health services, and systemic diseases and their treatment rather than the simple passage of time [5, 7, 58-62].

Dysfunctions related to salivary supply may negatively influence the masticatory and swallowing process by making them impossible for individuals to prepare food into a bolus before swallowing adequately. It has been frequently reported that salivation mechanisms seem to be affected with the advancing age. Indeed, mouth dryness (xerostomia) promoted by hyposalivation in older individuals is the most common complaint among the elderly. However, it has been demonstrated that in healthy older individuals there is not a significant alteration in volume and composition of saliva compared to a younger adult. Therefore, hyposalivation in older persons seems to be more associated with age-related diseases, masticatory disturbances, and use of certain therapeutic drugs [36, 63, 64].

Masticatory motor performance function is frequently affected in older individuals, especially those with poor subjective (self-perception of oral health) and normative (decay, periodontal disease, tooth loss) conditions of oral health. Older individuals exhibit a reduced bite which, in turn, determines a higher number of cycles needed to chew a standard piece of food, with increased particle size reduction and longer chewing sequence duration. Due to this, elderly frequently avoid highly textured foods, which are one of the important masticatory muscle activators, and might reduce the salivary flow. Other factors reported to affect masticatory performance in elderly persons include loss and restoration of posterior teeth, number of residual teeth, occlusal force, stimulated salivary flow rate, and oral motor function, which seem to accelerate masticatory dysfunction with ageing. However, it has become increasingly evident that masticatory performance need not decline with age if natural dentition is maintained. Therefore, if tooth loss and hyposalivation are not considered as characteristics of physiological ageing, ageing by itself may not be a risk factor for masticatory dysfunction. With increasing age, maintaining an adequate number of healthy natural teeth is the best guarantee to maintain adequate masticatory ability. Although the loss of teeth may be compensated for by dentures, and the dentures contribute to breaking down of food, it has been noted that prosthetic treatments seem to be unsuccessful for approaching the efficiency of a complete natural dentition, and so, of the masticatory mechanism [49, 65, 66].

Regarding swallowing, older healthy persons do not seem to experience major changes in this mechanism. However, the participation of certain risk factors, such as use of depressor central nervous system drugs or neurological diseases, might increase risk for dysphagia in aged persons. During mastication and swallowing, tongue activity creates a pressure that facilitates the manipulation of food particles and transport of the bolus. Older individuals exhibit a lower isometric swallowing (palate-tongue) pressure compared to younger persons. However, the influence of swallowing changes attributable to age appear to be important only for deglutition of certain types of food with different physical characteristics (consistency, texture). Generally, age does not seem to influence swallowing pressure. Moreover, healthy elderly individual exhibit a higher oral transit time with a prolonged oropharyngeal phase, upper esophageal sphincter relaxation, reduced pharyngolaryngeal sensory discrimination, and a higher threshold to trigger the pharyngeal phase of swallowing [55, 67].

A high occurrence of dysphagia in elderly persons has been documented although it is frequently neglected by health professionals and patients themselves. Clinical signs of dysphagia are not specific in geriatric patients and the clinical manifestation of swallowing disorder in these individuals may fluctuate over time, and therefore needs repeated clinical evaluation. In that population, the occurrence of dysphagia has been associated with malnutrition and/or dehydration while compromised safety increases the risk of aspiration pneumonia. With regards to oral health, elderly persons with oropharyngeal dysphagia frequently present with high prevalence of dental caries, periodontal diseases, and edentulism. Moreover, the occurrence of dysphagia in older persons has significant social and psychological consequences. Other health problems such as modifications of respiration or coughing at mealtime, reduction or refusal of food intake, changes in types of meal texture, recurrent pulmonary infections and unexplained bouts of fever or unintentional weight loss correlate with dysphagia in older individuals [7, 61, 68].

In this way, many of the pathological conditions that affect salivation, chewing, and swallowing therefore can cause dysphagia in an older population, but are not an inevitable consequence of advancing age of individuals. Early recognition and appropriate management of dysphagia in elderly patients is pivotal.

4.2. Congenital and traumatic anatomic abnormalities

A series of primary congenital anatomic abnormalities (such as laryngeal, palate and lip clefts, tracheoesophageal fistula, and jaw micrognathia) and traumatic injuries (such as fibrosis of the upper aerodigestive tract mucosa for physical and chemical etiologic factors, and post-operatory insults after surgical procedures) can affect the oral cavity and oropharynx and have been associated with immobility of organs/structures or respiratory difficulty during feeding. These congenital disturbances manifest early in childhood, occurring independently or in combination with other anatomic abnormalities, associated or not with syndromes. Traumatic anatomic abnormalities are typically caused by direct injury. All these types of abnormalities can lead to significant oropharyngeal dysphagia [69, 70].

4.3. Medication

Drugs that directly or indirectly affect the mechanisms of protection of normal oropharyngeal mucosa (antibiotics, cytotoxics/immunossupressors), production of saliva (anxiolytics, anticholinergics/antireflux, anticonvulsants, antidepressants, antihypertensives, antipsychotics, antihistamines/decongestants, diuretics, and opiates), and chewing (botulinum toxin type A) and swallowing (antipsychotics, antihypertensives, local anesthetic agents) mechanisms may potentiate the development of dysphagia. The dimensions and impact of these side effects vary depending on the response of the individual patient and the duration of medication use [71-73].

4.4. Neurological disorders

Chewing and swallowing are complex motor tasks characterized by a coordinated and synchronized activation of an afferent system (cortical and subcortical areas and oropharyngeal afferents), the brain stem swallowing center (interneuronal network organizer) and the efferent system (motoneurons). Some cerebrovascular diseases that affect the motor control of the cranio-cervical region may interfere with the appropriate performance of chewing and swallowing mechanisms, which can explain the occurrence of dysphagia. To date, dysphagia is found in about 50% of individuals with dementia and cerebrovascular accident (stroke), 30% with deconditioning, and 90% with Parkinson disease [74].

Dementia is a condition in which there is progressive deterioration in cognition that affects day to day function of patients. All types of neurodegenerative or vascular dementia (vascular,

http://dx.doi.org/10.5772/60766

multi-infarct, Lewy body dementia, Alzheimer's disease, and Parkinson's disease), may affect cortical regions involved in chewing and swallowing. Development of deglutition disorders differs with the type of dementia, but most frequently they occur during late stages. The most drastic complication in patients with dementia is the aspiration pneumonia [75]. Alzheimer's disease (AD) represents the most frequent form of dementia. In AD, brain areas underlying swallowing function show early compromise, probably before clinical dysphagia diagnosis. In these patients there occurs a delayed oral transit time due to deficits in the sensory aspects of swallowing. The common reported symptoms in these patients would be pocketing of food in the mouth, difficulties with mastication, coughing or choking with food or fluid, and the need for reminders to swallow food. In Parkinson disease (PD), drooling, persistent food residues, slow transit and repeated tongue movements can be observed during the oral phase. Delayed triggering of the pharyngeal swallow, prolonged opening of the upper esophageal sphincter and vallecular stasis are also reported. In less frequent extrapyramidal disorders (progressive supranuclear palsy, corticobasal degeneration, dementia with Lewy bodies, and multiple system atrophy), deglutition may be severely impaired even at early stages of the disease [76, 77].

Stroke is a devastating group of neurological diseases responsible for high rates of disabilities and death worldwide. Patients with stroke frequently exhibit a need for artificial feeding and higher length of hospital stay. Swallowing aspiration is reported in up to 50% of patients with stroke, with the major complication being pneumonia, a likely consequence of bacteria-infected secretions or ingested food repeatedly transgressing into the airway. Stroke patients have a worse outcome in terms of mortality and length of hospital stay when dysphagia is present [74, 78].

4.5. Neurodegenerative disorders of the motor system

Muscles need a patent motor innervation to maintain their functionality and trophism. In diseases characterized with progressive degeneration of motor neurons (both higher, cortical, and the brain stem and spinal cord), denervation atrophy occurs with consequent muscle wasting, progressive difficulty in performing movements, and loss of muscle strength. Many neurodegenerative disorders that affect the motor system exhibit a genetic etiology. However, it has been evidenced that immune system disturbances also contribute for development of that group of diseases [79]. Amyotrophic lateral sclerosis (ALS) is a neurodegenerative disorder that causes muscle spasticity and rapidly progressive muscle weakness and atrophy throughout the body due to the degeneration of the upper and lower motor neurons, which is often asymmetric at least in the early stages. Individuals affected by the disorder may ultimately lose the ability to initiate and control all voluntary movement. With respect to neuromuscular function occurring in the upper aerodigestive tract, ALS patients usually present with difficulty in speaking, swallowing, and breathing. Up to 30% of patients with ALS present with muscle bulbar (jaw, face, tongue, soft palate, pharynx, and larynx) symptoms, such as dysphagia and dysarthria (poor articulation of phonemes due to neurological injury of the motor component of the motor-speech system) at the onset of the disease, while almost all patients develop such symptoms at later stages of the disease. These patients often lose weight in part because of dysphagia, but also because there is denervation of limb muscles and significant reduction of appendicular muscle mass. Aspiration pneumonia and respiratory difficulties are severe complications of ALS. Bulbospinal muscular atrophy or Kennedy's disease is an X-linked chronic motor neuron disease that also promotes progressive degeneration of bulbar motor neurons. Other chronic motor neuron disorders such as spinal muscular atrophy sometimes affect the muscles of swallowing [80, 81].

4.6. Other muscle disorders

Dystonia represents an involuntary sustained (tonic) or spasmodic (rapid or clonic) muscle contraction that can occur in various regions of the body producing twisting, repetitive, and patterned movements, or abnormal postures. Its etiology is complex and includes genetic predisposition, peripheral or central nervous system injuries, drug induced or metabolic disturbances, paraneoplastic syndromes, and neurodegenerative or cerebrovascular diseases. Oromandibular dystonia (OD) manifests as focal disturbances on perioral movements performed by masticatory, lower facial, and tongue muscles which may result in trismus, bruxism, involuntary jaw opening or closure, involuntary tongue movement, dysphonia, difficulty with chewing, and dysphagia. OD can manifest alone or in association with other motor control disturbances, such as Meige's syndrome and Brueghel's síndrome [80, 82].

Muscular dystrophies are a group of muscle diseases that have in common a progressive weakening in the musculoskeletal system, defects in muscle proteins, and the death of muscle cells and tissue. Although it has been suggested that this could be caused by environmental factors, the muscular dystrophies are caused by a mutation of the dystrophin gene. Among the muscular dystrophies, oculopharyngeal muscular dystrophy (OMD), myotonic dystrophy (Steinert's disease), and advanced stages of Duchenne muscular dystrophia (DMD) are most commonly associated with dysphagia. Frequently, all phases of swallowing (oral, pharyngeal, and esophageal) are impaired in these disorders. As a consequence, these patients have a delayed onset of swallowing and slowed bolus transit times. Moreover, in these dystrophic diseases, dysphagia occurs as a consequence of a progressive weakness of the tongue, palatal, and pharyngeal muscles. In the onset of OMD, dysphagia is mainly pharyngeal, but the lingual and oral phases are also affected. In DMD, the occurrence of macroglossia complicates the oral phase of swallowing [75, 83, 84].

The primary inflammatory myopathies are polymyositis (generalized and chronic inflammatory myopathy), dermatomyositis (microangiopathy that affects skin and muscle), and inclusion body myositis (progressive acquired myopathy of late stage and slow progression). They all have in common infiltration of chronic inflammatory cells within muscle tissue and tissue destruction. It has been hypothesized that the presence of specific autoantigen(s) in the muscle tissue initiates the disease, though this has not yet been identified in each disease. These diseases can promote the progressive weakening of the oropharyngeal musculature. Consequently, dysphagia occurs in about in 60% of patients with primary inflammatory myopathies. Swallowing disorders may be severe in these patients, and complicate significantly any respiratory dysfunction they may have (aspiration, interstitial lung disease, respiratory muscle deficiency). In inclusion body myositis the inflammatory process can promote a prominent cricopharyngeus and inferior constrictor muscles [85, 86].

Myositis ossificans (MO) is a disease that is characterized by non-neoplastic, heterotopic bone formation within a muscle. MO is divided broadly into progressive and traumatic forms. The progressive form of MO is an autosomal dominant disease in which multiple heterotopic ossifications develop in the systemic muscle, fascia, tendons, and ligaments, sometimes within families. Traumatic MO is a disease in which muscles are ossified presumably following acute trauma, burns, surgical manipulation, or repeated injury. When affecting the masticatory muscles, MO exhibits higher frequency of involvement in the masseter, followed by the medial pterygoid, lateral pterygoid, and temporal muscle. In these cases, MO might cause swelling, trismus, pain, and dysphagia [87, 88].

In certain mitochondrial myopathies (Kearns-Sayre disease, chronic progressive external ophthalmoplegia, and mitochondrial myopathy, peripheral neuropathy, gastrointestinal disease, and encephalopathy syndrome), patients present with dysphagia owing to the weakness of the pharyngeal constrictor muscles that, in turn, impairs swallowing mechanisms. Peripheral neuropathy seldom involves the pharyngeal muscles, given the short length of the pharyngeal nerve fibers. However, disorders that are independent of fiber nerve length (Guillain-Barré syndrome and chronic inflammatory demyelinating polyradiculoneuropathy) tend to affect the bulbar muscles. In these cases, dysphagia usually involves the pharyngeal phase, but oral manipulation mainly for solid food is also compromised [89, 90].

4.7. Autoimmune diseases

The autoimmune diseases represent a broad spectrum of diseases that occur when the immune system turns against components of the body itself, attacking as if it were a foreign molecule. The autoimmune human diseases comprise more than 50 distinct diseases in which oral manifestations are encountered with high frequency, sometimes as the first clinical signs or symptoms of the autoimmune disease [91].

Sjögren's syndrome (SS) is a human chronic autoimmune disorder of the exocrine glands, with a population prevalence of about 0.5% and most commonly found in postmenopausal females. SS may clinically manifest as primary (primary SS, exocrinopathy form) or in the context of underlying connective tissue disease (secondary SS). Secondary SS exhibits connective tissue disorders that can affect the skin, ears, nose and throat, joints, lungs, heart, kidneys, liver, and the neurologic (peripheral and central), haematological, and lymphoproliferative systems [92]. The etiology of SS remains unknown but probably it is multifactorial. Exogenous and endogenous factors (virus infections, stress, and hormonal factors) are thought to trigger chronic inflammation in individuals with a genetic predisposition to the disorder. The initial steps in pathogenesis of SS probably involve disturbances in endothelial, acinar, stromal, and dendritic cells, with consequent upregulation of adhesive proteins that appear to drive the migration and retention of lymphocytes into the gland. The progressive accumulation of lymphocytes is associated with subsequent activation of cytotoxic cells and release of metalloproteinases that are responsible for the tissue destruction [93]. Lesions that affect lacrimal and salivary glands characterize both primary and secondary clinical forms of SS. In the oral cavity, the hallmark of SS is the lymphocytic infiltration of the salivary glands, particularly in the periductal areas, promoting a progressive destruction of the glandular tissues. The development of SS in the salivary gland results in dysfunction in glandular secretion with consequent hyposalivation (xerostomia). SS patients with hyposalivation exhibit loss of the lubricating, buffering, and antimicrobial capacities of saliva with an increased incidence of oral/dental infection, mucosal friability, objective and subjective findings of dryness, irritation, burning sensation, higher difficulty for dry and water bolus swallows, and significantly prolonged pharyngeal transit times as compared to controls. Another important factor that might increase the perception of dysphagia in SS patients is the occurrence of gastrotracheal reflux. Since saliva has high pH that normally neutralizes acid refluxed from the stomach, SS patients can be predisposed not only to gastro-oesophageal reflux but also to reflux into the trachea, which can mimic upper respiratory-tract infection [94, 95].

Major bullous conditions that involve the oral cavity (such as pemphigus vulgaris, cicatricial pemphigoid, bullous pemphigoid, and oral lichen planus) and idiopathic chronic inflammatory conditions (recurrent aphtous ulcers, Behçet's disease, Crohn's disease, ulcerative colitis, chronic graft-versus-host-disease) clinically manifest as painful and bleeding chronic ulcers in the oral mucosa. These ulcerative alterations may promote adverse affects on taste and smell sensation and impair mastication and swallowing by disrupting the integrity of oral mucosa without specifically affecting the anatomical structures directly related to salivary function and swallowing mechanisms [91].

Myasthenia gravis is an autoimmune disease in which self-antibodies are produced against nicotinic acetylcholine receptors on the neuromuscular junctions that connect the nervous system to the muscular system. This results in modification of the synaptic cleft and destruction of the postsynaptic neuromuscular membrane. In this way, myasthenia gravis is also considered a disorder of the neuromuscular junction [96]. Patients with this disease frequently exhibit fatigable muscle weakness that is clinically the hallmark of this disease. The clinical severity ranges from mild, purely ocular forms to severe generalized weakness and respiratory failure. Progressive destruction of neuromuscular junctions in muscles involved in masticatory swallowing mechanisms leads to disordered oral, masticatory, and pharyngeal phases, with consequent dysphagia. Clinically, due to progressive muscle weakness promoted by the disease, patients present with problems with manipulation and transport of food, whereas others have difficulties restricted to the pharyngeal phase. Some patients have greater problems with chewing food or moving it in their mouth, whereas others have difficulties restricted to the pharyngeal phase. About one third of myasthenia gravis patients with dysphagia aspirate food particles [97, 98].

4.8. Cysts and primary neoplasms in the head and neck

The initial dysphagia associated with hyperplastic and neoplastic lesions located on the upper aerodigestive tract mucosa is attributed to the combination of disrupted normal anatomy secondary to exophytic or infiltrative nature of the tumor growth, along with any muscle, vascular, and nerve involvements, soft tissue tethering, or tumor induced pain. In this way, the presence and development of hyperplastic lesions, large cysts and benign or malignant tumors might potentially promote disturbances in salivation (adenomas, adenocarcinomas, and carcinomas of the major salivary glands), chewing (large cysts, or benign or malignant tumors that occur in the jaws or in soft tissues of the oral cavity and oropharynx, such as dentigerous cysts, ameloblastomas, and infiltrative carcinomas), as well as swallowing mechanisms. Dysphagia also can occur in these patients as a consequence of therapeutics [70].

4.9. Treatment of the upper aerodigestive tract cancer

Upper aerodigestive tract cancer (UADTC), also known as head and neck cancer, represents a broad term, which encompasses a group of human malignancies that arise in the epithelial lining of the upper aerodigestive tract mucosa. Approximately 90% of UADC are diagnosed as squamous cell carcinoma and it represents the sixth most common type of human cancer, and is responsible for high morbidity and mortality rates worldwide every year. A plethora of socio-demographical, economic, and cultural factors associated with a background of genetic and epigenetic molecular disturbances are pivotal to progression of UADTC [99-102].

All UADTC patients will undergo surgery, chemotherapy, radiotherapy, or a combination of any of these three therapeutic modalities. The choice of modality is dependent on patient and tumor variables (presence of physical disabilities of patients, clinical stage, primary site, type, and resectability of tumor). Patients presenting with early-stage malignancy can be managed by curative surgery or radiotherapy. Frequently, patients diagnosed with a late stage tumor might be treated with complete surgical excision followed by post-operative radiotherapy or with concomitant chemoradiotherapy. The uses of organ-sparing treatments have been recommended in recent years; however, they have not necessarily translated into functional preservation of head and neck tissues. Dysphagia is recognized as a potentially devastating UADC post-treatment complication, occurring in up to 50% of UADTC survivors. The most significant consequences of dysphagia in UADTC patients are alteration of the sense of taste (dysgeusia), xerostomia, malnutrition, dehydration, weight loss, reduced functional abilities, fear of eating and drinking socially, anxiety, depression, reduced quality of life, and food aspiration [103].

During reconstruction or surgical procedures for treatment of tumors located in the head and neck (enucleation of primary tumor, tracheostomy, endoscopic laser surgery on the larynx, partial/supraglottic/supracricoid/total laryngectomy, hypopharyngeal surgery and skull base surgeries), notably for malignant tumors in late stages, the structure and function of specific cranial nerves (CN V, VII, IX, X, XII) or other specific anatomic structures related to salivation, chewing, and swallowing mechanisms are often affected and, therefore, patients might present with site-specific patterns of dysphagia. Surgical resection can have devastating effects on swallowing. When surgical resection extends beyond the tongue to laryngeal or pharyngeal structures the patients may never be functional oral eaters and always have dysphagia [104, 105].

Radiation therapy disrupts cell division in healthy tissue as well as in tumors and also affects the normal structure and function of upper aerodigestive tract tissues, including the oral and pharyngeal mucosa, salivary glands and bones. Frequent and distressing acute and chronic side-effects might occur in UADTC patients during and after radiotherapy. Acute side-effects of radiotherapy are mucositis, xerostomia, dysphagia, hoarseness, erythema and desquamation of the skin (dermatitis). Other late complications that frequently are observed in radiotherapy post-treatment are dental decay, trismus, hypogeusia, subcutaneous fibrosis, thyroid dysfunction, esophageal stenosis, hoarseness, damage to the middle or inner ear, and osteoradionecrosis (infection in a hypovascularized tissue with consequent tissue destruction). These post-radiotherapy sequelae are dependent on radiation field, radiation dose, use of anti-xerostomic medication, and post-radiotherapy time. In xerostomic patients, irreversible damage can occur to the salivary glands, resulting in dramatic hyposalivation and increases in oral and systemic infections. Moreover, oral mucositis induced by radiation therapy frequently occurs, leading to painful oral ulcerations and local and systemic infection. In patients treated with high dose radiation, swallowing can be affected several years after treatment due to a series of complications such as fixation of the hyolaryngeal complex, reduced range of tongue motion, reduced glottic closure, and cricopharyngeal relaxation, resulting in the potential for aspiration. Irradiated patients have longer oral transit times, increased pharyngeal residue, and reduced cricopharyngeal opening times [106].

Concurrent chemoradiation was introduced to improve prognosis of UADTC patients by increase the tumor cell killing with chemotherapy, which also acts as a radiosensitizer. However, although inoperable tumors showed a better prognosis, the toxicity of the two modalities combined resulted in more significant side-effects. Various side-effects like nausea, vomiting, mucositis induced by chemotherapy, dysphagia, neutropenia, and generalized weakness might occur. The anti-metabolites such as methotrexate and 5-fluorouracil are the cytotoxic agents most commonly associated with oropharyngeal and esophageal dysphagia. Chemotherapeutic agents can impact the ability of UADTC patients to swallow. Severe dysfunction of the base of the tongue, larynx and pharyngeal muscles are observed after chemoradiation, leading to stasis of the bolus, vallecular residue, dysmotility of the epiglottis, and food aspiration [106-108].

5. The role of the dentist in an interdisciplinary effort to manage oropharyngeal dysphagia

Oropharyngeal dysphagia arises as a result of so many types of endogenous or exogenous injuries that affect, isolated or combined, the salivation, chewing, and swallowing mechanisms. Injuries in these mechanisms usually impair the physical and mental health and quality of life of individuals. Undoubtedly, successful management requires an interdisciplinary collaboration among health professionals, which need to promote an accurate diagnostic workup, promote effective therapeutic strategies, and formulate an adequate management strategy of dysphagic patients in cases where cure of that condition is not currently possible.

The dentist is a health professional that clinically evaluates the oral health of patients at frequent intervals. However, in most curriculums of dental schools, very little is presented and discussed about chewing and swallowing disturbances regarding the diagnosis, management, and treatment of these conditions. Moreover, nor is it strongly discussed about salivary gland dysfunction (hyposalivation) and its interrelation as an important risk factor for swallowing disorders. However, as dysphagia is affected by salivation, chewing, and swallowing disturbances, it is clear to realize that the dentist can perform proper educational and clinical activities that might provide preventive approaches, fast and accurate diagnosis, and participate in treatment decisions in a multidisciplinary health care team. Moreover, the dentist may be the health professional with whom patients feel comfortable in reporting their salivation, chewing, and swallowing disorders.

With regards to the role of the dentist, the maintenance of oral health conditions in healthy individuals or the restoration of an adequate oral health in those individuals where these conditions are unfavorable (such as presence of dental caries, periodontal disease, oral candidiasis) must be prioritized before or during the treatment of oropharyngeal dysphagia. In addition, due to the high prevalence of edentulism (especially in older individuals), the replacement of missing teeth should be provided through the use of dental implants or dentures. The control of oral infections is mandatory. The aspiration of the pathogenic bacteria populations (mostly gram-negative) by dysphagic patients is responsible for development of pneumonia, the worse consequence of dysphagia. In healthy oral conditions, oral biofilm is colonized by commensal microflora, which acts as a barrier against the colonization of respiratory pathogens. However, poor oral health conditions reduce that commensal microflora, allowing the colonization and growth of pathogenic bacteria populations. Concerning the management of dysphagia due to hyposalivation, the dentist must identify the underlying cause, minimize or eliminate the effect of the underlying cause and, therefore, its effect on dental health and quality of life. In the same way, the dentist must prevent, identify, and treat many dental occlusion, articular (temporomandibular) and neuromuscular diseases that promote parafunction of masticatory muscles. Maintenance of oral health is fundamental for hospitalized patients and its impact appears to be more significant in medically compromised or long-stay hospitalized patients. Hospital-based dentistry might play an important role in the delivery of oral health care to long-term hospital dysphagic patients with disabilities (such as traumatic and congenital anatomical abnormalities and neurological and neuromotor disorders) who are unable to receive their required dental care in their community practice settings. In patients with deglutive disorders promoted by the side-effects of the usual oncologic treatments (surgical, chemotherapy, and radiotherapy) the oral care programs aim to remove mucosal irritating factors, cleanse the oral mucosa, maintain the moisture of the lips and the oral cavity, relieve mucosal inflammation and prevent and treat the inflammation.

In this way, a policy of systematic evaluation of dysphagic patients by oral health professionals is highly recommended, with routine assessment of oral health, improvement of oral hygiene, and appropriate treatment of diseases related to salivation, chewing, and swallowing mechanisms.

6. Conclusions

The different parts of the oral cavity and oropharynx are made up of several cell types of tissues (nerves, fibrovascular tissues, cartilaginous tissues, lining and salivary gland epithelium, and smooth and striated muscles) along withenamel and dentin tissues of the teeth and the supporting bones. The morphophysiology of the oral cavity and oropharynx components is responsible for preservation and maintenance of oral health which contributes to systemic health and a better quality of life to individuals. These components are parts of the body that are highly accessible, sensitive to the action of environmental factors and, at the same time, are able to reflect changes occurring internally in the body. Oropharyngeal dysphagia represents a neuromuscular disorder which characterizes individuals with a difficulty in swallowing. That disorder may result from an accumulation of many factors caused by both endogenous and exogenous etiologic agents which compromise, directly or indirectly, mechanisms of salivation, chewing, and swallowing. The dentist is the health professional that clinically evaluates the oral health conditions of individuals regularly. That health professional must be considered as an integral component of the multidisciplinary health team in order to perform proper educational and preventive approaches, management, and therapeutical actions that might restore oral health to their patients.

Acknowledgements

This work was supported by the Fundação de Amparo à Pesquisa do Estado de Minas Gerais (FAPEMIG) and Coordenação de Aperfeiçoamento de Pessoal de Nível Superior (CAPES). LR Souza is post-doc fellow of the Conselho Nacional de Desenvolvimento Cientifico e Tecnológico (CNPq. Proc. 150998/2014-7). AMB De-Paula is post-doc fellow of the Capes (Science without Borders Program. Proc. 10438/13-0) and researcher fellow of the CNPq.

Author details

Ludmilla R. Souza[1], Marcos V. M. Oliveira[1], John R. Basile[2], Leandro N. Souza[3], Ana C. R. Souza[4], Desiree S. Haikal[1,5] and Alfredo M. B. De-Paula[1,5*]

*Address all correspondence to: ambpatologi@gmail.com

1 Nucleus of Epidemiological and Molecular Research Catrumano. Health Research Laboratory. Health Science Post-graduate Programme. Universidade Estadual de Montes Claros, Montes Claros, Minas Gerais, Brazil

2 Department of Oncology and Diagnostic Sciences. University of Maryland School of Dentistry, Baltimore, Maryland, USA

3 Department of Oral Pathology and Surgery, Dentistry School, Universiadade Federal de Minas Gerais, Belo Horizonte, Minas Gerais, Brazil

4 Department of Dentistry, Centro Universitário Newton Paiva, Belo Horizonte, Minas Gerais, Brazil

5 Department of Dentistry. Universidade Estadual de Montes Claros, Montes Claros, Minas Gerais, Brazil

Authors declare no conlfict of interest.

References

[1] Cook IJ. Oropharyngeal dysphagia. Gastroenterol Clin North Am. 2009;38(3):411-31.

[2] Ekberg O, Hamdy S, Woisard V, Wuttge-Hannig A, Ortega P. Social and psychological burden of dysphagia: its impact on diagnosis and treatment. Dysphagia. 2002;17(2):139-46.

[3] Speyer R. Oropharyngeal dysphagia: screening and assessment. Otolaryngologic clinics of North America. 2013;46(6):989-1008.

[4] Hughes CV BJB, Philip C. Fox, Yitzhak Marmary, Chih-Ko Yeh, Barbara C. Sonies. Oral pharyngeal dysphagia: a common sequela of salivary gland dysfunction. Dysphagia. 1989;4:12.

[5] Dylan F. Roden KWA. Causes of Dysphagia Among Different Age Groups: A Systematic Review of the Literature. Otolaryngologic clinics of North America. 2013;46(6):23.

[6] Furuta M, Yamashita Y. Oral Health and Swallowing Problems. Curr Phys Med Rehabil Rep. 2013;1:216-22.

[7] Ortega O, Parra C, Zarcero S, Nart J, Sakwinska O, Clave P. Oral health in older patients with oropharyngeal dysphagia. Age and ageing. 2014;43(1):132-7.

[8] Lenz M, Greess H, Baum U, Dobritz M, Kersting-Sommerhoff B. Oropharynx, oral cavity, floor of the mouth: CT and MRI. Eur J Radiol. 2000;33(3):203-15.

[9] Yousem DM, Chalian AA. Oral cavity and pharynx. Radiol Clin North Am. 1998;36(5):967-81, vii.

[10] de Almeida Pdel V, Gregio AM, Machado MA, de Lima AA, Azevedo LR. Saliva composition and functions: a comprehensive review. J Contemp Dent Pract. 2008;9(3):72-80.

[11] Hatch JP, Shinkai RS, Sakai S, Rugh JD, Paunovich ED. Determinants of masticatory performance in dentate adults. Archives of oral biology. 2001;46(7):641-8.

[12] Koolstra JH, van Eijden TM. Dynamics of the human masticatory muscles during a jaw open-close movement. J Biomech. 1997;30(9):883-9.

[13] van der Bilt A, Engelen L, Pereira LJ, van der Glas HW, Abbink JH. Oral physiology and mastication. Physiol Behav. 2006;89(1):22-7.

[14] Laitman JT, Reidenberg JS. The evolution and development of human swallowing: the most important function we least appreciate. Otolaryngologic clinics of North America. 2013;46(6):923-35.

[15] Shaw SM, Martino R. The normal swallow: muscular and neurophysiological control. Otolaryngologic clinics of North America. 2013;46(6):937-56.

[16] Marur T TY, Demirci S. Facial anatomy. Clinics in Dermatology. 2014;32(1):10.

[17] Koussoulakou DS, Margaritis LH, Koussoulakos SL. A curriculum vitae of teeth: evolution, generation, regeneration. Int J Biol Sci. 2009;5(3):226-43.

[18] Thesleff I. The genetic basis of tooth development and dental defects. Am J Med Genet A. 2006;140(23):2530-5.

[19] Denny PC, Ball WD, Redman RS. Salivary glands: a paradigm for diversity of gland development. Crit Rev Oral Biol Med. 1997;8(1):51-75.

[20] Holmberg KV, Hoffman MP. Anatomy, biogenesis and regeneration of salivary glands. Monogr Oral Sci. 2014;24:1-13.

[21] Lydiatt DD, Bucher GS. The historical evolution of the understanding of the submandibular and sublingual salivary glands. Clin Anat. 2012;25(1):2-11.

[22] Miletich I. Introduction to salivary glands: structure, function and embryonic development. Front Oral Biol. 2010;14:1-20.

[23] Le Reverend BJ, Edelson LR, Loret C. Anatomical, functional, physiological and behavioural aspects of the development of mastication in early childhood. Br J Nutr. 2014;111(3):403-14.

[24] Iwasaki S. Evolution of the structure and function of the vertebrate tongue. Journal of anatomy. 2002;201(1):1-13.

[25] Sanders I, Mu L, Amirali A, Su H, Sobotka S. The human tongue slows down to speak: muscle fibers of the human tongue. Anat Rec (Hoboken). 2013;296(10):1615-27.

[26] Takemoto H. Morphological analyses of the human tongue musculature for three-dimensional modeling. Journal of speech, language, and hearing research : JSLHR. 2001;44(1):95-107.

[27] Crum RJ, Loiselle RJ. Oral perception and proprioception: a review of the literature and its significance to prosthodontics. The Journal of prosthetic dentistry. 1972;28(2):215-30.

[28] Gauthier A, Lezy JP, Vacher C. Vascularization of the palate in maxillary osteotomies: anatomical study. Surgical and radiologic anatomy : SRA. 2002;24(1):13-7.

[29] Pinar YA, Bilge O, Govsa F. Anatomic study of the blood supply of perioral region. Clin Anat. 2005;18(5):330-9.

[30] Sirot'akova M, Schmidtova K, Kocisova M, Kuchta M. Adrenergic and acetylcholinesterase-positive innervation of palatine tonsils in mammals. Acta Histochem. 2002;104(4):349-52.

[31] Whetzel TP, Saunders CJ. Arterial anatomy of the oral cavity: an analysis of vascular territories. Plastic and reconstructive surgery. 1997;100(3):582-7; discussion 8-90.

[32] Wilson DB. Embryonic development of the head and neck: part 2, the branchial region. Head & neck surgery. 1979;2(1):59-66.

[33] Amerongen AV, Veerman EC. Saliva--the defender of the oral cavity. Oral diseases. 2002;8(1):12-22.

[34] Bergdahl J, Bergdahl M. Environmental illness: evaluation of salivary flow, symptoms, diseases, medications, and psychological factors. Acta Odontol Scand. 2001;59(2):104-10.

[35] Dawes C. Circadian rhythms in human salivary flow rate and composition. J Physiol. 1972;220(3):529-45.

[36] Nagler RM. Salivary glands and the aging process: mechanistic aspects, health-status and medicinal-efficacy monitoring. Biogerontology. 2004;5(4):223-33.

[37] Schipper RG, Silletti E, Vingerhoeds MH. Saliva as research material: biochemical, physicochemical and practical aspects. Archives of oral biology. 2007;52(12):1114-35.

[38] Ghezzi EM, Wagner-Lange LA, Schork MA, Metter EJ, Baum BJ, Streckfus CF, et al. Longitudinal influence of age, menopause, hormone replacement therapy, and other medications on parotid flow rates in healthy women. The journals of gerontology Series A, Biological sciences and medical sciences. 2000;55(1):M34-42.

[39] Ishijima T, Koshino H, Hirai T, Takasaki H. The relationship between salivary secretion rate and masticatory efficiency. Journal of oral rehabilitation. 2004;31(1):3-6.

[40] Li TL, Gleeson M. The effect of single and repeated bouts of prolonged cycling and circadian variation on saliva flow rate, immunoglobulin A and alpha-amylase responses. J Sports Sci. 2004;22(11-12):1015-24.

[41] Enberg N, Alho H, Loimaranta V, Lenander-Lumikari M. Saliva flow rate, amylase activity, and protein and electrolyte concentrations in saliva after acute alcohol consumption. Oral surgery, oral medicine, oral pathology, oral radiology, and endodontics. 2001;92(3):292-8.

[42] Guggenheimer J, Moore PA. Xerostomia: etiology, recognition and treatment. J Am Dent Assoc. 2003;134(1):61-9; quiz 118-9.

[43] Pedersen AM, Bardow A, Jensen SB, Nauntofte B. Saliva and gastrointestinal functions of taste, mastication, swallowing and digestion. Oral diseases. 2002;8(3):117-29.

[44] Rad M, Kakoie S, Niliye Brojeni F, Pourdamghan N. Effect of Long-term Smoking on Whole-mouth Salivary Flow Rate and Oral Health. J Dent Res Dent Clin Dent Prospects. 2010;4(4):110-4.

[45] Lund JP, Kolta A. Generation of the central masticatory pattern and its modification by sensory feedback. Dysphagia. 2006;21(3):167-74.

[46] Turker KS, Sowman PF, Tuncer M, Tucker KJ, Brinkworth RS. The role of periodontal mechanoreceptors in mastication. Archives of oral biology. 2007;52(4):361-4.

[47] Zakir HM, Kitagawa J, Yamada Y, Kurose M, Mostafeezur RM, Yamamura K. Modulation of spindle discharge from jaw-closing muscles during chewing foods of different hardness in awake rabbits. Brain Res Bull. 2010;83(6):380-6.

[48] HIIEMAE K. Mechanisms of food reduction, transport and deglutition: how the texture of food affects feeding behavior. J Texture Stud. 2004;35(2):30.

[49] Ikebe K, Matsuda K, Morii K, Furuya-Yoshinaka M, Nokubi T, Renner RP. Association of masticatory performance with age, posterior occlusal contacts, occlusal force, and salivary flow in older adults. Int J Prosthodont. 2006;19(5):475-81.

[50] Okiyama S, Ikebe K, Nokubi T. Association between masticatory performance and maximal occlusal force in young men. Journal of oral rehabilitation. 2003;30(3): 278-82.

[51] Fueki K, Yoshida E, Igarashi Y. A structural equation model relating objective and subjective masticatory function and oral health-related quality of life in patients with removable partial dentures. Journal of oral rehabilitation. 2011;38(2):86-94.

[52] Persic S, Palac A, Bunjevac T, Celebic A. Development of a new chewing function questionnaire for assessment of a self-perceived chewing function. Community Dent Oral Epidemiol. 2013;41(6):565-73.

[53] Ertekin C, Keskin A, Kiylioglu N, Kirazli Y, On AY, Tarlaci S, et al. The effect of head and neck positions on oropharyngeal swallowing: a clinical and electrophysiologic study. Archives of physical medicine and rehabilitation. 2001;82(9):1255-60.

[54] Martin-Harris B, Brodsky MB, Michel Y, Ford CL, Walters B, Heffner J. Breathing and swallowing dynamics across the adult lifespan. Arch Otolaryngol Head Neck Surg. 2005;131(9):762-70.

[55] Plant RL. Anatomy and physiology of swallowing in adults and geriatrics. Otolaryngologic clinics of North America. 1998;31(3):477-88.

[56] Humbert IA, German RZ. New directions for understanding neural control in swallowing: the potential and promise of motor learning. Dysphagia. 2013;28(1):1-10.

[57] Jean A. Brain stem control of swallowing: neuronal network and cellular mechanisms. Physiol Rev. 2001;81(2):929-69.

[58] Ikebe K, Matsuda K, Kagawa R, Enoki K, Yoshida M, Maeda Y, et al. Association of masticatory performance with age, gender, number of teeth, occlusal force and salivary flow in Japanese older adults: is ageing a risk factor for masticatory dysfunction? Archives of oral biology. 2011;56(10):991-6.

[59] Mendes DC, Silva TF, Barros Lde O, de Oliveira MV, Vieira LT, Haikal DS, et al. Analysis of the normative conditions of oral health, depression and serotonin-transporter-linked promoter region polymorphisms in an elderly population. Geriatrics & gerontology international. 2013;13(1):98-106.

[60] Somsak K, Kaewplung O. The effects of the number of natural teeth and posterior occluding pairs on the oral health-related quality of life in elderly dental patients. Gerodontology. 2014.

[61] Yellowitz JA, Schneiderman MT. Elder's oral health crisis. The journal of evidence-based dental practice. 2014;14 Suppl:191-200.

[62] EF HDdPAMAMAF. Autopercepção da saúde bucal e impacto na qualidade de vida do idoso: uma abordagem quanti-qualitativa. Ciênc saúde coletiva. 2011;16(7).

[63] Enoki K, Matsuda KI, Ikebe K, Murai S, Yoshida M, Maeda Y, et al. Influence of xerostomia on oral health-related quality of life in the elderly: a 5-year longitudinal study. Oral surgery, oral medicine, oral pathology and oral radiology. 2014;117(6): 716-21.

[64] Morzel M, Jeannin A, Lucchi G, Truntzer C, Pecqueur D, Nicklaus S, et al. Human infant saliva peptidome is modified with age and diet transition. Journal of proteomics. 2012;75(12):3665-73.

[65] Fontijn-Tekamp FA, Slagter AP, Van Der Bilt A, Van THMA, Witter DJ, Kalk W, et al. Biting and chewing in overdentures, full dentures, and natural dentitions. Journal of dental research. 2000;79(7):1519-24.

[66] Hsu KJ, Lee HE, Wu YM, Lan SJ, Huang ST, Yen YY. Masticatory factors as predictors of oral health-related quality of life among elderly people in Kaohsiung City, Taiwan. Quality of life research : an international journal of quality of life aspects of treatment, care and rehabilitation. 2014;23(4):1395-405.

[67] Nicosia MA, Hind JA, Roecker EB, Carnes M, Doyle J, Dengel GA, et al. Age effects on the temporal evolution of isometric and swallowing pressure. The journals of gerontology Series A, Biological sciences and medical sciences. 2000;55(11):M634-40.

[68] Poisson P, Laffond T, Campos S, Dupuis V, Bourdel-Marchasson I. Relationships between oral health, dysphagia and undernutrition in hospitalised elderly patients. Gerodontology. 2014.

[69] Leder SB, Ross DA. Investigation of the causal relationship between tracheotomy and aspiration in the acute care setting. The Laryngoscope. 2000;110(4):641-4.

[70] TM M. Head and neck disorders affecting swallowing. GI Motility online. 2006.

[71] Dziewas R, Warnecke T, Schnabel M, Ritter M, Nabavi DG, Schilling M, et al. Neuroleptic-induced dysphagia: case report and literature review. Dysphagia. 2007;22(1): 63-7.

[72] Lo Russo L, Guida L, Di Masi M, Buccelli C, Giannatempo G, Di Fede O, et al. Adverse drug reactions in the oral cavity. Current pharmaceutical design. 2012;18(34): 5481-96.

[73] Rudolph JL, Gardner KF, Gramigna GD, McGlinchey RE. Antipsychotics and oropharyngeal dysphagia in hospitalized older patients. Journal of clinical psychopharmacology. 2008;28(5):532-5.

[74] Altman KW, Richards A, Goldberg L, Frucht S, McCabe DJ. Dysphagia in stroke, neurodegenerative disease, and advanced dementia. Otolaryngologic clinics of North America. 2013;46(6):1137-49.

[75] Alagiakrishnan K, Bhanji RA, Kurian M. Evaluation and management of oropharyngeal dysphagia in different types of dementia: a systematic review. Archives of gerontology and geriatrics. 2013;56(1):1-9.

[76] Kalf JG, de Swart BJ, Bloem BR, Munneke M. Prevalence of oropharyngeal dysphagia in Parkinson's disease: a meta-analysis. Parkinsonism & related disorders. 2012;18(4): 311-5.

[77] Poorjavad M, Derakhshandeh F, Etemadifar M, Soleymani B, Minagar A, Maghzi AH. Oropharyngeal dysphagia in multiple sclerosis. Mult Scler. 2010;16(3):362-5.

[78] Martino R, Foley N, Bhogal S, Diamant N, Speechley M, Teasell R. Dysphagia after stroke: incidence, diagnosis, and pulmonary complications. Stroke; a journal of cerebral circulation. 2005;36(12):2756-63.

[79] Reiter S, Goldsmith C, Emodi-Perlman A, Friedman-Rubin P, Winocur E. Masticatory muscle disorders diagnostic criteria: the American Academy of Orofacial Pain versus the research diagnostic criteria/temporomandibular disorders (RDC/TMD). Journal of oral rehabilitation. 2012;39(12):941-7.

[80] Gandhi YR. Oro-mandibular dystonia. National journal of maxillofacial surgery. 2010;1(2):150-2.

[81] Jaradeh S. Muscle disorders affecting oral and pharyngeal swallowing. GI Motility online. 2006.

[82] de Carvalho Aguiar PM, Ozelius LJ. Classification and genetics of dystonia. The Lancet Neurology. 2002;1(5):316-25.

[83] Kuhnlein P, Gdynia HJ, Sperfeld AD, Lindner-Pfleghar B, Ludolph AC, Prosiegel M, et al. Diagnosis and treatment of bulbar symptoms in amyotrophic lateral sclerosis. Nature clinical practice Neurology. 2008;4(7):366-74.

[84] Mascia MM, Valls-Sole J, Marti MJ, Sanz S. Chewing pattern in patients with Meige's syndrome. Movement disorders : official journal of the Movement Disorder Society. 2005;20(1):26-33.

[85] Ertekin C, Secil Y, Yuceyar N, Aydogdu I. Oropharyngeal dysphagia in polymyositis/dermatomyositis. Clinical neurology and neurosurgery. 2004;107(1):32-7.

[86] Nagano H, Yoshifuku K, Kurono Y. Polymyositis with dysphagia treated with endoscopic balloon dilatation. Auris, nasus, larynx. 2009;36(6):705-8.

[87] Boffano P, Zavattero E, Bosco G, Berrone S. Myositis ossificans of the left medial pterygoid muscle: case report and review of the literature of myositis ossificans of masticatory muscles. Craniomaxillofacial trauma & reconstruction. 2014;7(1):43-50.

[88] Godhi SS, Singh A, Kukreja P, Singh V. Myositis ossificans circumscripta involving bilateral masticatory muscles. The Journal of craniofacial surgery. 2011;22(6):e11-3.

[89] Petty RK, Harding AE, Morgan-Hughes JA. The clinical features of mitochondrial myopathy. Brain : a journal of neurology. 1986;109 (Pt 5):915-38.

[90] Sonies BC. Evaluation and treatment of speech and swallowing disorders associated with myopathies. Current opinion in rheumatology. 1997;9(6):486-95.

[91] Mays JW, Sarmadi M, Moutsopoulos NM. Oral manifestations of systemic autoimmune and inflammatory diseases: diagnosis and clinical management. The journal of evidence-based dental practice. 2012;12(3 Suppl):265-82.

[92] Galvez J, Saiz E, Lopez P, Pina MF, Carrillo A, Nieto A, et al. Diagnostic evaluation and classification criteria in Sjogren's Syndrome. Joint, bone, spine : revue du rhumatisme. 2009;76(1):44-9.

[93] Salomonsson S, Larsson P, Tengner P, Mellquist E, Hjelmstrom P, Wahren-Herlenius M. Expression of the B cell-attracting chemokine CXCL13 in the target organ and autoantibody production in ectopic lymphoid tissue in the chronic inflammatory disease Sjogren's syndrome. Scandinavian journal of immunology. 2002;55(4):336-42.

[94] Mavragani CP, Moutsopoulos NM, Moutsopoulos HM. The management of Sjogren's syndrome. Nature clinical practice Rheumatology. 2006;2(5):252-61.

[95] Rhodus NL, Colby S, Moller K, Bereuter J. Quantitative assessment of dysphagia in patients with primary and secondary Sjogren's syndrome. Oral surgery, oral medicine, oral pathology, oral radiology, and endodontics. 1995;79(3):305-10.

[96] Vincent A, Bowen J, Newsom-Davis J, McConville J. Seronegative generalised myasthenia gravis: clinical features, antibodies, and their targets. The Lancet Neurology. 2003;2(2):99-106.

[97] Colton-Hudson A, Koopman WJ, Moosa T, Smith D, Bach D, Nicolle M. A prospective assessment of the characteristics of dysphagia in myasthenia gravis. Dysphagia. 2002;17(2):147-51.

[98] Higo R, Nito T, Tayama N. Videofluoroscopic assessment of swallowing function in patients with myasthenia gravis. Journal of the neurological sciences. 2005;231(1-2): 45-8.

[99] Correa GT, Bandeira GA, Cavalcanti BG, de Carvalho Fraga CA, dos Santos EP, Silva TF, et al. Association of -308 TNF-alpha promoter polymorphism with clinical aggressiveness in patients with head and neck squamous cell carcinoma. Oral oncology. 2011;47(9):888-94.

[100] De Paula AM, Souza LR, Farias LC, Correa GT, Fraga CA, Eleuterio NB, et al. Analysis of 724 cases of primary head and neck squamous cell carcinoma (HNSCC) with a focus on young patients and p53 immunolocalization. Oral oncology. 2009;45(9): 777-82.

[101] Rothenberg SM, Ellisen LW. The molecular pathogenesis of head and neck squamous cell carcinoma. The Journal of clinical investigation. 2012;122(6):1951-7.

[102] Warnakulasuriya S. Global epidemiology of oral and oropharyngeal cancer. Oral oncology. 2009;45(4-5):309-16.

[103] Manikantan K, Khode S, Sayed SI, Roe J, Nutting CM, Rhys-Evans P, et al. Dysphagia in head and neck cancer. Cancer treatment reviews. 2009;35(8):724-32.

[104] Pauloski BR, Logemann JA, Rademaker AW, McConnel FM, Stein D, Beery Q, et al. Speech and swallowing function after oral and oropharyngeal resections: one-year follow-up. Head & neck. 1994;16(4):313-22.

[105] Zuydam AC, Rogers SN, Brown JS, Vaughan ED, Magennis P. Swallowing rehabilitation after oro-pharyngeal resection for squamous cell carcinoma. The British journal of oral & maxillofacial surgery. 2000;38(5):513-8.

[106] Dirix P, Nuyts S, Van den Bogaert W. Radiation-induced xerostomia in patients with head and neck cancer: a literature review. Cancer. 2006;107(11):2525-34.

[107] Logemann JA, Smith CH, Pauloski BR, Rademaker AW, Lazarus CL, Colangelo LA, et al. Effects of xerostomia on perception and performance of swallow function. Head & neck. 2001;23(4):317-21.

[108] Rosenthal DI, Lewin JS, Eisbruch A. Prevention and treatment of dysphagia and aspiration after chemoradiation for head and neck cancer. Journal of clinical oncology : official journal of the American Society of Clinical Oncology. 2006;24(17):2636-43.

Chapter 2

Impact of Polypharmacy on Deglutition in Patients with Coronary and Cardiac Diseases

Hadeer Akram Abdul Razzaq and
Syed Azhar Syed Sulaiman

Additional information is available at the end of the chapter

http://dx.doi.org/10.5772/61085

1. Introduction

Dysphagia relates to swallowing problems due to physiological changes in aging people or such factors as diseases and medications [1]. Previous studies stated that world prevalence of dysphagia ranged between 16% and 22% [2]. Dysphagia can be classified into two types: oropharyngeal and esophageal. Oropharyngeal dysphagia includes cerebrovascular disorders (like stroke), central nervous system disorders (like Parkinson's disease), and others (like thyroid disorders). Esophageal dysphagia includes aging, alcoholism, diabetes mellitus (DM), cancers, and medications [3]. Several symptoms detected to determine the type of dysphagia (i.e. swallowing problems) included gastrointestinal symptoms (such as heartburn, indigestion, and gastro-esophageal reflux disease), respiratory symptoms (like cough), and musculoskeletal chest pain [4].

Many medications are known to induce dysphagia by affecting smooth and striated muscle via increasing the sensitivity of mucosa resulting in swallowing difficulty. There are two different ways in which this occurs. First, there is the normal adverse effect (or the indirect effect) due to pharmacological action and complications such as dysphagia induced by antibiotics as well as immunosuppressive and anti-cancer agents. Second, there is the direct effect of medications irritating the mucosa, which is more observed in the elderly [5]. The aortic arch is the area most susceptible to injuries induced by pills. Medications with a pH less than 3 (such as doxycycline and tetracycline) as well as certain slow-release anticholinergic dosage medications were more caustic resulting in moderate and severe injuries [6]. The severity of injuries depended on chronic irritation, high osmolarity, and the dissolution rate of dosage forms [7]. Medications that are known to induce dysphagia can be categorized into four groups [8]: (1) medications affecting smooth muscle such as theophylline and calcium channel blockers; (2) medications reducing esophageal sphincter pressure such as nitrates and atropine; (3) medications inducing xerostomia such as antihypertensive agents and antiarrhythmics; and (4) medications inducing esophageal injury such as aspirin and non-steroidal anti-inflammatory medications.

Polypharmacy is defined as patient use of five or more medications [9]. Polypharmacy contributes to the high incidence of adverse effects as a consequence of possible drug interactions between medications [10, 11]. Although some studies state that polypharmacy should be considered a significant predictor for dysphagia [2, 12], they have weaknesses in that they were either case reports or mainly dealt with specific dysphagia type. Thus, the aims of the current study are, first, to describe the incidence, severity, and predictors of dysphagia; second, to determine the relationship between polypharmacy and dysphagia; and, third, to describe the association between types of dysphagia (depending on concurrent symptoms) and polypharmacy.

2. Methodology

2.1. Study design

The cross-sectional design based on patients self-reporting was used in the current study to determine the incidence of dysphagia and its concurrent symptoms. The reason this study was carried out at the Cardiac Clinic of Penang General Hospital was because polypharmacy is more detectable in cardiac patients as a result of their treatment by chronic and multiple therapies. There were 576 cardiac outpatients involved in the current study. Approval for this study was granted by the Ministry of Health of Malaysia and consent forms were collected from patients. All patients involved in the current study were aged 18 years or above, used medications dispensed from the pharmacy of the hospital, and were able to understand and fill in the questionnaire form in Standard Malay (Bahasa Malaysia) or English.

2.2. Self-reporting questionnaire and assessment of polypharmacy

The self-reporting questionnaire used in the current study had the purpose of counting the incidence and severity of dysphagia and its symptoms. The validity of the questionnaire was established after conducting language, panel, and statistical validity, after conducting a pilot study, and after settling on an appropriate coefficient of reliability (Cronbach's α = 0.92). Statistical advanced logistic regression was used to measure the specificity and sensitivity of dysphagia and its symptoms, which had fixed in the questionnaire form. Patients were asked to answer "yes" or "no" to questions about the existence of dysphagia and its symptoms. Patients were also asked to report the severity of the symptoms as "mild", "moderate", or "severe". Mild referred to symptoms that did not bother the patient who had no need for assistance. Moderate referred to patients who were bothered by symptoms but had no need for assistance. Severe referred to patients who were seriously bothered by these symptoms and had urgent need for assistance. Other information such as demographic data, medical history, and concurrent medications and diseases were taken from the progress files of patients.

The patients included in this study were classified into three groups: (1) patients taking no medications who were referred from other clinics for a follow-up; (2) patients already known to the department taking fewer than 5 medications and (3) patients known to the department taking 5 or more medications. All patients on medication had been in chronic therapy for at least one year.

2.3. Statistical analysis

The Statistical Package for the Social Sciences (SPSS) software program was used to analyze the results of the current study. The incidence and severity of dysphagia and its symptoms were measured descriptively. The correlation between dysphagia and its symptoms was tested using Spearman's rank correlation. Multiple logistic regression was used, first, to find out the effect of predictors' interaction on the incidence of dysphagia; second, to discover how polypharmacy impacted dysphagia; and, third, to determine the association between polypharmacy and type of dysphagia (oropharyngeal and esophageal). All the results of this study were considered significant if their p values were less than 0.05.

3. Results

3.1. Demographic characteristics and medical information

The highest incidence of disease was found in males with a mean age of 59.11±10.14 years. The most common diseases found in the current study were hypertension, DM, and ischemic heart disease (IHD). The medications used the most were statins, aspirin, beta-blockers, and angiotensin-converting enzyme inhibitors (ACE-Is). Other demographic characteristics and medical information are illustrated in Table 1.

3.2. Severity of dysphagia types and its symptoms

The incidence (and percentage) of current patients complaining of dysphagia and its symptoms during therapy were 122 (21.2%), 177 (30.7%), 265 (46%), and 286 (49.7%) for dysphagia, indigestion, cough, and chest pain, respectively. Mild symptoms were the highest incidences followed by moderate and severe (as shown in Figure 1).

Spearman's rank correlation showed a positive significant (2-tailed, $p< 0.001$) relationship between dysphagia and its symptoms. The correlation coefficient between dysphagia and its symptoms was 0.322, 0.146, and 0.126 for indigestion, cough, and chest pain, respectively. This result showed that the incidence of esophageal dysphagia was more frequent than that of oropharyngeal dysphagia.

Demographic data and diseases		% (No.)	Medications	% (No.)
Gender (male)		74.3 (428)	Statins	87.8 (506)
Age (≤65)		68.9 (397)	Aspirin	67.4 (388)
Race	Malay	39.6 (228)	Beta-blockers	70.8 (408)
	Chinese	28.5 (164)	Calcium channel blockers	24.5 (141)
	Indian	29.7 (171)	ACE-Is	54 (311)
	Other	2.3 (13)	Angiotensin receptor blockers (ARBs)	10.6 (61)
Smoking		14.8 (85)	Trimetazidine	29.2 (168)
Alcohol consumption		9.4 (54)	Isosorbide dinitrate	23.1 (133)
Hypertension		65.8 (379)	Thiazides	6.8 (39)
DM		39.9 (230)	Furosemide	18.9 (109)
IHD		39.8 (229)	Spironolactone	6.3 (36)
Arrhythmia		3.3 (19)	Gliclazide	22.2 (128)
Renal disease		2.4 (14)	Metformin	25 (144)
Thyroid diseases		2.3 (13)	Digoxin	4.3 (25)
Myocardial infarction		2.3 (13)	Warfarin	5.6 (32)
			Clopidogrel	17.7 (102)
			Ticlopidine	11.3 (65)
			Prazosin	2.3 (13)

Table 1. Demographic characteristics and medical information of patients

3.3. Predictors of dysphagia

Gender, IHD, and statins were the most significant factors that must be involved in the regression model to insure the predictors of dysphagia could be determined (as shown in Table 2).

Categorical variables	χ^2	*df*	*p*
Gender	6.181	1	0.013
IHD	7.909	1	0.005
Statins	4.539	1	0.033

χ^2 = chi-square test; *df* = degrees of freedom; *p* = calculated probability

Table 2. Categorical variables included in the regression model

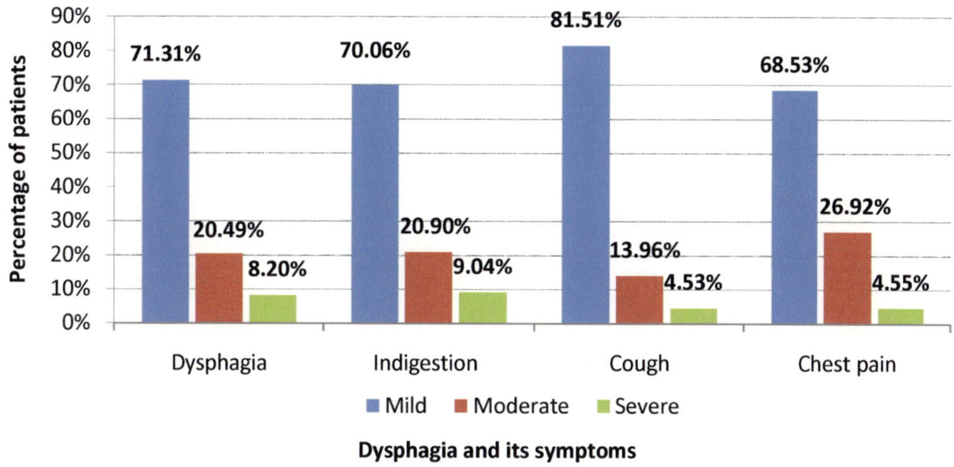

Figure 1. Incidence and severity of dysphagia and its symptoms

As a result of logistic regression, gender and IHD were found to be the significant risk factors involved in the high incidence of dysphagia. Female cardiac patients had incidences of dysphagia that were approximately 1.8 times higher than those of males. Patients with IHD had incidences of dysphagia that were 1.8 times higher than those without (as shown in Table 3).

Variable		*β*	*SE*	*OR*	*95% CI*	*p*
Gender	Female	0.575	0.233	1.777	(1.148, 2.750)	0.010
	Male (ref.)					
IHD	Yes	0.599	0.207	1.820	(1.212, 2.731)	0.004
	No (ref.)					

The reference category for the model is no dysphagia. The backward stepwise logistic regression test was used. The Hosmer and Lemeshow goodness-of-fit test with χ^2 (N = 576) = 3.365 and p =0.186

Table 3. Predictors of dysphagia in cardiac outpatients

3.4. Polypharmacy and its impact on dysphagia

Patients with polypharmacy (i.e. those using 5 or more medications) have a higher incidence (45.84%) of dysphagia than other patients (as shown in Figure 2).

Binary logistic regression showed that medication use was a risk factor in the incidence of dysphagia in cardiac outpatients. The incidence of dysphagia was about 2.8 and 3.2 times higher for patients taking 1–4 drugs and those taking ≥ 5 drugs (polypharmacy), respectively, than those taking no medications. However, the incidence of dysphagia in patients with polypharmacy was found to be higher than those taking fewer than 5 medications (as shown in Table 4).

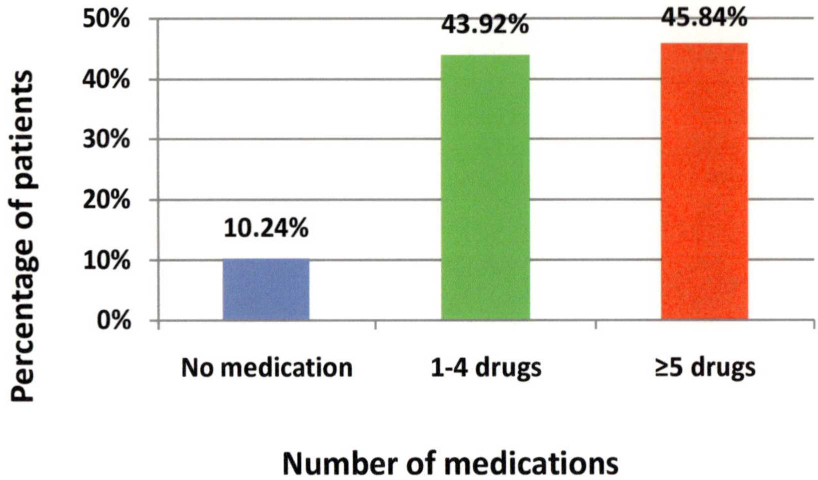

Figure 2. Percentage of medications used

Category	β	*SE*	*OR*	*95% CI*	*p*
1–4 drugs	1.144	0.491	2.842	(1.200, 8.223)	0.020
≥ 5 drugs	1.156	0.490	3.176	(1.216, 8.299)	0.018
No medications (ref.)					

The reference category for the model is no dysphagia.

Table 4. The association between polypharmacy and dysphagia

3.5. Predictor interaction and impact on dysphagia

The impact of predictor interaction on the incidence of dysphagia according to binary logistic regression showed gender and IHD to be two significant predictors. Patients taking 5 medications or more (i.e. polypharmacy) were more susceptible to the incidence of dysphagia, especially female patients and those with IHD.

Female cardiac patients taking 5 or more medications were about 2.2 times more prone to a high incidence of dysphagia than males taking no medications, while there was no significant impact on females taking fewer than 5 medications. This proved the impact polypharmacy has on females complaining of dysphagia (as shown in Table 5).

IHD patients taking 5 medications or more had a significantly higher (about 1.9 times) incidence of dysphagia than those free of IHD and taking no medications. However, no impact was found for IHD patients taking less than 5 medications (as shown in Table 6).

These tables show the impact of polypharmacy is going to increase the incidence of dysphagia when the interactions between predictors are taken into consideration. However, gender (female) was a higher predictor effect for dysphagia than the IHD predictor.

Category	*β*	*SE*	*OR*	*95% CI*	*p*
No. of drugs (gender)					0.012
1–4 drugs (female)	0.555	0.280	1.741	(1.006-3.015)	0.050
≥ 5 drugs (female)	0.770	0.306	2.159	(1.186-3.930)	0.012

The reference category is males taking no medications

The reference category for the model is no dysphagia

Table 5. Impact of polypharmacy and gender on dysphagia

Category	*β*	*SE*	*OR*	*95% CI*	*p*
No. of drugs (IHD)					0.022
1–4 drugs (IHD)	0.484	0.271	1.623	(0.954, 2.761)	0.074
≥ 5 drugs (IHD)	0.617	0.242	1.854	(1.154, 2.978)	0.011

The reference category is no medications and no IHD

The reference category for the model is no dysphagia

Table 6. Impact of polypharmacy and IHD on dysphagia

3.6. Polypharmacy and type of dysphagia

Dysphagia was classified according to symptoms of cardiac patients taking part in the study. Chest pain is the only symptom that showed a significant association with polypharmacy. Patients taking 5 or more medications had a significantly higher incidence of chest pain (about 2.1 times) than those without medications. Moreover, no significant effect was found for chest pain in patients taking fewer than 5 medications. Thus, polypharmacy has a greater effect on esophageal dysphagia than oropharyngeal dysphagia (as shown in Table 7).

4. Discussion

Many different results have been reported on the incidence of dysphagia in different areas of the world as a consequence of the number of diseases and medications that bring it about. Moreover, some studies have restricted themselves to different age groups; for example, some relate to childhood dysphagia while others relate to geriatrics [13]. Many physicians fail to take these symptoms into account either because they do not take dysphagia seriously or are unfamiliar with the factors that bring it about [14]. Siebens *et al* [15] and Croghan *et al* [16] found that morbidity and mortality were significantly higher in those with dysphagia than those without because of malnutrition and/or low quality of life [17]. Speyer *et al* [18] and Wallace *et al* [19] found that patients' self-reporting was the most effective tool for identifying dysphagia symptoms. This led to many studies being conducted on patients self-reporting with the aim of determining the incidence of dysphagia [20–22]. This was because patients were considered the main source of information to get at the data needed to conduct clinical

Indigestion	*β*	*SE*	*OR*	*95% CI*	*p*
1–4 drugs	-0.099	0.315	0.906	(0.488, 1.681)	0.754
≥ 5 drugs	0.130	0.311	1.139	(0.619, 2,079)	0.676
No medications (ref.)					
Cough					
1–4 drugs	0.040	0.291	1.041	(0.588, 1.842)	0.890
≥ 5 drugs	0.132	0.290	1.141	(0.647, 2.014)	0.648
No medications (ref.)					
Chest pain					
1–4 drugs	0.369	0.297	1.447	(0.808, 2.591)	0.214
≥ 5 drugs	0.748	0.296	2.113	(1.182, 3.777)	0.012
No medications (ref.)					

The reference category is no dysphagia.

Table 7. Association between polypharmacy and type of dysphagia

studies. Unfortunately, very few studies have reported on the risk factors relating to dysphagia.

There are a number of benefits stemming from the current study: first, establishing a new method to count the incidence of dysphagia by getting cardiac outpatients to fill in a validated, acceptable, and feasible questionnaire, especially because until now there has been no standard validated tool to report dysphagia and its symptoms capable of meeting clinical requirements [23]. Second, this study can be used to determine the type of dysphagia based on the types of symptoms by statistically correlating them into oropharyngeal and esophageal types; up until now all previous studies either depended on one type or using scales for the classification. Moreover, no study has ever been assigned to a specific clinical case such as the one here for cardiovascular diseases or investigated the interactions of dysphagia predictors.

The survey carried out by Barczi *et al* [24] stated the incidence of adult patients complaining of dysphagia ranged from 10 to 30%. The dysphagia incidence (21.2%) of the present study was in the normal range, which was considered to be a good level of incidence when other risks were taken into consideration; for example, the subjects involved in the current study were elderly cardiac patients complaining of serious diseases and using chronic multiple therapies. There is variance in the incidence of dysphagia symptoms such as cough, chest pain, and indigestion. Such differences have also been reported in previous studies [25, 26]. The reason for such differences is because the diseases affecting patients and the medications they take differ from one patient to another. Compared with other studies, cough had a higher incidence of dysphagia in the current study (46.7%), which was higher than incidence of dysphagia, and this case was similar to the compared results of Eslick *et al* [27] who reported dysphagia (16%), cough (27%) and chest pain (23%). Their study was based on different explanations of different mechanisms of dysphagia [28, 29]. The incidence of mild, moderate, and severe dysphagia in the present study was 71.31, 20.49, and 8.20%, respectively, which was similar to the results of Eslick *et al* who reported 65, 30, and 5% for mild, moderate, and severe, respectively [27].

http://dx.doi.org/10.5772/61085

Dobrzycki *et al* found a significant association between IHDs and dysphagia, because the shifting of parasympathetic levels increases the incidence of gastric reflex and induces cardiac problems [30]. Similarly, cardiac patients in the current study considered IHDs to be the main risk factors of dysphagia, where the incidence of dysphagia increased approximately 1.8 times in patients complaining of IHDs. Alves *et al* found gender had a significant impact on the incidence of dysphagia by measuring swallowing parameters such as velocity, intervals, number, and volume capacity. The velocity at which females swallow was found to be slower than for males, the volume capacity of females was found to be less than males, and females were found to need more time to swallow [31]. There are two reasons for this. First, males have larger oral and pharyngeal cavities than females; hence, they find it easier to swallow. Second, some studies have reported that it takes longer for the esophageal sphincter to open in females than in males [32, 33]. However, the results of the current study are in agreement with previous studies regarding the relationship between gender and dysphagia; for example, there is a higher incidence (approximately 1.8 times) of dysphagia in females than in males.

The reason polypharmacy can be considered a significant risk factor to the high incidence of mortalities, morbidities, and serious adverse reactions, is because drug interactions increase the potential toxicity of medications, especially in elderly patients [34]. The incidence of polypharmacy detected varies widely between studies (22–82%) [35–39] as a result not only of the way in which medications are prescribed in different countries but also awareness about the risks of medications. The incidence of polypharmacy reported in the present study was considered good (45.84%) when compared with other studies. Moreover, none of these studies compared the incidence of dysphagia in healthy individuals and ill patients. Some patients in the current study were not taking any medications because they had came from other clinics for checking purposes only, making them a good standard group for comparison with those with polypharmacy and those without polypharmacy.

Previous studies have found that polypharmacy has an effect on the incidence of dysphagia and swallowing problems. However, these studies either were reports focused on types of dosage forms, or conducted at community pharmacies for primary care patients [4, 40, 41]. The present study has demonstrated significant clinical outcomes for the relationship between polypharmacy and dysphagia, and provided evidence to show that number of medications elevates the incidence of dysphagia in cardiac outpatients. In addition to these results, the interactions of predictors were also investigated with significant positive outcomes. Females with polypharmacy had a higher incidence of dysphagia than females without polypharmacy, due to females with polypharmacy being more susceptible to adverse reactions of medications [42]. Patients complaining of IHDs had a high incidence of polypharmacy, which elevates the incidence of adverse drug reactions including dysphagia [43]. Thus, the present study has shown that the incidence of patients with polypharmacy complaining of IHDs and reporting dysphagia is high. The present study has satisfied theories about the interactions between predictors and their impact on the incidence of adverse reactions. Few studies have investigated the synergistic effect of predictors on the incidence of dysphagia, which gives the current study importance in providing a new clinical viewpoint.

A final novel result concerns the classification of dysphagia induced by polypharmacy in cardiac outpatients. There has yet to be a study determining the effects of polypharmacy on the incidence of dysphagia, let alone the type of dysphagia. The present study found that chest pain had a greater association with polypharmacy than other symptoms. By correlating the symptoms of dysphagia, the study found that polypharmacy is likely to induce a higher incidence of esophageal dysphagia due to the significant irritation (e.g. of the mucosa) of medications and physiological changes with aging. Despite being unable to pinpoint a specific medication as the main causative agent for inducing a high incidence of dysphagia, the cumulative impact of polypharmacy was a prime candidate. Therefore, the current study suggests that the effect of total number of medications (polypharmacy) is greater than the effect of the medication itself, possibly due to the interactions and adverse reactions of medications.

5. Conclusion

Patients' self-reporting was considered the optimal method to gather information on adverse symptomatic effects like dysphagia. Polypharmacy, female patients, and IHDs are the main predictors for dysphagia. Despite these predictors being non-preventable, polypharmacy control can minimize the incidence and severity of dysphagia induced by medications. The authors of the present study recommend healthcare professionals (especially pharmacists) to do their utmost to reduce the number of prescribed medications (according to the guidelines of polypharmacy), because they are more aware than most of adverse drug reactions and drug interactions.

Author details

Hadeer Akram Abdul Razzaq* and Syed Azhar Syed Sulaiman

*Address all correspondence to: hadproof@yahoo.com

Department of Clinical Pharmacy, School of Pharmaceutical Sciences, Universiti Sains Malaysia (USM), Penang, Malaysia

References

[1] Sura L, Madhavan A, Carnaby G, Crary MA (2012). Dysphagia in the elderly: management and nutritional considerations. Clin Interv Aging, 7: 287–98. doi: 10.2147/CIA.S23404.

[2] Eslick GD, Talley NJ (2008). Dysphagia: epidemiology, risk factors and impact on quality of life—a population-based study. Aliment Pharmacol Ther, 27(10): 971–9. doi: 10.1111/j.1365-2036.2008.03664.x.

[3] Prasse JE, Kikano GE (2004). An overview of dysphagia in the elderly. Adv Stud Med, 4: 527–33.

[4] Aslam M, Vaezi MF (2013). Dysphagia in the elderly. Gastroenterol Hepatol, 9(12): 784–95.

[5] Stoschus B, Allescher HD (1993). Drug-induced dysphagia. Dysphagia, 8(2):154–9.

[6] Morris TJ, Davis TP (2000). Doxycycline-induced esophageal ulceration in the U.S. military service. Mil Med, 165(4): 316–9.

[7] Helm JF, Dodds WJ, Riedel DR, Teeter BC, Hogan WJ, Arndorfer RC (1983). Determinants of esophageal acid clearance in normal subjects. Gastroenterology, 85: 607–12.

[8] Al-Shehri A (2001). Dysphagia as a drug side effect. Internet J Otorhinolaryngol, 1: 2.

[9] Najjar MF, Abd Aziz N, Hassan Y, Ghazali R, Abdul AlRazzaq HA, Zalila A (2010). Predictors of polypharmacy and adverse drug reactions among geriatric inpatients at Malaysian hospital. HealthMED, 4(2): 273–83.

[10] Shah BM, Hajjar ER (2012). Polypharmacy, adverse drug reactions, and geriatric syndromes. Clin Geriatr Med, 28(2): 173–86.

[11] Bushardt RL, Massey EB, Simpson TW, Ariail JC, Simpson KN (2008). Polypharmacy: misleading, but manageable. Clin Interv Aging, 3(2): 383–9.

[12] Chaumartin N, Monville M, Lachaux B (2012). Dysphagia or dysphagias during neuroleptic medication? Encephale, 38(4): 351–5. doi: 10.1016/j.encep.2011.07.002.

[13] World Gastroenterology Organisation Practice Guidelines: Dysphagia (2007). World Gastroenterology Organisation.

[14] Paterson WG (1996). Dysphagia in the elderly. Can Fam Physician, 42: 925–32.

[15] Siebens H, Trupe E, Siebens A, Cook F, Anshen S, Hanauer R *et al* (1986). Correlates and consequences of eating dependency in institutionalized elderly. Am J Geriatr Soc, 34: 192–8.

[16] Croghan E, Burke EM, Caplan S, Denman S (1994). Pilot study of 12-month outcomes of nursing home patients with aspiration on videofluoroscopy. Dysphagia, 9: 141–6.

[17] Groher ME, Crary MA (2010). Dysphagia: Clinical Management in Adults and Children. Maryland Heights, MO: Mosby Elsevier.

[18] Speyer R, Cordier R, Kertscher B, Heijnen BJ (2014). Psychometric properties of questionnaires on functional health status in oropharyngeal dysphagia: a systematic literature review. Biomed Res Int, 458678. doi: 10.1155/2014/458678.

[19] Wallace KL, Middleton S, Cook IJ (2000). Development and validation of a self-report symptom inventory to assess the severity of oral-pharyngeal dysphagia. Gastroenterology, 118(4): 678–87.

[20] Sales DS, Alvarenga RM, Vasconcelos CC, Silva RG, Thuler LC (2013). Translation, cross-cultural adaptation and validation of the Portuguese version of the DYMUS questionnaire for the assessment of dysphagia in multiple sclerosis. Springerplus, 2: 332. doi: 10.1186/2193-1801-2-332.

[21] Holland G, Jayasersekeran V, Pendleton N, Horan M, Jones M, Hamdy S (2011). Prevalence and symptom profiling of oropharyngeal dysphagia in a community dwelling of an elderly population: self-reporting questionnaire survey. Dis Esophagus, 24(7): 476–80.

[22] Kawashima K, Motohashi Y, Fujishima I (2004). Prevalence of dysphagia among community-dwelling elderly individuals as estimated using a questionnaire for dysphagia screening. Dysphagia, 19: 266–71.

[23] Sallum RA, Duarte AF, Cecconello I (2012). Analytic review of dysphagia scales. Arq Bras Cir Dig, 25(4): 279–82.

[24] Barczi SR, Sullivan PA, Robbins J (2000). How should dysphagia care of older adults differ? Establishing optimal practice patterns. Semin Speech Lang, 21: 347–61.

[25] Wiesner W, Wetzel SG, Kappos L, Hoshi MM, Witte U, Radue EW *et al* (2002). Swallowing abnormalities in multiple sclerosis: correlation between videofluoroscopy and subjective symptoms. Eur Radiol, 12(4): 789–92.

[26] Cook AJ (2008). Diagnostic evaluation of dysphagia. Nat Clin Pract Gastroenterol Hepatol, 5: 393–403.

[27] Eslick GD, Talley NJ (2008). Dysphagia: epidemiology, risk factors and impact on quality of life—a population-based study. Aliment Pharmacol Ther, 27(10): 971–9. doi: 10.1111/j.1365-2036.2008.03664.x.

[28] Kikendall JW, Friedman AC, Oyewole MA, Fleischer D, Johnson LF (1983). Pill-induced esophageal injury. Dig Dis Sci, 28: 174–82.

[29] Agha PP, Wilson JAP, Notstrand TT (1986). Medication-induced esophagitis. Gastrointest Radiol, 11: 7–11.

[30] Dobrzycki S, Skrodzka D, Musiał WJ, Go M, Korecki J, Gugała K *et al* (2004). Relationship between gastroesophageal reflux disease and myocardial ischemia. Effect of reflux on temporary activity of autonomic nervous system. Rocz Akad Med Bialymst, 49: 93–7.

[31] Alves LM, Cassiani Ride A, Santos CM, Dantas RO (2007) Gender effect on the clinical measurement of swallowing. Arq Gastroenterol 44: 227–9. doi: 10.1590/s0004-28032007000300009.

[32] Logemann JA, Pauloski BR, Rademaker AW, Kahrilas PJ (2002). Oropharyngeal swallow in younger and older women: videofluoroscopic analysis. J Speech Lang Hear Res, 45: 434–45.

[33] Robbins JA, Hamilton JW, Lof GL, Kempster GB (1992). Oropharyngeal swallowing in normal adults of different ages. Gastroenterology, 103: 823–9.

[34] Abdulraheem IS (2013). Polypharmacy: a risk factor for geriatric syndrome, morbidity and mortality. Aging Sci, 1: e103. doi: 10.4172/23298847.1000e103.

[35] Nobili A, Marengoni A, Tettamanti M, Salerno F, Pasina L, Franchi C *et al* (2011). Association between clusters of diseases and polypharmacy in hospitalized elderly patients: results from the REPOSI study. Eur J Intern Med, 22(6): 597–602. doi: 10.1016/j.ejim.2011.08.029.

[36] Leiss W, Méan M, Limacher A, Righini M, Jaeger K, Beer HJ *et al* (2014). Polypharmacy is associated with an increased risk of bleeding in elderly patients with venous thromboembolism. J Gen Intern Med,30(1):17–24 doi: 10.1007/s11606-014-3000-0.

[37] Al-Arifi MN, Al-Husein HO, Al Shamiri MO, Said R, Wajid S, Babelghaith SD (2014). Prevalence of polypharmacy in elderly cardiac patients at King Fahad Cardiac Center KFCC in King Khalid University Hospital, Riyadh, Saudi Arabia. Int J Rec Sci Res, 5(6): 1053–7.

[38] Banerjee A, Mbamalu D, Ebrahimi S, Khan AA, Chan TF (2011). The prevalence of polypharmacy in elderly attenders to an emergency department—a problem with a need for an effective solution. Int J Emerg Med, 4: 22.

[39] Weiss CO, Boyd CM, Wolff JL, Leff B (2012). Prevalence of diabetes treatment effect modifiers: the external validity of trials to older adults. Aging Clin Exp Res, 24(4): 370–6.

[40] Hey H, Jørgensen F, Sørensen K, Hasselbalch H, Wamberg T (1982). Oesophageal transit of six commonly used tablets and capsules. Br Med J (Clin Res Ed), 285(6356): 1717–9.

[41] Marquis J, Schneider MP, Payot V, Cordonier AC, Bugnon O, Hersberger KE *et al* (2013). Swallowing difficulties with oral drugs among polypharmacy patients attending community pharmacies. Int J Clin Pharm, 35(6): 1130–6. doi: 10.1007/s11096-013-9836-2.

[42] Tharpe N (2011). Adverse drug reactions in women's health care. J Midwifery Wom Heal, 56(3): 205–13. doi: 10.1111/j.1542-2011.2010.00050.x.

[43] Trumic E, Pranjic N, Begic L, Becic F, Asceric M (2012). Idiosyncratic adverse reactions of most frequent drug combinations: long-term use among hospitalized patients with polypharmacy. Med Arch, 66(4): 243–8.

Chapter 3

Presbyphagia

Marian Dejaeger, Claudia Liesenborghs and
Eddy Dejaeger

Additional information is available at the end of the chapter

http://dx.doi.org/10.5772/60780

1. Introduction

Everybody is eager to attain old age while preserving as much of their capabilities as possible. The lifespan has indeed increased considerably but is this also true for the disease-free period? Dealing with geriatric patients, there is growing awareness of the importance of the link between old age and swallowing problems. Although the severity and the nature of the swallowing problems are variable, deglutition in the elderly is somewhat compromised due to a decreased functional reserve [1]. However, it is important to distinguish between changes due to normal aging (i.e., presbyphagia) and changes due to pathologic conditions (i.e., dysphagia) caused by age-related diseases and their treatment. In primary aging a number of functions stay preserved, a number of functions deteriorate, and some compensatory mechanisms are evident.

Though a number of physiological, anatomical, and functional changes take place in the process of aging inducing an increased risk for dysphagia in older patients, the swallowing of a healthy older adult in not per se impaired. *Presbyphagia* refers to characteristic changes in the swallowing mechanism of otherwise healthy older adults [2].

While presbyphagia remains largely asymptomatic, as in contrast to presbyopia or presbyacousis [3], dysphagia implies the presence of a symptomatic swallowing problem. In healthy aging there seems to be no reduction of the quality of life linked to deglutition [4]. Dysphagia arises from the combination of presbyphagia and a pathologic condition such as a stroke [5], Parkinson's disease [6], or dementia [7], just to mention the three most frequently encountered ones. Moreover, the geriatric patient with a diminished functional reserve, admitted in hospital with an acute illness, may develop a delirious state and subsequently a swallowing problem. There is also an increased likelihood that iatrogenic causes such as medication, surgical interventions, or radiotherapy are involved and finally the so-called frail elderly may be reaching the lower limits of his physiological reserves, which may induce a swallowing problem.

2. Changes due to normal aging

Swallowing is an integrated neuromuscular process in which volitional and relatively automatic movements successively are controlled. Normal swallowing consists of 5 phases: an anticipating phase, an oral preparatory phase, an oral phase, a pharyngeal phase, and finally an esophageal phase [2].

The act of swallowing starts with the anticipation when seeing and smelling the food and in a cognitively adequate elderly person with normal eyesight there are no changes whatsoever in this first phase.

In the second phase or *oral preparatory phase*, the solid bolus needs preparation to be swallowed. Of course the dentures play an important role here; elderly who are often lacking teeth or who are wearing ill-fitted dentures may experience problems in chewing and as a consequence they may have made some spontaneous adaptations as far as their diet is concerned, and they are, for example, likely to avoid raw vegetables and certain meats. It has also been established that with ill-fitted dentures the masticating muscles function less well, thereby leading to a prolongation of the chewing process and to a larger number of chewing movements [8, 9]. The saliva production, a factor strongly related to subjective comfort during swallowing, on the other hand, will remain intact with aging, with xerostomia in old age being mostly due to medication [10].

2.1. Oral phase

This phase comprises the manipulation and transportation of the food in the mouth; the tongue propels the food in one fluid movement into the pharynx. When reaching the "trigger zone" near the faucial pillars, the reflexively pharyngeal phase will be initiated. Labial, buccal, and lingual actions, in combination with saliva, all work together to manipulate the food and to ultimately mechanically formulate a bolus. This bolus is then moved to the posterior side of the mouth into the inlet of the superior aspect of the pharynx. With aging the tongue strength declines, yet during swallowing itself the tongue strength is similar as in young people probably indicating a compensation for a diminished functional reserve [11]. The duration of the oral phase increases while there is also an increase of residue in the mouth post swallowing [12]. Here, it is important to have a good evacuation of the bolus because food that rests lingering in the oral cavity may lead to bacterial overgrowth and to aspiration as well.

2.2. Pharyngeal phase

The oral cavity and pharynx contains an enormous amount of sensory receptors, represented by dense intricate nerve supply to the oral cavity, pharynx, and larynx. The exact timing of the onset of the pharyngeal swallow is triggered by reflexes based on the input from these sensory receptors in such a way that even a one-second delay in initiation can result in airway invasion of ingested material or aspiration.

This phase starts with the initiation of the swallowing reflex, and the triggering of this reflex is somewhat delayed in the elderly [13], which again points to a reduced functional reserve although there is still sufficient time to close the airway.

In the elderly, there is an increased distance between the hyoid bone and the larynx [14, 15]. This leads in combination with sarcopenia to a larger pharyngeal space that needs clearing at deglutition [14]. The hyoidal movement in the superior and anterior direction plays a crucial role as it is important not only for safety reasons as it moves the entrance of the airway further away from the bolus but also for reasons of efficiency as this movement is responsible for the opening of the upper esophageal sphincter (UES). This movement declines with aging and is even in healthy elderly already significantly reduced compared with younger individuals.

The safety of swallowing is further bolstered by the movement of the epiglottis and by active approximation of the vocal cords and both mechanisms remain intact [16, 17].

The opening of the UES, as observed on videofluoroscopy, is unchanged but in approximately 30% of the healthy elderly one can observe the presence of a so-called cricopharyngeal bar, a posterior impression at the pharyngoesophageal segment [15]. The cricopharyngeal bar is a frequent incidental radiologic finding, which in many cases does not cause any symptoms.

When the UES is investigated in the elderly with manometry, it shows a decreased relaxation of the UES often in combination with increased amplitude of the pharyngeal contraction [2, 18-22]. The intrabolus pressure measured at the level of the UES is also elevated. And to be complete in the description of this phase we see that at the top of the pharynx the velopharyngeal closure remains intact.

Due to these physiological changes normal in aging, the pharyngeal transit time is significantly increased in old age [2].

Swallow safety and swallow efficiency not only imply an adequate motor function but also a preserved sensibility. Increasing age is often associated with a declined perception of spatial tactile recognition on the lip and tongue [23] and the rest of the oral cavity.

A study that used air pulses at the posterior pharyngeal wall at the level of the piriform sinuses showed a decreased sensibility in old age and as a consequence the amount of pharyngeal residue required to initiate a so-called clearing swallow proved to be significantly higher than in young persons [24-26].

In older healthy adults, it is not uncommon for the bolus to spend a greater length of time next to an open airway, by pooling in the piriform sinuses and in the valleculae, than in younger adults. This senescent change may be associated with greater risk for airway penetration or aspiration.

Swallow safety means that no material enters the airway; one distinguishes between penetration and aspiration. While in penetration nothing descends beyond the level of the true vocal cords, one speaks of aspiration when this is indeed the case with material ending up in the tracheal structures. In healthy elderly, there seems to be an increased incidence of penetration but not of aspiration [2, 27]. Another important clinical parameter consists of swallow efficiency, that is, the possibility to transport a bolus through the pharynx without leaving residue. Several studies have shown that residue both at the vallecular and the piriform sinuses level is frequently encountered in healthy asymptomatic elderly [22, 28]. With a new technique (Automated Impedance Manometry or AIM), it is possible to measure a Swallow Risk Index (SRI) [22]. This index is based on a number of manometric and impedance parameters and is clearly higher in the elderly pointing at an elevated level of swallowing dysfunction.

2.3. The esophageal phase

In 1974, it was shown that in elderly men above 80 years of age without comorbidities the peristaltic amplitude was significantly lower than in younger controls, but without changes in the speed or duration of the peristaltic wave [29]. The authors stated that aging results in a weaker esophageal muscle but with intact innervation. Later on the technique to perform manometric studies was further improved facilitating the discovery that the duration of the peristaltic wave increases in the aged population [30, 31].

Another manometric study of healthy Japanese volunteers showed that the elderly population (>60 years) had decreased peristaltic contraction amplitude compared to the young control group (<49 years) [32]. But in a similarly large study comparing older (>65 years) and younger (<45 years) patients with dysphagia, they could not find any significant difference in peristaltic amplitude, duration, and LES (lower esophageal sphincter) pressure [33].

Finally several studies have indicated an increase in both the amount of failed peristaltic events as well as in synchronous contractions [34].

To summarize, most studies in healthy elderly indicated that approximately 90% of these subjects had impaired peristaltic activity, while no peristalsis at all was observed in one third of them. Moreover the incidence of non-peristaltic contractions of the esophagus increases with age.

In conclusion, it is not easy to compare the preceding studies due to differences in subject population, average ages, and degree of comorbidities as well as differences in manometric and radiographic techniques. It appears that in subjects older than 90, the majority have comorbidities that would possibly predispose them to an esophageal motility disorder making it difficult to distinguish whether dysmotility in this group is due to age and disease or disease alone. In subjects aged 60 to 80, the duration of peristalsis is prolonged and the amplitude may be lessened, although whether these findings are clinically significant remains unclear. In healthy subjects aged from 80 to 90, esophageal muscle weakness exists but the swallow function remains intact. Although certain parameters change significantly with aging, the swallow safety and swallow efficiency are still adequately preserved in normal aging.

A summary of the changes can be found in Table 1.

ORAL PREPARATORY PHASE	
Altered function	Loss of teeth Chewing problems [9]
No change	Saliva production [10]
Compensatory functions	Increased duration [8] Increased number of chewing movements [9]
ORAL PHASE	
Altered functions	Decreased functional reserve of the tongue strength [11] Increased oral residue [12]
No changes	Tongue strength during swallowing [11]
PHARYNGEAL PHASE	
Altered functions	*At the motor level* Decreased movement of the hyoid [16] Decreased pharyngeal constriction [15] Decreased relaxation of the UES [18-21] Reduced opening of the UES [22] Increased duration [2, 15]
	At the sensory level Delayed swallow reflex [1, 9, 13, 16] Decreased sensibility of the posterior pharyngeal wall [24, 25]
No changes	Downward movement of the epiglottis [16] Active closure of the vocal cords [17] Velopharyngeal closure [2]
Compensatory function	Increased pharyngeal contractility [18, 19]
Deglutition in general	
Altered functions	Increased incidence of penetration [18,26] increased pharyngeal residue [22, 28]
No change	No aspiration [2, 27]

3. Changes associated with normal aging, which might influence swallowing

A holistic approach is required while studying swallowing in the elderly. Swallowing cannot be regarded as an isolated action; one has to take into account the age-related functional decline occurring in several body-functions and its repercussions on swallowing (figure 1).

First of all there is an age-related decrease of sense of smell and taste, which are important for the pleasure we enjoy while eating [35-37].

Also, some anatomical differences arise in the older person such as a smaller cross-sectional area of masticatory muscles (masseter and medial pterygoid) and an increased lingual atrophy [38]. Next to the anatomical changes also, functional alterations occur in the muscle activity of the masseter, orbicularis oris, the supra- and infra-hyoidal muscles [39], and the thyroarytenoid muscle [39].

The respiratory system undergoes some changes as well; there is a decreased cough reflex, a diminished ciliary clearing, and a weakening of the respiratory muscles. These changes in combination with a deterioration of the immune system make the elderly more prone to developing an aspiration pneumonia.

As far as the digestive system is concerned, a delayed gastric emptying may lead to an earlier feeling of fullness at mealtime. Recent studies have shown a decreased sensibility and an increased stiffness of the esophagus in old age [40].

Another important issue is fatigue [41]. Fatigue, being a very common complaint in the elderly, is often associated with functional decline and may, as well as sleeping disturbances and depression, lead to a reduced food intake [42-44]. The elderly also often experience a declined perception of thirst and subsequently they have a low fluid intake. Tongue strength and endurance decline during a meal and this in combination with a diminished reserve may negatively influence deglutition especially in already weakened elderly [45].

As people get older, the slower swallowing act may actually also be a benefit as it can allow greater time to recruit the necessary number of muscle fibers to generate the necessary pressures for adequate bolus propulsion through the oropharynx. Hence, speeding up an elderly patient's swallow may induce contradictory results, as it may lead to insufficient swallow pressures and therefore may be contraindicated as a therapy technique.

Cognitive changes are also considered to be part of the normal aging process and cognitive processes such as concentration, attention, and double-tasking are influenced by age. A decline in concentration and attention together with a reduced reserve may lead to aspiration. Moreover as eating is a social event, people tend to talk during mealtime further increasing the risk of penetration and aspiration.

Staying physically active is associated with healthy aging, therefore elderly who are bedridden are additionally exposed to a number of important risk factors due to the sedative life style such as a diminished lung capacity and a weaker cough, a greater risk to develop a pneumonia, muscle weakness, and a loss of appetite [46].

Finally, medication may also negatively influence deglutition [47]. Drugs with an anticholinergic effect may cause xerostomia while some may lead to a diminished (e.g., allopurinol, carbamazepine, and penicillamine) or an altered (e.g., captopril lithium) taste perception. Sedatives can reduce the level of alertness and neuroleptics may mimic the swallowing problems encountered in Parkinson's disease. Nitrates are relatively contraindicated in gastro-esophageal, reflux disease as they lower the pressure in the lower gastro-esophageal sphincter and steroids can not only induce a Candida infection orally but they can also provoke a steroid myopathy. Moreover, 40% of already weakened elderly take at least one medication that is completely superfluous [48].

http://dx.doi.org/10.5772/60780

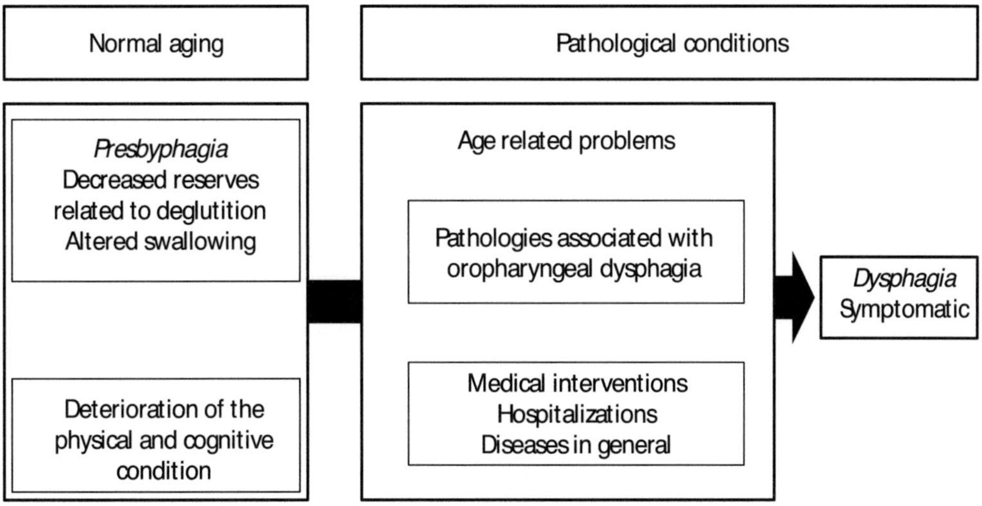

Figure 1. The relationship between presbyphagia and dysphagia

4. Implications for the clinical practice: prevention and detection of swallowing problems

a. Detection

In view of the high prevalence of dysphagia in the elderly and its important consequences such as malnutrition, dehydration, aspiration pneumonia, acute food impaction, and a reduced quality of life, it is crucial to detect swallowing problems at an early stage. Moreover, the elderly themselves are not always aware of their deglutition problems [49]. In a study on 47 elderly women living at home a questionnaire was used to assess swallowing problems. Participants were all observed while drinking water. Only 44% of those in whom a clinical problem was observed admitted having experienced a deglutition problem [50]. The personnel in nursing homes is often not well trained to detect these problems [51], while for isolated elderly living at home this can be a challenge for their GP. When an elderly is admitted to a geriatric ward, the geriatrician as well as the nursing staff plays a key role in detecting a swallow problem.

In Table 2 some tips are given as to when presbyphagia is suspected and when there might be a pathologic condition.

b. Prevention

As prevention is always preferred over cure, an overview is here presented with the most common preventative measures to allow a safe oral intake in the elderly.

Symptoms indicating the presence of presbyphagia	Symptoms indicating the presence of dysphagia
Prolonged chewing in a person with no teeth or ill-fitted dentures	Significantly prolonged duration of a meal
Diminished taste	No taste
Less appetite	Important lack of appetite
The elder drinks less	Drinking fluids has become so difficult that he avoids it
The elder chokes seldom when his attention decreases (e.g., when talking during mealtime)	He often chokes at mealtime, coughs frequently, and/or develops a wet voice during or after a meal
In general there are no problems with eating, only hard consistencies might be a challenge	He avoids several foods and the difficulties at swallowing may influence his quality of life
He chokes seldom on his own saliva	He is continuously coughing and has a wet voice

Advices
Pay attention to a good hygiene of the mouth
Clean your dentures adequately, make them fit well
Discard any food residue from your mouth after mealtime
Keep your mouth moist by rinsing or drinking at regular intervals
Pay attention to eat and drink moments
Avoid eating and drinking when you are extremely tired or when your concentration is diminished.
Do not speak during mealtime but start a conversation afterward.
Do not eat just prior going to sleep.
Remain in an upright position at least 5 to 10 min following a meal.
Adaptations of food
When experiencing difficulties chewing raw vegetables or some meat, you may cut it in very small pieces.
When your food tastes insufficiently, you may add some spices.
When you aspirate now and then on fluids, chilling it and adding some flavor could be a good idea.
When you aspirate now and then on your own saliva try to think to swallow it on a regular base for instance whenever you look for the time thereby making it a habit.
Medication
Take your pills only when you are perfectly alert and sitting upright.
Remain in a prone position, at least 5 to 10 minutes.
Drink sufficient water during and after the medication.
When swallowing medication proves difficult mention it to your physician so that he can look for an alternative route of administration (sublingual, transdermal).
General advice
Stay active
When to consult a physician in case of deglutition problems?
When you are worried
When you choke regularly
When you cough regularly during and between meals
When you eat a lot slower
When you stop enjoying to eat and drink
When you lose weight

http://dx.doi.org/10.5772/60780

5. Conclusions

Swallow safety is preserved in normal aging. Yet there are a number of changes, which bring the elderly in a more vulnerable position. Moreover, the elderly are more frequently confronted with events likely to provoke a deglutition problem.

All medical personnel dealing with the elderly should be alert not to miss any sign that might suggest the presence of a swallowing problem. Finally, the elderly should receive proper advice on how to cope with changes due to normal aging.

Acknowledgements

We hereby acknowledge that the tables in this manuscript are based on the following article: Presbyfagie: de invloed van het primair verouderingsproces op de slikfunctie. Liesenborghs C, Dejaeger E, Liesenborghs L, Tack J, Rommel N.Tijdschr Gerontol Geriatr 2014; 45: 261-272.

Author details

Marian Dejaeger[1], Claudia Liesenborghs[2] and Eddy Dejaeger[3*]

*Address all correspondence to: eddy.dejaeger@uzleuven.be

1 Laboratory of Skeletal Cell Biology and Physiology (SCEBP), Skeletal Biology and Engineering Research Center (SBE), Department of Development and Regeneration, KU Leuven, Leuven, Belgium

2 Translational Research Center for Gastrointestinal Disorders (TARGID), Leuven, Belgium

3 Department of Gerontology and Geriatrics, UZ Leuven, Leuven, Belgium

References

[1] Logemann J. Slikstoornissen: Onderzoek en Behandeling Amsterdam: Harcourt. 2000.

[2] Robbins J, Hamilton JW, Lof GL, Kempster GB. Oropharyngeal swallowing in normal adults of different ages. Gastroenterology. 1992 Sep;103(3):823-9. PubMed PMID: 1499933.

[3] Van Den Noortgate N. Lichamelijke veranderingen en de gevolgen van veroudering. Lannoo Leuven. 2006.

[4] Cassol K, Galli JF, Zamberlan NE, Dassie-Leite AP. Quality of life in swallowing in healthy elderly. Jornal da Sociedade Brasileira de Fonoaudiologia. 2012;24(3):223-32. PubMed PMID: 23128170.

[5] Truelsen T, Piechowski-Jozwiak B, Bonita R, Mathers C, Bogousslavsky J, Boysen G. Stroke incidence and prevalence in Europe: a review of available data. European journal of neurology : the official journal of the European Federation of Neurological Societies. 2006 Jun;13(6):581-98. PubMed PMID: 16796582.

[6] Willis AW. Parkinson disease in the elderly adult. Missouri medicine. 2013 Sep-Oct; 110(5):406-10. PubMed PMID: 24279192.

[7] Berr C, Wancata J, Ritchie K. Prevalence of dementia in the elderly in Europe. European neuropsychopharmacology : the journal of the European College of Neuropsychopharmacology. 2005 Aug;15(4):463-71. PubMed PMID: 15955676.

[8] Chichero J MB. Dysphagia Foundation, theory and practice. Chichester: John Wiley &Sons Ltd 2006.

[9] Mioche L, Bourdiol P, Monier S, Martin JF, Cormier D. Changes in jaw muscles activity with age: effects on food bolus properties. Physiology & behavior. 2004 Sep 30;82(4):621-7. PubMed PMID: 15327909.

[10] Ship JA, Pillemer SR, Baum BJ. Xerostomia and the geriatric patient. Journal of the American Geriatrics Society. 2002 Mar;50(3):535-43. PubMed PMID: 11943053.

[11] Todd JT, Lintzenich CR, Butler SG. Isometric and swallowing tongue strength in healthy adults. The Laryngoscope. 2013 Oct;123(10):2469-73. PubMed PMID: 23918664.

[12] Logemann JA, Pauloski BR, Rademaker AW, Kahrilas PJ. Oropharyngeal swallow in younger and older women: videofluoroscopic analysis. Journal of speech, language, and hearing research : JSLHR. 2002 Jun;45(3):434-45. PubMed PMID: 12068997.

[13] Leonard R, McKenzie S. Hyoid-bolus transit latencies in normal swallow. Dysphagia. 2006 Jul;21(3):183-90. PubMed PMID: 16897323.

[14] Leonard RJ SR. Effect of aging on the pharynx and the UES Principles of Deglutition: A Multidisciplinary Text for Swallowing and its Disorders. New York: Springer. 2013..

[15] Leonard R, Kendall K, McKenzie S. UES opening and cricopharyngeal bar in nondysphagic elderly and nonelderly adults. Dysphagia. 2004 Summer;19(3):182-91. PubMed PMID: 15383948.

[16] Logemann JA, Pauloski BR, Rademaker AW, Colangelo LA, Kahrilas PJ, Smith CH. Temporal and biomechanical characteristics of oropharyngeal swallow in younger and older men. Journal of speech, language, and hearing research : JSLHR. 2000 Oct; 43(5):1264-74. PubMed PMID: 11063246.

[17] Shaker R, Ren J, Bardan E, Easterling C, Dua K, Xie P, et al. Pharyngoglottal closure reflex: characterization in healthy young, elderly and dysphagic patients with predeglutitive aspiration. Gerontology. 2003 Jan-Feb;49(1):12-20. PubMed PMID: 12457045.

[18] Shaker R, Ren J, Podvrsan B, Dodds WJ, Hogan WJ, Kern M, et al. Effect of aging and bolus variables on pharyngeal and upper esophageal sphincter motor function. The American journal of physiology. 1993 Mar;264(3 Pt 1):G427-32. PubMed PMID: 8460698.

[19] van Herwaarden MA, Katz PO, Gideon RM, Barrett J, Castell JA, Achem S, et al. Are manometric parameters of the upper esophageal sphincter and pharynx affected by age and gender? Dysphagia. 2003 Summer;18(3):211-7. PubMed PMID: 14506987.

[20] Shaw DW, Cook IJ, Gabb M, Holloway RH, Simula ME, Panagopoulos V, et al. Influence of normal aging on oral-pharyngeal and upper esophageal sphincter function during swallowing. The American journal of physiology. 1995 Mar;268(3 Pt 1):G389-96. PubMed PMID: 7900799.

[21] Kern M, Bardan E, Arndorfer R, Hofmann C, Ren J, Shaker R. Comparison of upper esophageal sphincter opening in healthy asymptomatic young and elderly volunteers. The Annals of otology, rhinology, and laryngology. 1999 Oct;108(10):982-9. PubMed PMID: 10526854.

[22] Omari TI, Kritas S, Cock C, Besanko L, Burgstad C, Thompson A, et al. Swallowing dysfunction in healthy older people using pharyngeal pressure-flow analysis. Neurogastroenterology and motility : the official journal of the European Gastrointestinal Motility Society. 2014 Jan;26(1):59-68. PubMed PMID: 24011430.

[23] Wohlert AB. Tactile perception of spatial stimuli on the lip surface by young and older adults. Journal of speech and hearing research. 1996 Dec;39(6):1191-8. PubMed PMID: 8959604.

[24] Aviv JE, Martin JH, Jones ME, Wee TA, Diamond B, Keen MS, et al. Age-related changes in pharyngeal and supraglottic sensation. The Annals of otology, rhinology, and laryngology. 1994 Oct;103(10):749-52. PubMed PMID: 7944164.

[25] Aviv JE. Effects of aging on sensitivity of the pharyngeal and supraglottic areas. The American journal of medicine. 1997 Nov 24;103(5A):74S-6S. PubMed PMID: 9422628.

[26] Shaker R, Ren J, Zamir Z, Sarna A, Liu J, Sui Z. Effect of aging, position, and temperature on the threshold volume triggering pharyngeal swallows. Gastroenterology. 1994 Aug;107(2):396-402. PubMed PMID: 8039616.

[27] Almirall J, Rofes L, Serra-Prat M, Icart R, Palomera E, Arreola V, et al. Oropharyngeal dysphagia is a risk factor for community-acquired pneumonia in the elderly. The European respiratory journal. 2013 Apr;41(4):923-8. PubMed PMID: 22835620.

[28] Dejaeger E, Pelemans W, Bibau G, Ponette E. Manofluorographic analysis of swallowing in the elderly. Dysphagia. 1994 Summer;9(3):156-61. PubMed PMID: 8082323.

[29] Hollis JB, Castell DO. Esophageal function in elderly man. A new look at "presbyesophagus". Annals of internal medicine. 1974 Mar;80(3):371-4. PubMed PMID: 4816179.

[30] Ren J, Shaker R, Kusano M, Podvrsan B, Metwally N, Dua KS, et al. Effect of aging on the secondary esophageal peristalsis: presbyesophagus revisited. The American journal of physiology. 1995 May;268(5 Pt 1):G772-9. PubMed PMID: 7762661.

[31] Aly YA, Abdel-Aty H. Normal oesophageal transit time on digital radiography. Clinical radiology. 1999 Aug;54(8):545-9. PubMed PMID: 10484223.

[32] Nishimura N, Hongo M, Yamada M, Kawakami H, Ueno M, Okuno Y, et al. Effect of aging on the esophageal motor functions. Journal of smooth muscle research = Nihon Heikatsukin Gakkai kikanshi. 1996 Apr;32(2):43-50. PubMed PMID: 8845565.

[33] Robson KM, Glick ME. Dysphagia and advancing age: are manometric abnormalities more common in older patients? Digestive diseases and sciences. 2003 Sep;48(9): 1709-12. PubMed PMID: 14560988.

[34] Grande L, Lacima G, Ros E, Pera M, Ascaso C, Visa J, et al. Deterioration of esophageal motility with age: a manometric study of 79 healthy subjects. The American journal of gastroenterology. 1999 Jul;94(7):1795-801. PubMed PMID: 10406237.

[35] Doty RL, Kamath V. The influences of age on olfaction: a review. Frontiers in psychology. 2014;5:20. PubMed PMID: 24570664. Pubmed Central PMCID: 3916729.

[36] Baruch P. D-PL, Feenstra R., Roos R., Sterk C.,. Zintuigen en communicatie uit: Inleiding gerontologie en geriatrie. Houten: Bohn Stafleu von Loghum. 2004.

[37] Methven L, Allen VJ, Withers CA, Gosney MA. Ageing and taste. The Proceedings of the Nutrition Society. 2012 Nov;71(4):556-65. PubMed PMID: 22883349.

[38] Nakayama M. [Histological study on aging changes in the human tongue]. Nihon Jibiinkoka Gakkai kaiho. 1991 Apr;94(4):541-55. PubMed PMID: 2061734.

[39] Takeda N, Thomas GR, Ludlow CL. Aging effects on motor units in the human thyroarytenoid muscle. The Laryngoscope. 2000 Jun;110(6):1018-25. PubMed PMID: 10852524.

[40] Menard-Katcher P. FG. Normal aging and the esophagus from: Principles of Deglutition: A multidisciplinary text for swallowing and its disorders.. New York: Springer. 2013.

[41] Poluri A, Mores J, Cook DB, Findley TW, Cristian A. Fatigue in the elderly population. Physical medicine and rehabilitation clinics of North America. 2005 Feb;16(1): 91-108. PubMed PMID: 15561546.

[42] Forlani C, Morri M, Ferrari B, Dalmonte E, Menchetti M, De Ronchi D, et al. Prevalence and gender differences in late-life depression: a population-based study. The American journal of geriatric psychiatry : official journal of the American Association for Geriatric Psychiatry. 2014 Apr;22(4):370-80. PubMed PMID: 23567427.

[43] Phillips PA, Rolls BJ, Ledingham JG, Forsling ML, Morton JJ, Crowe MJ, et al. Reduced thirst after water deprivation in healthy elderly men. The New England journal of medicine. 1984 Sep 20;311(12):753-9. PubMed PMID: 6472364.

[44] Brownie S. Why are elderly individuals at risk of nutritional deficiency? International journal of nursing practice. 2006 Apr;12(2):110-8. PubMed PMID: 16529597.

[45] Kays SA, Hind JA, Gangnon RE, Robbins J. Effects of dining on tongue endurance and swallowing-related outcomes. Journal of speech, language, and hearing research : JSLHR. 2010 Aug;53(4):898-907. PubMed PMID: 20689047. Pubmed Central PMCID: 3077124.

[46] Rousseau P. Immobility in the aged. Archives of family medicine. 1993 Feb;2(2): 169-77; discussion 78. PubMed PMID: 8275186.

[47] Dejaeger E. Slikstoornissen. Leuven: Acco. 2007.

[48] Hajjar ER, Hanlon JT, Sloane RJ, Lindblad CI, Pieper CF, Ruby CM, et al. Unnecessary drug use in frail older people at hospital discharge. Journal of the American Geriatrics Society. 2005 Sep;53(9):1518-23. PubMed PMID: 16137281.

[49] Gonzalez-Fernandez M, Humbert I, Winegrad H, Cappola AR, Fried LP. Dysphagia in old-old women: prevalence as determined according to self-report and the 3-ounce water swallowing test. Journal of the American Geriatrics Society. 2014 Apr;62(4): 716-20. PubMed PMID: 24635053.

[50] DePippo KL, Holas MA, Reding MJ. Validation of the 3-oz water swallow test for aspiration following stroke. Archives of neurology. 1992 Dec;49(12):1259-61. PubMed PMID: 1449405.

[51] Pelletier CA. What do certified nurse assistants actually know about dysphagia and feeding nursing home residents? American journal of speech-language pathology / American Speech-Language-Hearing Association. 2004 May;13(2):99-113. PubMed PMID: 15198630.

Section 2

Assessment of Dysphagia

Chapter 4

Endoscopic Criteria in Assessing Severity of Swallowing Disorders

Farneti Daniele and Genovese Elisabetta

Additional information is available at the end of the chapter

http://dx.doi.org/10.5772/60836

1. Introduction

The management of patients with swallowing disorders must involve a team of specialists whose work is aimed at preventing complications, ensuring a proper hydration and nutrition; as well as the the best quality of life to the patient [1]. This is an axiom that has guided our clinical activity for over 25 years. The goals of the team [2], in fact, can be summarized as follows:

- Diagnostic assessment (impairment)
- Define severity (development of complications)
- Treatment options
- Rapid and usable exchange of information
- Monitoring of results achieved (also considering complications, worsening)
- Improve the quality of life of the patient (disability and handicap):
- Collection of self-assessment questionnaires of the symptom and results.

The first three goals require an instrumental assessment. In other words the definition of the bio-mechanical events that are responsible of the deglutition disorder, have to be assessed with one or more instrumental tools, able to define the altered or mistimed movements, or muscular patterns, that compromise the passage of the bolus through the oral and pharyngeal cavities [3].

Simplifying such an approach, the evaluation of the clinical severity of a swallowing disorder remains a crucial aspect to determine, when managing patients with diseases or co-morbidities that may predispose them to respiratory or nutritional complications. The evaluation of the risk of complications, as just mentioned earlier, is a value that synthesizes data regarding the patient in his/her totality, in relation to physical parameters (age, sex, race), the main pathology or other co-morbidities, the possibilities of an ecological management of the deglutition disorders (ie the possibility to effect behavioral strategies), also considering the wish of the patient and of the family [1].

The systematic method of the FEES (fiberoptic endoscopic evaluation of swallowing) evaluation is reported elsewhere in this book.

In this chapter the utility of endoscopy in the evaluation of dysphagic patients, new ways to conceive endoscopy and the correlations of endoscopy with a whole clinical context in the attempt to determine severity, will be discussed.

2. Instruments and settings

In daily practice, an instrumental procedure is indicated in the face of any suspected dysphagia or when a definition in differential diagnostic terms of the oro-pharyngeal situation is required. An instrumental procedure is also indicated for patients with pathologies that carry a high risk of complications even if they are apparently asymptomatic or when there is a discrepancy between the subjective signs and the outcome of a bedside evaluation. Even the clinical onset of dysphagia with complications makes an instrumental investigation of swallowing necessary [4-13].

So: which tool ?

The local availability of resources conditions the management of these patients but the possibility of a specialistic evaluation (carried out by a deglutologist) or the evaluation by trained carers has to be guaranteed in all the settings where elderly or dysphagic patients are recovered [1]. The tools, which are chosen, will be the available ones in our setting, aware that the "human factor" is the key to the success or failure of the clinical outcome. In our experience, the best way to manage dysphagic patients is represented by the evaluation of their swallowing abilities by means of a non instrumental clinical evaluation (clinical swallowing assessment, CSA) [14] and an instrumental endoscopic evaluation [15].

3. The endoscopic evaluation

Since 1988, when Susan Langmore first proposed the FEES protocol [16], the use of endoscopy in the evaluation of swallowing, has become an extraordinary tool in the hand of clinicians, offering a revolutionary way to observe the pharynx and the larynx during dynamic tasks (respiration, phonation and swallowing) and during the passage of the bolus. The possibility to test sensation is another extraordinary potentiality of the procedure. Subsequently, various standardized protocols for the dynamic study of swallowing have been proposed [17,18] but another advantage of endoscopy, in addition to those shown in Table 1, is exactly that of the possibility to adapt the evaluation to any kind of patient and in any kind of setting [19].

	ADVANTAGES	DISADVANTAGES
FEES	Less invasive Easy to perform Well tolerated Possible for a long time (fatigue viewing) Portable (acute and sub-acute patients) Routine Economic Therapeutic feed-back Decision making of oral feeding Natural foods Direct visualization of structures Motor and sensory activities Three-dimensional similar view Optimal pooling evaluation Pooling management viewing	Pharyngeal phase only White-out Indirect consideration about - Oral - Esophageal phase Fear and discomfort Poor vision in repeated swallowing acts Not possible if changes in upper airway
VFSS	Whole deglutition evaluation Time parameterization	Invasive (radiological exposure) Uncomfortable execution Environment and suitable personnel Expensive Bi-dimensional view (under estimation of pooling matter) Motor activity only (reaction to aspiration, if documented) Fatigue evaluation missing

Table 1. Advantages and disadvantages comparison between VFSS and FEES [19]

Firstly FEES has been compared and contrasted to VFSS (video-fluoroscopic study of swallowing) proposed by J. Logemann [20], an examination nowadays considered the instrumental gold standard for the study of swallowing. Compared to VFSS, FEES redeemed itself in terms of sensitivity, specificity and predictive values, if we consider its ability to identify aspiration as the main sensory-motor event linked to dysphagia and the leading cause of airway complications [21,19]. In a more recent period, the role of VFSS, as the instrumental gold standard, has been questioned [22].

Studies that have compared VFSS and FEES show that both procedures are comparable and have equivalent values of sensitivity, specificity and predictive abilities [23-30]. A more proper approach is to consider these two examinations as complementary [21]. The availability of both, allows the clinician to choose the method most appropriate to each case, relating to the required information. FEES also shows a considerable versatility in the management of the patients, of the multidisciplinary team and of the therapeutic process. The fact that it can be performed at the bedside, in any clinical condition and repeated over time, according to changing clinical needs, makes it an optimal method in the follow-up of any patient (Table 1).

4. The procedure

As previously said, the systematic method of FEES evaluation is reported elsewhere in this book. In the following paragraph, there is only a reference to the main steps of the evaluation that are summarized in Table 2. The most important step, in the endoscopic procedure, is the evaluation of the correlations existing between the morphological and functional findings; a few considerations follow. What must be remembered is that the anatomy influences the function, and the function influences the behavior of the structure to the passage of the bolus. In other words the safe functioning of the effectors of swallowing can be inferred evaluating the anatomical shaping of the effectors and the ability of the structure to support the passage of the bolus through the pharynx subsequently inferred by their functional abilities.

EVALUATION		SITE
Morphological	- Tumor - Ulcer - Erythema - Morphological defects - Hypertrophy - Hypotrophy - Atrophy - Asymmetry - Pathological events at rest	Epi-pharynx (soft palate) Meso-pharynx (tongue base) Hypo-pharynx (larynx)
Functional	- Symmetry - Reduced speed of movement - Reduced range of movement - Altered coordination	
Motor activities	- Velo-pharyngeal closure - Base of tongue retraction - Pharyngeal movements - True vocal cords movements - Sphincterial activity	
Pooling - dry swallows	- Color - Viscosity - Awareness - Patient reaction - Dry swallow frequency	
Sensation	- Reaction to the endoscope - Reaction to light touch of structures	

Table 2. Main parameters of anatomical and functional assessment.

http://dx.doi.org/10.5772/60836

Sensation is a crucial factor, strongly influencing the safe passage of the bolus through the cavities. A copy of the peripheral sensation is sent in parallel to the cortex and to the brainstem, to coordinate the neuro-motor activity of the muscular effectors of the oral cavity, pharynx and supra-hyoid muscles. Table 3 and Fig.1 represent the central and peripheral interaction between sensation and motor activities.

Subglottic Pressure Thermal Gustative Proprioceptive		ANATOMY
SENSIBILITY	CORTEX BRAINSTEM	- The position at rest of the epiglottis affects the volume of the vallecule, predisposing to anterior penetration - The position at rest of the arytenoids conditions the volume of retro-cricoid space, predisposing to posterior episodes of penetration - The height of the aryepiglottic folds conditions the volume of the pyriform sinuses, predisposing to lateral episodes of penetration - The anterior-posterior and traverse diameters of the hypo-pharynx (in relation to the dimension of the larynx), condition the volume of the hypo-pharynx and in general the maximum volume through which the bolus passes.
		MOTOR ACTIVATION

Table 3. Central and peripheral interaction between sensation and motor activities.

The stimulation of sub-glottic receptors may possibly act as a signal for the central nervous system that the larynx is "ready" (that is protected) for the bolus passage into the pharynx and this signal may, at the same time, influence the low motoneurons of the brainstem innervating

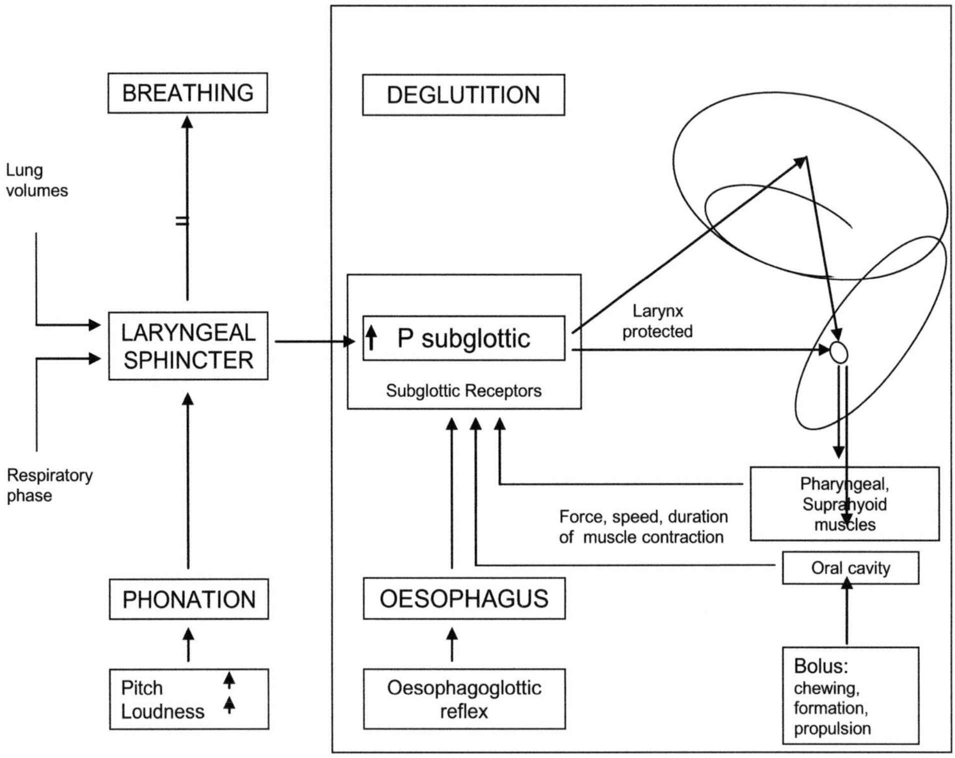

Figure 1. Interaction of subglottic pressure among respiration, deglutition and phonation.

the pharynx ("on line" processing) [31]. As a result of the neuro-anatomical connection between subglottic receptors and motor neurons for pharynx and larynx, the feedback from subglottic receptors may presumably affect the recruitment of motor neurons in the brainstem capable of activating the pharyngeal muscles during swallowing so that the force, speed and duration of the muscular contractions are regulated by the closing of the larynx. This feed-forward system may detect that a sensory input (subglottic pressure) has not been received and control a function (swallowing) by increasing the cortical processing thereby ensuring a safe passage of the bolus into the esophagus. Cortical processing would thus account for a prolonged muscular contraction [32].

5. New ways to conceive endoscopy

As previously mentioned, the role of VFSS as the instrumental gold standard, has been questioned. This in relation to the possibility of a direct endoscopical evaluation of the oral and esophageal stages of swallowing [22].

Oral FEES (O-FEES) and the esophageal FEES (E-FEES) have been introduced. The E-FEES is possible by means of the introduction of a 70 cm endoscope into the esophageal cavity (endoscope in deep position) (Table 4). In this stage the procedure, with the same morphological and functional goals of FEES for the pharynx, has been known since 1994 (trans-nasal pharyngo-esophago-gastroduodenoscopy: T-EGD) [33]. Later Hermann first performed the test with bolus [34]. With shorter instruments, and where the study of the stomach or duodenum is not required, a trans-nasal examination of the esophagus is possible (trans-nasal esophagoscopy – TNE). TNE as a procedure also used for many years in the instrumental evaluation of patients with ENT complaints [35]. In a short time it became an office practice, performed on outpatients without anesthesia. Several protocols have been proposed [36-38] for patients with bolus or other complaints of gastroesophageal reflux diseases. The application of the procedure in patients with voice problems or other signs of laryngopharyngeal reflux (LPR) and swallowing disorders is limited [39]. The procedure allows for a perfect viewing of the esophageal wall and its movements, up to the cardias and of the functioning of the esophageal sphincters. With the tip of the endoscope in a retrograde position, retracting the instrument close to the upper part, a direct back viewing of the upper esophageal sphincter and its dynamics during different tasks (swallowing, belching, Valsalva) is possible. TNE also permits the evaluation of the role of saliva, bile and gas during swallowing and digestion, aside from testing the effects of reflux on the upper digestive and respiratory tracts. Finally, it allows for the proper placement of catheters before functional pharyngeal or esophageal assessment [22, 34].

The term E-FEES could be used in similarity to the new term of O-FEES, proposed for the endoscopic evaluation of the oral stage of swallowing.

O-FEES is performed using an endoscope with a reversible tip of 180°, starting from a position intermediate between the high and low (in relation to the anatomy of the patient). In this position it is possible to intercept the soft palate and introduce the tip of the instrument into the oral cavity (*anterior position or retrograde position*) (Fig. 2). From this position, it is possible to see an inverted image of the oral cavity and its content, up to the teeth and lips, if kept open. With the tip retroflexed and by retracting the endoscope by a few centimeters (*anterior posterior position*) (Fig. 3), the coana with the instrument emerging from the nasal cavity, can be seen. The glosso-palatal port is, thus, visible in a dorsal viewing. Even from the tip in these positions, it is possible to obtain static (anatomical) and dynamic (phono-articulatory) information and test sensation. More information is collected during the bolus tests: bolus preparation (Fig. 4) and propulsion (Fig. 5) can be checked directly, as well as bolus entering into the pharyngeal cavity. Any kind of consistency can be tested, checking oral preparation and propulsion. The passage of the bolus through the fauces is not visible, because of the presence of the white-out, as happens during pharyngeal transit as viewed with the tip in the high position. After the tests with bolus and with the tip in the anterior position, the presence and location of residue (on the hard palate, gums, alveoli, tongue) can be verified (Fig. 6) [22].

With O-FEES and E-FEES variations, the functional assessment of the effectors of swallowing is complete. A trace of the functional assessment is reported in Table 4.

	Static evaluation	Dynamic evaluation	Sensation
Endoscope position			
NASAL-RHINOPHARYNGEAL ***(naso-rhino-pharynx)***	*Morphology of:* - Nasal cavities - Rhinopharynx - Pathological muscular activities *Pooling site:* . Nasal cavities . Rhynopharynx . Tubal ostium	*Speech* Velo-pharyngeal sphincter : - Velum deviation - Gap of closure - /s/ forced *Deglutition* - Nasal regurgitation	*General of the area:* - Reaction to the endoscope - Reaction to light touch of structures *Pooling* - Perception - Cleaning efforts - Cleaning effectiveness
HIGH ***(meso-pharynx)***	*Morphology of:* - Base of tongue - Pharyngeal wall - Pathological muscular activities *Pooling site:* . Valleculae . Pyriform synus . Post-pharyngeal wall . Retro-cricoidal space	*Speech* - Base of tongue: retraction . /l/ ball . /k/ cocco - Pharyngeal wall deviation: . /e/ strained . /e/ repeated *Deglutition (dry swallowing)* - Base of tongue movements - Pharyngeal movements	*General of the area:* - Reaction to the endoscope - Reaction to light touch of structures - Gag reflex (base of tongue) *Pooling* - Perception - Cleaning efforts - Cleaning effectiveness
ANTERIOR (retrograde) ***(oral cavity)***	*Morphology of:* - Tip, medium and base of tongue - Hard palate and gums/teeth - Lips *Pooling site:* . Hard palate . Tongue: tip, medium, base	*Speech* - Tongue movements: . /ka/ repeated - Lips movements : . /pa/ repeated *Deglutition (dry swallowing)* - Medium, base of tongue movements	*General of the area:* - Reaction to the endoscope - Reaction to light touch of structures - Gag reflex (tongue) *Pooling* - Perception - Cleaning efforts - Cleaning effectiveness
ANTERIOR POSTERIOR ***(oral cavity)***	*Morphology of:* - Base of tongue - Soft palate (superior face) - Glosso-palatal seal - Coana *Pooling site:* . Hard palate . Tongue: body, base	*Speech* - Tongue movements: . ka/ repeated - Palate movements . /ma/ repeated *Deglutition (dry swallowing)* - Tongue movements - Palate movements - Pharyngeal movements	*General of the area:* - Reaction to the endoscope - Reaction to light touch of structures - Gag reflex (tongue) *Pooling* - Perception - Cleaning efforts - Cleaning effectiveness
LOW ***(hypo-pharynx)***	*Morphology of* - Hypo-pharynx - Larynx during respiration - Pathological muscular activities *Pooling site:* . Sopra-glottic . Glottic . Sub-glottic . Cervical trachea	*Speech* - Glottic closure: . /a/ strained . /a/ repeated - Posterior commissure deviation . /a/ strained . /a/ repeated - Glottic opening: . Sniff - Vocal quality *Sphincterial activities* - True vocal cords closure: /a/ strained (time) - False vocal cord closure: . /a/ forced . Glide up /ee/ . Valsalva . Cough - Epiglottis inversion: . Dry swallows	*General of the area:* - Reaction to the endoscope - Reaction to light touch of: . Aryepiglottic folds . Arytenoids . True vocal folds . False vocal cords *Pooling* - Perception - Cleaning efforts - Cleaning effectiveness
DEEP ***(esophagus)***	*Morphology of* - UES - Body - LES	*Sphincterial activities* - UES . Valsalva . Cough . Belching . Dry swallows - LES *Muscular activity* - Body	*General of the area:* - Reaction to the endoscope

Table 4. The main steps of the anatomo-functional evaluation

Also the tests with bolus can be modified and enriched by O-FEES and E-FEES, as synthesized in Table 5. (UEP: upper esophageal sphincter; LES: lower esophageal sphincter)

PHASE	SENSORY-MOTOR EVENT
Bolus tests: different volumes and consistencies	
ORAL Endoscope in anterior position Endoscope in anterior-posterior position Endoscope in high position	**WHITE OUT**
Linguo-palatal sphincter competence Tongue movements Tongue propulsion Oral transport Total time	Spillage (premature bolus falling) Bolus preparation Bolus propulsion Bolus flow Site of pharyngeal reflex onset Pre-swallow penetration Pre-swallow aspiration
PHARYNGEAL Endoscope in high and low position	**WHITE OUT**
Velo-pharyngeal closure Vocal cords closure Laryngeal elevation Epiglottic inversion	Bolus flow Site of pharyngeal reflex onset Pre/intra-swallow penetration Pre/intra-swallow aspiration
Laryngeal returns low Epiglottis returns to rest	Pooling evaluation (site, amount, management): Post-swallow penetration Post-swallow aspiration Awareness Dry swallows Clearing Gurgling Cough with/without emission residues Effective management (larynx/trachea cleaned)
ESOPHAGEAL Endoscope in deep position Endoscope in deep retrograde position	**WHITE OUT**
Peristaltic activity Sphincters activity	Bolus flow Bolus delivery Bolus pooling

Table 5. Main sensory motor events of swallowing induced by the bolus [22, modified]

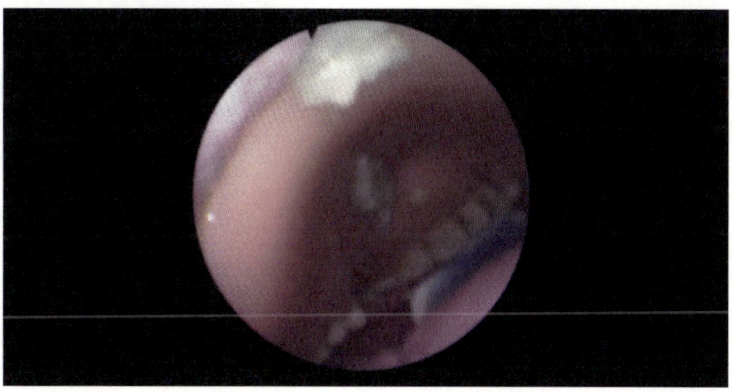

Figure 2. Anterior or retrograde position: the oral cavity is directly visible (all the following photographs have been rotated 180° to obtain viewing equal to the real one and make the images more easily interpretable).

Figure 3. Antero-posterior position: the soft palate is lifted from the base of the tongue or lowered.

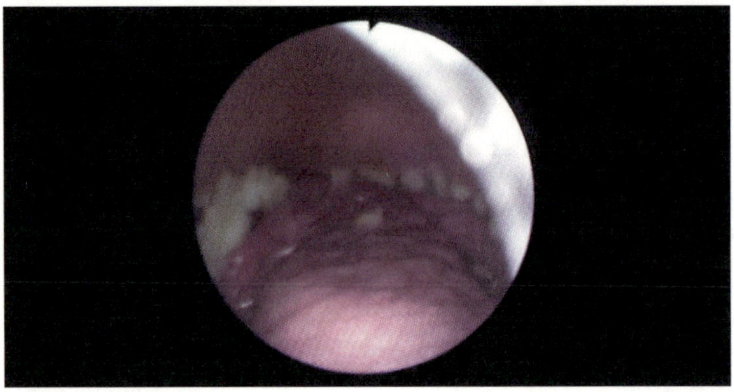

Figure 4. Anterior or retrograde position: bolus preparation.

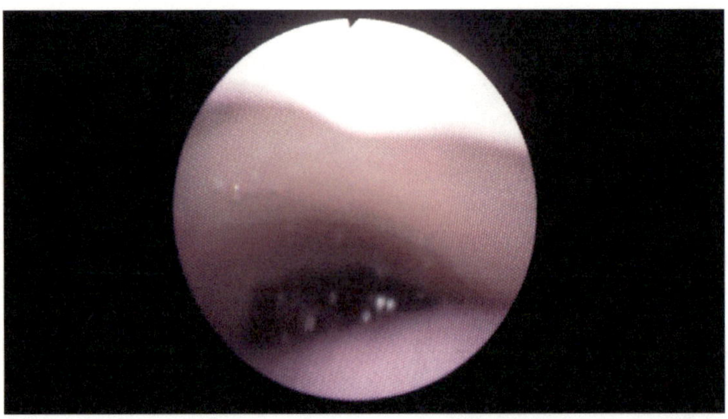

Figure 5. Anterior position: bolus propulsion.

Figure 6. Anterior position: tongue clearing of material coating the oral cavity.

6. Endoscopy with a whole clinical context and severity

Returning to our topic, it can be assumed that those parameters that express inefficient or unsafe swallowing are markers of severity: respectively residue and false routes (airway invasion). An efficient and safe swallowing expresses the perfect balance between events that occur in the domain of time and space, domains in which vector forces guarantee that defensive strategies are put in place to protect the airways, or cleanse the containment cavities from the bolus passing through them [40]. The anatomo-functional evaluation and the tests with bolus, resumed earlier, offer several points for reflection. Residue or material pooling into cavities (before or after the tests with bolus) are powerful indicators of disturbed swallowing, predisposing the patient to airway invasion [41]. Material pooling and residue were used to develop scores, variously used in clinical practice. There are several scores in the literature, with severity criteria divided into 4 or 5 levels and this division does not seem to interfere with the inter-intra rater reliability of those scores [42, 43]. In 2008 the P-score was introduced [44]. In the development of this score, pooling is considered in a broader sense, as any material that is present in the containment cavities of the hypo-pharynx and larynx, before and after the act of swallowing. The severity criterion proposed by the score (Table 6) takes into account anatomical parameters: site, identified by anatomical landmarks; amount: determined in a semi-quantitative way by the amount of pooling materials (coating, more or less than 50% of cavity containment capacity); management, as well as the efficiency of secretion management, considering the number of dry swallowings performed by the patient, either spontaneously or upon request of the clinician involved in the assessment. The effectiveness of gargling, throat clearing or coughing is considered in the same way.

In clinical practice, the P-score may be integrated with other parameters of the clinical swallowing evaluation (CSE), that are more easily determined: age, sensation of the pharynx, patient collaboration. These parameters are considered in the P-SCA score (pooling-sensation, collaboration and age score) as those able to mitigate the severity criteria expressed by the endoscopic evaluation alone (see earlier and [44]). The inter-rater and intra-rater reliability of the P-score has recently been determined [40]. Four judges with long-standing experience in the use of endoscopy, and after a training session, evaluated 30 films (the pharyngeal transit of boluses with different consistency) of 23 subjects with swallowing disorders. The films, randomly recorded on two different CDs, were viewed three times: a first time, after 24 hours and after 7 days. Inter and intra-rater reliability was calculated through the intra-class correlation coefficient ICC(3,k) individually for site, amount, management and the total score. As for the items site, amount, management and total P-score, the ICC(3,k) was 0.999, 0.997, 1.00, and 0.999, respectively. The analysis of variance showed no statistically significant dependency determined by the consistency in the differences detected.

As regards the domains previously mentioned, we have that in the time domain, the score may identify events that occur before or after swallowing; indeed, part of the material pooling that has not been swallowed during the previous swallow, becomes a bolus for the next swallow, with a different volume. The P-score considers the sequence of swallowing in the "management", evaluating the fate of a bolus that persists in the pharynx after five empty swallows. In the space domain, where forces are in action, the P-score identifies the pathway and the flow of the bolus: the pathway is identified by the direction along the digestive or respiratory tracts, as well as false route (penetration or aspiration); the flow is indicated by the amount of bolus that does not cross the pharynx while swallowing.

The events that occur in these domains together with vectorial forces, may be integrated in different ways, generating a very wide range of possibilities. For instance, the dynamic vectors and volumetric aspects, considered by the score, allow for information to be obtained on the reaction of the patient to airway invasion (management): the occurrence, or absence, of dry swallowing, cough or throat clearing, in response to the transit of the bolus in the larynx or in the cervical trachea before, during or after swallowing is considered.

Pooling	Endoscopic landmarks		Bedside parameters		
			Sensation	**Collaboration**	**Age (years)**
Site	Valleculae	1			
	Marginal zone	1			
	Pyriform sinus	2			
	Vestibule/vocal cords	3			
	Lower vocal cords	4			+1 (<65)
Amount	Coating	1	Presence = - 1	Presence = - 1	+2 (65-75)
	Minimum	2	Absence = +1	Absence = +1	+3 (>75)
	Maximum	3			
Management	< 2	2			
	2 ><5	3			
	> 5	4			
Score	P 4-11		P-SCA 3-16		

Table 6. P-score and P-SCA score

The P-score expresses, as a numerical value, a continuum of severity that in clinical practice may be used in different ways, with correlations that still have to be verified (Table 6).

Therefore, a minimum score (P-score 4_5) may indicate the absence of endoscopic signs of dysphagia. A low score (P-score 6_7) may identify mild dysphagia, a medium score (P-score 8_9) moderate dysphagia, and a high score (P-score 10_11), severe dysphagia. The score refers to a specific type of consistency and volume, and may change according to these. A similar subdivision can be made for the P-SCA score (for more details see [44]). In this way, it is possible to give clear indications with reference to treatment, or make comparisons before and after treatment.

Anatomical landmarks and bedside parameters with relative values.

P: pooling P-SCA: pooling _ sensation, collaboration, age

P score:

45 = minimum score, corresponding to no dysphagia

6_7 = low score, corresponding to a mild dysphagia

8_9 = middle score, corresponding to a moderate dysphagia

10_11 = high score, corresponding to a severe dysphagia

P-SCA score:

3_4 = minimum score, corresponding to no dysphagia

5_8 = low score, corresponding to a mild dysphagia

9_12 = middle score, corresponding to a moderate dysphagia

13_16 = high score, corresponding to a severe dysphagia.

7. The integrated clinical evaluation

The instrumental criterion of severity (endoscopic or radiological) needs to be contextualised according to a more general clinical criterion of severity, of the patient and of the swallowing disorder, considering that the non-instrumental assessment tends to underestimate the risk of aspiration, whereas the instrumental assessment tends to overestimate it [45].

It is therefore a relative criterion, which is identified through its parametrization. In clinical practice, aspiration is the most significant event that marks a swallowing disorder, yet it is not the only one. It is worth considering that during an instrumental assessment, we check the outcome of a very low number of swallowing acts, compared to the number of swallowings that are performed, for instance, during a meal or a whole day. It should be considered that many variables affect the successful outcome of pharyngeal transit of a bolus (Table 3). Swallowing patterns may be modified in real time in response to the functional status of swallowing effectors, in their turn related to sensation, volume, consistency and position of the bolus in the mouth when the pharyngeal reflex is elicited.

In 2008 [46], in a perspective study, the P-score and the P-SCA score (Table 6) were applied to a sample of 556 consecutive patients (inpatients and outpatients, 318M/238F, mean age 65.56±10.36 years), seen at our Swallowing Centre.

The correlation between the two tests was determined by the Spearman correlation coefficient. The agreement between the two scores has been calculated (Cohen's Kappa) considering the categories of risk corresponding to the totalized scores (no dysphagia, mild, moderate, severe). The categories of risk individualized with the two scores have been studied with the aim to underline possible systematic divergences in the attribution of the severity to the cases. Subsequently, the P-score and the P-SCA score were dichotomized, dividing the patients without risk from those with middle and high risk of aspiration. By the comparison of the dichotomic scores with the result of the FEES evaluation (considered as gold standard), the values of sensitivity and specificity have been obtained.

The results of this study documented a close correlation between the P-score and P-SCA score (rho=0.88) (Table7): The correlation is significant (p<0,001).

The agreement among the scores as regards the categories of risk attributed results discrete (Cohen's Kappa=0,46 p <0,001).

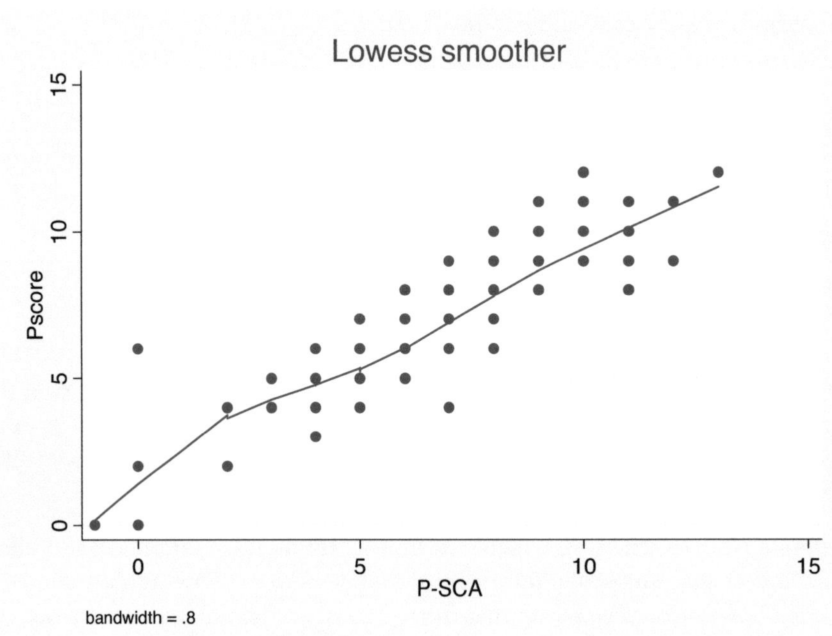

Table 7. Correlation between P-score and P-SCA score

The double Table 8 shows how the two scores have classified the patients in the different categories of risk.

	P-SCA score				
P-score	No	Mild	Moderate	Severe	Total
No	163 61.98	100 38.02	0 0.00	0 0.00	263 100.00
Mild	11 7.33	139 92.67	0 0.00	0 0.00	150 100.00
Moderate	0 0.00	43 55.18	35 44.87	0 0.00	78 100.00
Severe	0 00.0	12 36.36	20 60.61	1 3.03	33 100.00
Total	174 33.21	294 55.61	55 10.50	1 0.19	524 100.00

Table 8. Double table comparing the P-score and the P-SCA score and the classification of risk.

The table shows that the P-SCA score tends to "increase" the severity in the category with lower risk, while in those with higher risk it tends to be more cautious, attributing a category with lower severity in comparison to P-score. Overall the patients classified as at risk of aspiration by the P-score are 50%, while the P-SCA score considers at risk 67% of the patients. Comparing the two scores it is shown that the P-SCA score tends to have a lower value than the P-score (Wilcoxon signed-rank test p<0.001) (Table 9).

	Frequency	Percentage	
P-score			
No dysphagia		264	50.29
At risk		261	49.71
	Total	525	100.00
P-SCA score			
No dysphagia		174	33.21
At risk		350	66.79
	Total	524	100.00

Table 9. P-score and P-SCA score and risk of aspiration

The judgement expressed by the scores has been dichotomized setting the cut-off point between patients without risk and those with any kind of risk, with the purpose of comparing the evaluation of the scores with the result of the FEES (gold standard) regarding "aspiration" and to get for both, values of sensibility and specificity.

The P-score has reached values of sensibility of 96% and specificity of 60%, with an area underlying the ROC curves of 0.78, while the P-SCA score has reached values of sensibility of 98% and specificity of 40%, with an area underlying the ROC curves of 0.69. With such dichotomization, the P-SCA score recognizes more patients at risk, resulting more sensitive than the P-score, but also less specific (more false positive).

In conclusion, the assessment of patients with deglutition disorders has to consider as many elements as are available from the clinical and instrumental evaluation (integrated clinical evaluation).

The possibility of an instrumental evaluation sharpens the diagnostic precision with margins of error that vary for every procedure, but with the possibility of over estimating the risk of aspiration. In fact, patients with higher risk according to the P-score are attributed by P-SCA score to lower risk categories. Both have a high sensibility to individualize patients with a risk of inhalation from minimum to high. Nevertheless, the P-score is more specific, more skilled in recognizing the false positive and therefore more reliable in correctly classifying patients without dysphagia and patients with a risk of any degree of dysphagia.

In other words, while in patients considered without risk by the P-score, the clinical variable considered by the P-SCA-score increases the evaluation of the risk, in patients classified by P-score in the categories of higher severity, the evaluation of such clinical variables tends to mitigate the judgement expressed by the P-score and to put back patients into the categories with lower risk.

The association of endoscopy and elements of the CSE in the evaluation of the severity of dysphagia, tends to mitigate the gravity of the clinical case, allowing a more careful estimate in a routine clinical context.

8. Conclusions

In conclusion, some observations can be made.

The first consideration is that a criterion of severity must be a complete clinical criterion, which considers as many elements as possible from the clinical non-instrumental and instrumental evaluation. In general, any event leading the team to modify the treatment programme already decided, can become element of severity. As previously said, the only CSE, however well conducted, may underestimate the severity of a swallowing disorder in relation to the inability to directly see the effectors of swallowing and their behavior during the passage of the bolus. The contribution of the instrumental examination, in this issue, is essential: It shows the clinicians what happens inside the effectors during the passage of the bolus, but it tends to overestimate the severity of the disorder, inducing in the risk of generalization of patterns that may not reflect the real functional status of the effectors.

The endoscopic examination is a versatile and well-tolerated tool, which promptly facilitates and ratifies the team's activities. The latest developments of the endoscopic investigation with the possibility of a direct visualization of the oral (O-FEES) and the esophageal (E-FEES) phase of swallowing makes FEES more complete and brings it closer to the radiological gold standard.

Compared to VFSS, endoscopy allows for an optimal viewing of the effectors, making us appreciate all the anatomical variations that can affect the passage of the bolus. The interpretation of the biomechanical events resulting from this passage should enable the clinician to estimate behaviors useful for therapeutic purposes.

Taken together, all this information will provide us with a complete criterion of severity, able to guide the team towards effective activities and improve the QOL of the patient.

Author details

Farneti Daniele[1*] and Genovese Elisabetta[2]

*Address all correspondence to: lele_doc@libero.it

1 Audiology and Phoniatry Service, AUSL of Romagna - Infermi Hospital – Rimini, Italy

2 Audiology Service, University of Modena - Reggio Emilia, Modena, Italy

References

[1] Farneti D, Consolmagno P. The Swallowing Centre: rationale for a multidisciplinary management. Acta Otorhinolaryngol Ital. Aug 2007; 27(4): 200–207.

[2] Nan D. Musson. Dysphagia team management: continuous quality improvement in a long-term care setting. ASHA in the Winter 1994 Quality Improvement Digest.

[3] American Speech-Language-Hearing Association. (2001). Scope of practice in speech-language pathology. Rockville, MD: Author.

[4] Frederick MG, Ott DJ, Grishaw EK, Gelfand DW, Chen MYM. Functional abnormalities of the pharynx: a prospective analysis of radiographic abnormalities relative to age and symtoms. Am J Rad 1996;166:353-357.

[5] Pauloski BR, Logemann JA, Fox JC, Colangelo LA. Biomechanical analysis of the pharyngeal swallow in postsurgical patients with anterior tongue and floor of mouth resection and distal flap reconstruction. J Speech Hear Res 1995;39:110-123.

[6] Logemann JA. Screening, diagnosis, and management of neurogenic dysphagia. Semin Neurol 1996;16(4):319-327.

[7] Aviv JE, Martin JH, Sacco RL, Zagar D, Diamond B, Keen MS, Blitzer A. Supraglottic and pharyngeal sensory abnormalities in stroke patients with dysphagia. Ann Otol Rhinol Laryngol 1996;105:92-97.

[8] Kuhlemeier KV. Epidemiology and dysphagia (review). Dysphagia 1994;9:209217.

[9] Aviv JE, Sacco RL, Thomson J, Tandon R, Diamond B, Martin JH, Close GL. Silent laryngopharyngeal sensory deficits after stroke. Ann Otol Rhinol Laryngol 1997b; 106:87-93.

[10] St Giuly JL, Perie S, Willig TN, Chaussade S, Eymard B, Angelard B. Swallowing disorders in muscular disease: functional assessment of cricopharyngeal myotomy. Ear Nose Troat J 1994;73(1):34-40.

[11] Rademaker AW, Pauloski BR, Logemann JA, Shanahan TK. Oropharyngeal swallow efficiency as a representative measure of swallowing function. J Speech Hear Res 1994;37(2):314-325.

[12] Smithard DG, O'Neill PA, Park C, Renwik DS, Wyatt R, Morris J, Martin DF. Can bedside assessment reliably exclude aspiration following acute stroke? Age and Aging 1998;27:99-106.

[13] Backer BM, Fraser AM, Backer CD. Long-term postoperative dysphagia in oral-pharhyngeal patients: subjects perceptions vs. videofluoroscopic observations. Dysphagia 1991;6:11-16.

[14] American Speech-Language-Hearing Association. (2002). Ececutive summary: Roles os speech-language pathologists in swallowing and feeding disorders: technical report. ASHA. Supplement 2. Rockville, MD: Author.

[15] Farneti D, Consolmagno P. Aspiration: the predictive value of some clinical and endoscopy signs. Evaluation of our case series. Acta Otorhinolaryngol Ital. Feb 2005; 25(1): 36–42.

[16] Langmore SE, Schatz K, Olsen N. Fiberoptic endoscopic examination of swallowing safety: a new procedure. Dysphagia 1988; 2: 216-219.

[17] Bastian, RW. Contemporary diagnosis of the dysphagic patient. In: Dysphagia in children, adults, and geriatrics. Otolaryngologic Clinics of North America 1998;31(3): 489-506.

[18] Leder, S.B., Sasaki C.T., Burrel M.I. Fiberoptic endoscopic evaluation of dysphagia to identify silent aspiration. Dysphagia 1998;13(1):19-21.

[19] Langmore SE. Endoscopic evaluation of oral and pharyngeal phases of swallowing *GI Motility online* (2006).

[20] Logemann JA. Evaluation and treatment of swallowing disorders. Pro-Ed Publishers, Austin, Texas 1983.

[21] AHCPR Agency for Health Care Policy and Research. Diagnosis and treatment of swallowing disorders (dysphagia). Evidence Report Technology Assessement n. 8, 1999).

[22] Farneti D. The Instrumental gold standard: FEES. Journal of Gastroenterology and HepatologyResearch 2014; 3(10): 1281-1291.

[23] Wu CH, Hsiao TY, Chen JC, Chang YC, Lee SY. Evaluation of swallowing safety with fiberoptic endoscope: comparison with videofluoroscopic technique. Laryngoscope1997;107:396-401.

[24] Leder SB. Serial fiberoptic endoscopic swallowing evaluation in the management of patients with dysphagia. Arch Phys Med Rehabil 1998;79:1264-1269.

[25] Harnick CJ, Miller C, Hartley BEJ, Willging JP. Pediatric fiberoptic endoscopic evaluation of swallowing. *Ann OtolRhinol Laryngol* 2000;109:996–999.

[26] Lim SH, Lieu PK, Phua SY, Seshadri R, Venketasubramanian N, Lee SH, Choo PW. Accuracy of bedside clinical methods compared with fiberoptic endoscopic examination of swallowing (FEES) in determining the risk of aspiration in acute stroke patients. *Dysphagia* 2001;16:1–6.

[27] Ajemian MS, Nirmul GB, Anderson MT, Zirlen DM, Kwasnik EM. Routine fiberoptic endoscopic evaluation of swallowing following prolonged intubation: implications for management. *Arch Surg* 2001;136:434–437.

[28] Hiss SG, Postma GN. Fiberoptic endoscopic evaluation of swallowing. Laryngoscope 2003; 113: 1386-1393.

[29] Gomes GF, Rao N, Brady S, Chaudhuri G, Donzelli JJ, Wesling MW. Gold-Standard? Analysis of the videofluoroscopic and fiberoptic endoscopic swallow examinations. J Applied Res 2003; 3:89-96.

[30] Campos AC, Pisani JC, Macedo ED, Vieira MC. Diagnostic methods for the detection of anterograde aspiration in enterally fed patients. Curr Opin Clin Nutr Metab Care 2004; 7(3): 285-292.

[31] [31] Maddock DJ, Gilbert RJ. Quantitative relationship between liquid bolus flow and laringea closure during deglutition. Am J Physsiol 1993;265:G704-G711

[32] Diez Gross R, Mahlmann J, Grayhack JP. Physiologic effects of open and closed thacheostomy tubes on the pharyngeal swallow. Ann Otol Laryngol 2003;112:143-52.

[33] Shaker R. Unsedated transnasal pharyngoesophageal gastroduodenoscopy (TEGD) technique. *Gastrointest Endosc* 1994;40:346–348.

[34] [34] Herrmann IF, Recio SA. Functional pharyngoesophagoscopy: a new technique for diagnostics and analyzing deglutition. *Oper Tech Otolaryngol Head Neck Surg* 1997; 8:163-167.

[35] Thompson GH and Batch JG. Flexible oesophagogastroscopy in otolaryngology. The Journal of Laryngology and Otology 1989;1989:399-403.

[36] Belafsky PC, Postma GN. Koufman JA Normal transnasal esophagoscopy. *Ear, Nose & Throat Journal;* 2001; 80 (7):438.

[37] Postma GN, Bach KK; Belafsky PC, Koufman JA. The Role of transnasal esophagoscopy in head and neck oncology. Laryngoscope 2002;112:2242-2243.

[38] Hermann IF, Recio SA, Cirillo F., Bechi P. Trans-Nasal Esophagoscopy (TNE). In Nikki Johnston, Robert J. Toohill (Eds), Effects, Diagnosis and Management of Extra-Esophageal Reflux. Medical College of Wisconsin, Milwaukee, WI, 2012.

[39] Farneti D, Genovese E, Chiarello G, Pastore A. The usefulness of transnasal esophagoscopy in the evaluation of patients with deglutition disorders. Poster presentation at the 2nd Congress of the European Society for Swallowing Disorders (ESSD). Barcelona, 25-27 October 2012.

[40] Farneti D, Fattori B, Nacci A, Mancini V, Simonelli M, Ruoppolo G, Genovese E. The Pooling-score (P-score): inter-rater and intra-rater reliability in the endoscopic assessment of the severity of dysphagia. Acta Otorhinolaryngol Ital. Apr 2014; 34(2): 105–110.

[41] Murray J, Langmore SE, Ginsberg S, Dostie A. The significance of accumulated oropharyngeal secretions and swallowing frequency in predicting aspiration. Dysphagia 1996;11:99-103.

[42] Brady S. Use of dysphagia severity scales during fiberoptic endoscopic exam of swallowing: treatment decisions and planning". ASHA Special Interest Division 13 – Perspectives in Swallowing and Swallowing Disorders 2007;16 (2):10-13.

[43] Kaneoka AS, Langmore SE, Krisciunas GP, Field K, Scheel R, McNally E, Walsh MJ, O'Dea MB, Cabral H. The Boston residue and clearance scale: preliminary reliability and validity testing. Folia Phoniatr Logop. 2013;65(6):312-317.

[44] Farneti D. Pooling score: an endoscopic model for evaluating severity of dysphagia. Acta Otorhinolaryngol Ital 2008; 28: 135-140.

[45] Leder BS, Espinosa JF. Aspiration risk after acute stroke: comparison of clinical examination and fiberoptic fndoscopic fvaluation of swallowing. Dysphagia 2002;17:214-218.

[46] Farneti D, Turroni V, Scarponi L, Fabbri E, Panzini I, Genovese E. The integrated clinical evaluation. The correlation between non instrumental and endoscopic parameters in the evaluation of patients with deglutition disorders. Poster presentation at the The Dysphagia Research Society Annual Meeting, San Diego, California, March 3 - 6, 2010.

Chapter 5

Endoscopy for Diseases with Esophageal Dysphagia

Hiroshi Makino, Hiroshi Yoshida and Eiji Uchida

Additional information is available at the end of the chapter

http://dx.doi.org/10.5772/60909

1. Introduction

The Standards of Practice Committee of the ASGE prepared the data to update the previous ASGE guidelines [1]. Guidelines for the appropriate use of endoscopy are based on critical reviews of the available data and the expert consensus on the guidelines when they are drafted. Esophagogastroduodenoscopy (EGD) is an effective tool for the diagnostic evaluation and management of patients with dysphagia. Varadarajulu reported a diagnostic yield of 54% with EGD in the initial evaluation of patients aged >40 years who presented with dysphagia and concomitant heartburn, odynophagia, and weight loss [2]. The American Gastroenterological Association (AGA) previously reviewed the treatment of patients with dysphagia, which is caused by benign disorders of the distal esophagus [3,4]. The most important examination for these diseases is endoscopy. Specimens of esophageal lesions obtained by biopsy and brush cytology may be used to establish a diagnosis of neoplasms or specific infections [5]. Malignant esophageal tumors are also diagnosed by biopsy on endoscopy. Endoscopic evaluation is recommended for most patients with dysphagia of the esophageal origin as an effective means of establishing or confirming a diagnosis, seeking evidence of esophagitis (excluding malignancies), and implementing therapy when appropriate.

The AGA has recommended endoscopic dilation by both bougie and balloon for the endoscopic management of diseases involving dysphagia [3,4], but more recent reports also describe therapy by endoscopic injection of corticosteroid, triamcinolone, or botulinum, or endoscopic fundoplication for GERD. Peroral endoscopic myotomy (POEM) is another new endoscopic procedure used for the treatment of achalasia.

In this review we report the usefulness of endoscopy for the evaluation and management of diseases involving dysphagia.

2. Evaluation

The most common causes of esophageal dysphagia are listed in Table 1.

	Endoscopic dilation		Other endoscopic treatments
	Bougie	Balloon	
Benign diseases	Yes		
Peptic stricture	Yes		Transoral incisionless fundoplication
			Radiofrequency ablation
			Injection of corticosteroids or triamcinolone
Schatzki ring	Yes		Electrocautery incision with a needle-knife papillotome
Esophageal web	Yes		
Eosinophilic esophagitis	Yes		
Caustic injury	Yes		
Anastomotic stricture	Yes		Biodegradable stent
Radiation injury	Yes		
Drug-induced stricture	Yes		
Postendoscopic therapy stricture	Yes		
Malignant diseases			
Head and neck tumor	No		Self-expanding metal stents (SEMS)
Esophageal carcinoma (adeno and squamous cell)	Yes		Self-expanding metal stents (SEMS)
Extrinsic compression	No		Self-expanding metal stents (SEMS)
Motility disorders			
Achalasia	Yes		Peroral endoscopic myotomy (POEM)
			Injection of botulinum toxin
Diffuse esophageal spasm	No		

Table 1. Common diseases of esophageal dysphagia and endoscopic management

http://dx.doi.org/10.5772/60909

The acceptance of endoscopy as a gold standard for testing for mucosal disease may bias evaluations of the sensitivity of other diagnostic modalities. Given that endoscopy was used as the gold standard for mucosal disease, the sensitivity of radiology could not have exceeded that of endoscopy [3].

If the patient history, barium swallow, or both suggest achalasia, manometry to confirm the diagnosis should generally precede the endoscopic evaluation, to better prepare for endoscopic therapy.

2.1. GERD: Peptic esophageal stricture

White light endoscopy is now the standard investigation procedure for identifying esophageal injury. An experienced endoscopist who takes the time to methodically inspect the esophagus is generally expected to succeed in diagnosing reflux esophagitis. There has been evidence, however, of interindividual variability in the endoscopic diagnosis of erosive reflux esophagitis and other lesions of the upper gastrointestinal tract. Krugmann reported detailed endoscopic findings for GERD [4]. Peptic esophageal stricture as a consequence of gastroesophageal reflux disease is the most frequent among benign esophageal strictures [6]. The typical case of peptic esophageal stricture is shown in Figure 1. There are multiple etiologies for benign esophageal stricture or stenosis, but the most frequent is the peptic stricture resulting from pathologic acid exposure in GERD. Dysphagia is a common symptom. When dysphagia is encountered, accurate diagnostic procedures (barium esophagogram, upper endoscopy with biopsies) have to be performed to exclude malignant causes first. Strictures can be divided into two categories anatomically: "simplex" or "complex." The former are short, focal, nonangulated, and wide enough to allow an endoscope to easily pass through. The latter are long and angulated, with a severely narrowed diameter. The strictures are also sometimes scored based on three parameters to optimize the therapeutic decisions: the stricture diameter, stricture length, and degree of difficulty of stricture dilation [7]. After this scoring, the stricture can be classified as type I (mild), type II (moderate), or type III (severe or critical). This classification is also useful for predicting the most appropriate therapeutic option.

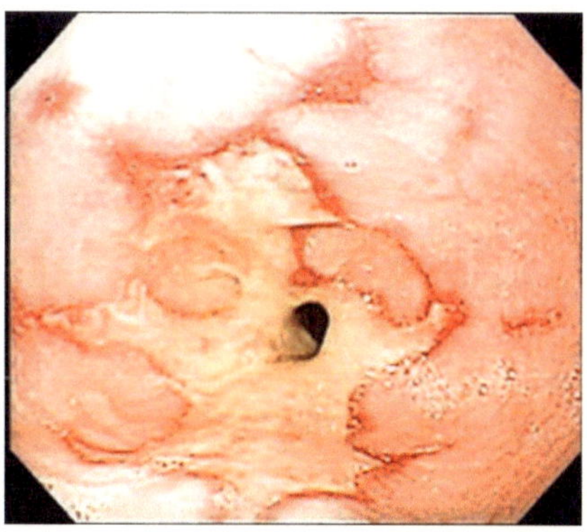

Figure 1. Peptic structure

2.2. NERD (Nonerosive Reflux Disease)

NERD is a subcategory of GERD characterized by troublesome reflux-related symptoms in the absence of esophageal mucosal erosions or breaks on conventional endoscopy, without recent acid-suppressive therapy [8]. Most patients with typical reflux symptoms show no evidence of erosive esophagitis on endoscopy. Upper gastrointestinal endoscopy is required to establish a diagnosis of NERD. Further investigation is required when alarming symptoms are present. Routine random biopsy is not currently recommended for the diagnosis of NERD. Additional diagnostic information is provided by ambulatory 24-hour intraesophageal pH-metry and impedance measurement with reflux-related symptom correlation.

2.3. Schatzki ring and esophageal web

Narrowing of the esophagus can be due to either a benign or malignant stricture formation, webs (mucosa or submucosa alone), or rings (mucosa, submucosa, and muscle). Esophageal rings and webs are both membranous structures in which a thin fold of tissue creates at least a partial obstruction of the esophageal lumen. Esophageal webs usually measure 2–3 mm wide. The obstruction is a smooth extension of normal esophageal tissue made up of mucosa or submucosa alone. Webs can be found anywhere along the esophagus, but classically they appear in the anterior postcricoid area of the upper esophagus. A web at this site constitutes the Paterson Brown–Kelly syndrome, otherwise known as Plummer–Vinson syndrome in the USA [9].

Esophageal rings are concentric, smooth, thin extensions of normal esophageal tissue, usually 3–5 mm thick. They consist of mucosa, submucosa, and muscle. Rings are often detected incidentally at barium studies or endoscopy. There is no sex difference in the incidence of rings overall, though multiple rings are usually found in young men. Rings are classified as types A, B, and C [9]. The A ring, an uncommon type located a few centimeters proximal to the esophagogastric squamocolumnar junction, is thought to be caused by normal physiologic smooth muscle contractions. The B ring (more commonly known as Schatzki ring) is actually a web, as it involves only mucosa and submucosa and tends to appear in the distal esophagus and as the proximal part of a hiatus hernia. The B ring is nonprogressive and usually presents in patients aged over 50 who experience intermittent dysphagia to solid food over periods spanning months or years. The C ring, another rare type, is found in the most distal portion of the esophagus. On X-ray, the C ring manifests as an indentation caused by diaphragmatic crural pressure. A and C rings are both unlikely to be readily seen on upper endoscopy. Hence, the B ring (Schatzki ring) is the most common esophageal ring found on either esophagogram or endoscopy. Schatzki rings rarely cause symptoms. Overall, esophageal rings with luminal narrowing significant enough to cause symptoms (13 mm or less) are seen in only about 0.5% of all esophagograms.

2.4. Head and neck tumor and esophageal tumor

A core cancer-specific symptom of head and neck tumors is difficulty in swallowing [10]. Most patients with tumors of the head and neck or esophagus present for medical attention because of dysphagia.

Among the many symptoms of esophageal cancer, dysphagia may have an especially adverse effect on quality of life (QOL) [11]. Dysphagia is the predominant symptom in more than 70% of patients with esophageal cancer. The optimum management of dysphagia caused by advanced primary EC has not yet been established, although continued progress toward this goal has been achieved in recent years.

Apart from the weight loss that may result, an inability to swallow comfortably or a tendency to regurgitate food may spoil meals shared with families and friends or induce patients to withdraw from social situations.

Granular cell tumors and solitary fibrous tumors of the cervical esophagus also cause dysphagia [12, 13].

2.5. Eosinophilic esophagitis and infection

The incidence of eosinophilic esophagitis (EoE) is registering an increase in adults. An allergic reaction to food is now established to play an important role in its etiology, and dietary interventions and biologic agents to block the inflammatory cascade are thought to hold promise as novel fields of clinical research. Biopsies should be obtained from the proximal and distal esophagus to evaluate for eosinophilic esophagitis in patients who present with dysphagia together with endoscopic findings suggestive or not suggestive of EoE, and also in patients without esophageal mechanical obstruction. Patients usually present with dysphagia, food impaction, and/or reflux-like symptoms, and biopsy of the esophagus typically shows more than 15 eosinophils per high-power field [14]. The dysphagia predominantly seen in EoE has been attributed to both organic and nonorganic (i.e., motility) disorders. Endoscopically, a normal-appearing esophagus is usually incompatible with a diagnosis of EE, although the findings can be subtle. EGD findings implicative of EoE include an attenuation of the subepithelial vascular pattern, linear furrowing (possibly extending along the whole length of the esophagus), surface exudates composed of eosinophils, or abscesses or strictures [15,16].

Endoscopic evaluation of the gastrointestinal tract remains a cornerstone of diagnosis, especially in patients with advanced immunodeficiency who are at risk for opportunistic infections (OIs) [17]. Infectious esophagitis may be caused by fungal, viral, bacterial, or even parasitic agents [18]. Acute onset of symptoms such as dysphagia and odynophagia is typical of this condition. Candida esophagitis most commonly appears in patients with hematologic malignancies or AIDS, or who use steroids for the treatment of disorders. Candida esophagitis is usually diagnosed when white mucosal plaque-like lesions are seen on esophagogastroduodenoscopy. HSV esophagitis occurs most frequently in solid organ and bone marrow transplant recipients.

The diagnosis of herpes simplex virus esophagitis is usually based on endoscopic findings confirmed by histopathological examination. Well-circumscribed ulcerous lesions with a "volcano-like" appearance may appear in the mucosa of the distal esophagus, typically with diameters of less than 2 cm. Diffuse erosive esophagitis may also be present.

Cytomegalovirus esophagitis is observed in patients who have undergone transplantation, are on long-term dialysis, are infected with HIV, or are receiving chronic steroid therapy. Esophagogastroduodenoscopy usually reveals large solitary ulcers or erosions in the distal esophagus.

2.6. Esophagitis induced by caustic injury, radiation injury, or drugs

A patient with a usual history of caustic substance ingestion and prolonged hospitalization for severe caustic damage was hospitalized again because of an increase in dysphagia and odynophagia [19]. The gold standard of safely assessing the depth, extent of caustic ingestion injury, and appropriate therapeutic regimen is EGD. The patients underwent EGD within 24 hours of admission and mucosal damage was graded using Zagar's modified endoscopic classification scheme [19].

Radiation therapy (RT), the primary modality for patients with tumors of the upper aero-digestive tract, allows larynx preservation [20]. Proximal esophageal strictures occur in 2–16% of patients after radiation therapy for cancers of the lung or head and neck. RT-induced laryngeal edema (due to inflammation and lymphatic disruption) is a common and expected side effect. Progressive edema and associated fibrosis detected by endoscope or barium swallowing can lead to long-term problems with phonation and swallowing. Aspiration pneumonia associated with dysphagia after intensive chemo radiation therapy has recently been reported at a growing frequency.

Drug-induced esophagitis mainly presents as chest pain, odynophagia, and dysphagia. In the agents known to induce esophagitis, antibiotics are the most common culprit. Other causative agents include nonsteroidal anti-inflammatory drugs, antihypertensive drugs, acetaminophen, oral hypoglycemic agents (glimepiride), bisphosphonates (alendronate, ibandronate), ascorbic acid, and warfarin [21]. The most frequent endoscopic site of drug-induced esophagitis is the middle third of the esophagus. On endoscopy, drug-induced esophagitis manifests as ulcers of various forms such as kissing ulcers, erosions, or ulcers with bleeding, as patchy sections coated with drug materials or impacted pill fragments, or sometimes as strictures.

2.7. Achalasia

Achalasia is regarded as a disease exclusively involving the smooth muscle. About 70–80% of patients have absent or incomplete lower esophageal sphincter (LES) relaxation with wet swallows, while the remainder have complete but shortened relaxation [22]. The typical endoscopic findings are shown in Figure 2A,B. Patients with esophageal stasis are often unaware of this condition. Heartburn, though not infrequent, bears little relationship to the esophageal acid exposure in achalasia, regardless of whether heartburn is elicited by GER or esophageal stasis. Endoscopic examination can readily differentiate these disorders in most cases, although manometry may sometimes be required to make the distinction in equivocal cases. Readers may find interest in the AGA's recent technical review of the clinical uses of esophageal manometry and detailed descriptions of the procedure. Esophageal manometry is the gold standard test for esophageal motility disorders [23]. Esophageal manometry has been shown to be especially useful for definitively diagnosing achalasia or diffuse esophageal spasm and for detecting esophageal motor abnormalities associated with collagen-vascular disease.

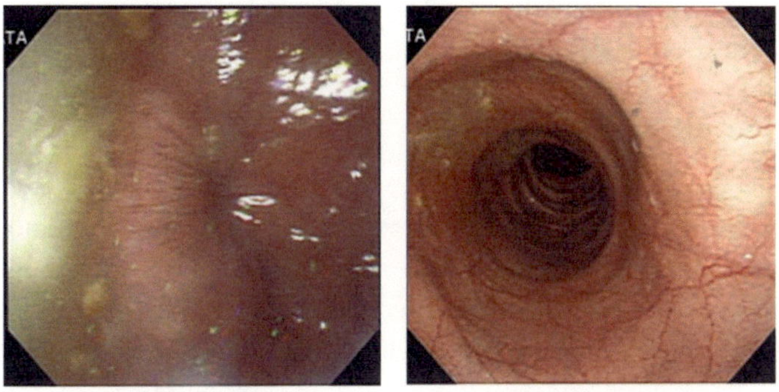

(a) Fluid-filled esophagus (b) Dilated esophagus

Figure 2. Achalasia

2.8. Diffuse esophageal spasm

Diffuse esophageal spasm (DES) is an uncommon disorder characterized by an impairment of ganglionic inhibition in the distal esophagus. Upper endoscopy should be performed as an initial evaluation of esophageal symptoms consistent with spastic disorders [24]. No specific endoscopic abnormality appears in most cases, but the endoscopist may notice disordered esophageal contractions. DES is defined by the presence of simultaneous contractions on conventional manometry. In higher resolution recordings by HRM with EPT, however, the propagation velocity varies greatly along the length of the esophagus and often progresses rapidly in some regions. Esophageal manometry, the putative gold standard in the diagnosis of achalasia, classically shows aperistalsis and failure of relaxation of the lower esophageal sphincter.

2.9. Extrinsic compression

Dysphagia is also caused by extrinsic compression of the esophagus associated with mediastinal diseases, tumors such as lung cancer and lymphoma, or infections such as tuberculosis or histoplasmosis [1,3].

3. Treatment method for diseases with dysphagia

A general approach to the treatment of adult patients with dysphagia caused by benign disorders of the distal esophagus is outlined in the "Medical Position Statement on Treatment of Patients with Dysphagia Caused by Benign Disorders of the Distal Esophagus" from the American Gastroenterological Association (AGA) [3]. The review describes the management of dysphagia, peptic stricture, lower esophageal mucosal rings, and achalasia. More recently, the Standards of Practice Committee of the American Society for Gastrointestinal Endoscopy (ASGE) updated its previous guideline. In sections covering the role of endoscopy in evaluation and management, the uses of endoscopy evaluating dysphagia and dilation techniques for various dysphagic diseases are discribed [1.3]. The endoscopic management of esophageal dysphagia is summarized in Table 1.

3.1. Preparation and dilation technique

Patients who have esophageal stasis because of underlying achalasia, diverticula, or tight strictures may require a prolonged nasogastric tube placement to minimize the risk of aspiration and are instructed to refrain from intake of solids for 6 hours and clear liquids for 2 hours before the procedure in the outpatient setting. The esophageal dilation procedure carries a high risk of adverse bleeding events. In patients considered low risk for thromboembolic events, oral anticoagulation with warfarin should be withheld for 5–7 days before the procedure. Bridging therapy with heparin before restarting warfarin is often recommended for patients at high risk for thromboembolic events. Thienopyridines (e.g., clopidogrel) are usually withheld for 7–10 days before the procedure.

Bougie dilators exert both radial and axial forces along the entire length of the stricture. In the technique of wire-guided bougie dilation, a guidewire is passed through the esophagus and its tip is positioned in the antrum.

Balloon dilators exert only a radial force along the length of the stricture. This circumferential pressure, called hoop stress, is a product of the diameter and pressure within the balloon.

3.2. GERD: Peptic strictures

Various methods for endoscopic management of peptic stricture were reported [25]. The AGA recommend progressive dilatation to 40–60 F using polyvinyl bougies or balloons for both simple (diameter<10 mm, not tortuous) and complicated (diameter >10 mm, tortuous) strictures, and mercury bougies for only simple strictures [3]. The ASGE reported that patients with peptic strictures may be treated with Maloney, push-type dilators and balloon dilators with similar efficacy. The degree of dilation in a session should be based on the severity of the stricture [1]. The first dilator that causes resistance to passage is counted as 1. The "rule of three" states that only two additional dilators of sequential size should be passed (three dilators in total). The "rule of three" for bougie dilation has been accepted but not formally studied for safety. The initial dilator is selected based on the stricture diameter. This is estimated to be about the same size as the lumen of the stricture, or not more than 1–2 mm larger than the lumen. Sequential dilation is then performed.

The AGA described the endoscopic therapy for GERD and concluded that radiofrequency ablation is generally effective for the treatment of GERD [26].

Endoscopic fundoplication is also successfully performed in many institutes [27]. Transoral incisionless fundoplication (TIF) with the EsophyX TM device is effective for creating a continent gastroesophageal valve and obtaining good functional results, as measured by pH impedance in patients with gastroesophageal reflux disease (GERD). TIF significantly improved both atypical and typical symptoms in patients: the corresponding GERD health-related quality of life (HRQL) and reflux symptom index (RSI) score was reduced by 50% or more compared to baseline on proton pump inhibitors (PPIs).

Several reports confirmed the beneficial effect of intralesionally administered corticosteroids or triamcinolone in benign esophageal strictures of different etiologies [6].

3.3. Lower esophageal mucosal ring

Large-bore endoscopic dilation or bougienage (15 mm/45 Fr or larger) is the mainstay therapy for both upper and lower esophageal lesions. The AGA recommends progressive dilatation to 45–60 F using mercury or polyvinyl bougies or balloons [3]. This procedure is frequently performed with either Savary or Maloney dilators, though balloon dilation has also been reported. The ASGE pointed out that dilation with a single large (16–20 mm) dilator leads to rupture of the Schatzki ring and symptomatic relief in almost all patients. Electrocautery incision with a needle-knife papillotome and four-quadrant biopsies of the ring has been performed together with dilation as adjunctive methods.

3.4. Head and neck and esophageal tumors: extrinsic compression

Bougie dilation and balloon dilation are both unavailable for malignant tumors of the esophagus and head and neck, as dilation is considered a high-risk procedure for adverse bleeding and perforation events. Endoscopic dilation is performed temporarily for nutritional support in patients who are to undergo tumor resections. Figure 3A,B showed the typical esophageal advanced cancer and endoscopic balloon dilation for its stricture.

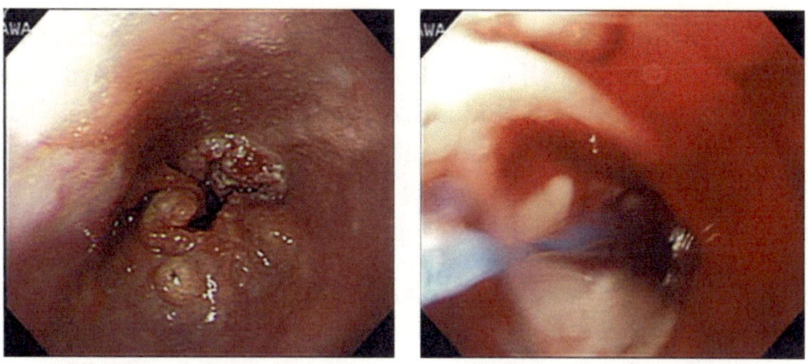

(a) Esophageal advanced cancer (b) Pneumatic balloon dilation

Figure 3. Endoscopic balloon dilation for esophageal cancer

Self-expanding metal stents (SEMS) are a well-established palliation modality for dysphagia in patients with tumors of the esophagus and head and neck [28]. Stenting is also temporarily effective for extrinsic compression. Health-related quality of life (HRQoL) is becoming a major issue in the evaluation of any therapeutic or palliative intervention.

3.5. Eosinophilic esophagitis and infection

Pharmacological, endoscopic, and dietary interventions are used as treatment modalities for patients with eosinophilic esophagitis (EE), either singly or in combination.

For endoscopic dilatation, the balloon is positioned across the gastro-esophageal junction and inflated to the smallest diameter. The endoscopist grasps the catheter to assess the tension during pull through and then slowly withdraws the endoscope to the proximal esophagus. The procedure is repeated using a sequentially larger diameter balloon until adequate dilation is achieved [3,14].

3.6. Postradiation stricture

Several sessions of bougie dilation may be necessary for adequate treatment for radiation-induced strictures because most strictures are complex. The ASGE report summarizes a combined antegrade–retrograde rendezvous approach described in case reports and case series for the management of severe radiation-induced strictures with complete occlusion of the proximal esophagus. After dilation, the endoscopist performing this technique passes a standard endoscope or small-caliber endoscope through the stomach into the esophagus via an existing gastrostromy tract.

3.7. Achalasia

Esophageal dilation for achalasia involves forceful disruption of the lower esophageal sphincter. This is usually accomplished with 30- to 40-mm-diameter pneumatic balloon dilators. Dilation is generally performed over a wire under fluoroscopic guidance, although nonfluoroscopically guided dilation using endoscopic visualization alone has been reported.

POEM is a new endoscopic procedure used for the treatment of achalasia [29]. This novel endoscopic esophagomyotomy method was first reported by Pasricha et al. in porcine models and then by Inoue et al. in humans. POEM is performed by dissection and division of the inner circular muscle layer of the esophagus through a submucosal tunnel created endoscopically by a small proximal opening of the esophageal mucosa. A study evaluating the role of POEM reported a significant improvement in dysphagia scores.

A further option is endoscopic botulinum toxin injection into the lower esophageal sphincter. This technique offers good short-term results.

Ham et al. identified the currently available biodegradable stents for benign esophageal strictures [30]. This technique will also be available for the treatment of achalasia.

3.8. Postesophagectomy anastomotic strictures

Anastomotic strictures have been reported in 9–48% of patients after esophagectomy for esophageal cancer. The strictures are diagnosed in patients with dysphagia in whom a standard flexible esophagoscope cannot be passed across the anastomosis. Both bougie and balloon dilation have been used for the treatment of anastomotic strictures with success rates of up to 93%. In Figure 4A,B showed the typical anastomotic stricture and endoscopic balloon dilation for it. There is a high recurrence rate, however, and patients often require frequent sessions.

http://dx.doi.org/10.5772/60909

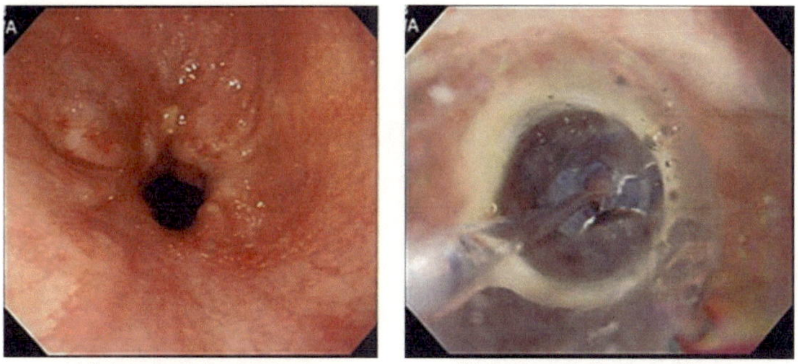

(a) Anastomotic stricture (b) Pneumatic balloon dilation

Figure 4. Endoscopic balloon dilation for Anastomotic stricture

4. Conclusion

This chapter is based on the ASGE guidelines and recommendations by AGA. Endoscopy is more sensitive than radiology for identifying subtle mucosal lesions of the esophagus such as mild esophagitis caused by gastroesophageal reflux or infection. A cost analysis also showed that EGD with therapeutic intent is more cost effective than an initial diagnostic approach with barium swallow in patients with histories suggestive of benign or malignant esophageal obstruction.

Various endoscopic treatments are useful for diseases with dysphagia and minimally invasive compared to surgical procedures.

Acknowledgements

The authors wish to thank Dr. Hiroshi Maruyama and Dr. Ichiro Akagi for their clinical support.

Author details

Hiroshi Makino[1*], Hiroshi Yoshida[1] and Eiji Uchida[2]

*Address all correspondence to: himiyumo@nms.ac.jp

1 Department of Surgery, Nippon Medical School, Tama-Nagayama Hospital, Japan

2 Department of Surgery, Nippon Medical School, Japan

References

[1] Pasha, S.F., Acosta, R.D., Chandrasekhara, V., Chathadi, K.V., Decker, G.A., Early, D.S., Evans, J.A., Fanelli, R.D., Fisher, D.A., Foley, K.Q., Fonkalsrud, L., Hwang, J.H., Jue, T.L., Khashab, M.A., Lightdale, J.R., Muthusamy, V.R., Sharaf, R., Saltzman, J.R., Shergill, A.K., Cash, B. The role of endoscopy in the evaluation and management of dysphagia. Guideline, ASGE Standards of Practice Committee, *Gastrointest. Endosc.*, 79(2014), 191–201.

[2] Varadarajulu, S., Eloubeidi, M. A., Patel,R. S., Mulcahy,H.E., Barkun, A., Jowell, P., Libby, E., Schutz, S., Nickl, N.J., Cotton, P.B. The yield and the predictors of esophageal pathology when upper endoscopy is used for the initial evaluation of dysphagia. *Gastrointest. Endosc.*, 61 (2005), 804–808.

[3] Spechler, S. J. AGA technical review on treatment of patients with dysphagia caused by benign disorders of the distal esophagus. *Gastroenterology*, 117 (1999), 233–254.

[4] Spechler, S. J. American gastroenterological association medical position statement on treatment of patients with dysphagia caused by benign disorders of the distal esophagus. *Gastroenterology*, 117 (1999), 229–232.

[5] Krugmann, J., Neumann, H, Vieth, M, Armstrong, D., What is the role of endoscopy and oesophageal biopsies in the management of GERD? *Best Practice Res. Clin. Gastroenterol.*, 27 (2013), 373–385.

[6] Chaitan, K. N, Jon, O.W, Hiran, C. F., Endoscopic management of gastroesophageal reflux disease: A review. *J. Thoracic Cardiovasc. Surgery*, 144, (2012), S74–S79.

[7] Pregun, I., Hritz, I., Tulassay, Z., HerszényiIstván, L., Peptic esophageal stricture: Medical treatment., *Digestive diseases.*, 27 (2009), 31– 37.

[8] Modlin, I. M., Hunt, R.H., Malfertheiner, P., Moayyedi, P., Quigley, E.M., Tytgat, G. N. J., Tack, J., Heading, R.C., Holtman, G.,. Moss, S.F., on behalf of the Vevey NERD Consensus Group, Diagnosis and Management of Non-Erosive Reflux Disease, *Digestion*, 80 (2009), 74–88.

[9] Smith, M. S., Diagnosis and management of esophageal rings and webs, *Gastroenterol. Hepatol.*, 6, (2010), 701–704.

[10] Chera, B. S., Eisbruch, A., Murphy, B. A., Ridge, J. A., Gavin, P., Reeve, B. B., Bruner, D. W., Movsas, B. Recommended patient-reported core set of symptoms to measure in head and neck cancer treatment trials, *JNCI*, 106 (2014). Brief Communication 1–4.

[11] Darling, G. E., Quality of life in patients with esophageal cancer. Review. *Thorac. Surg. Clin.*, 23 (2013) 569–575.

[12] Huang, A. T., Dominguez, L. M., Powers, C. N. Reiter, E. R. Granular cell tumor of the cervical esophagus: Case report and literature review of an unusual cause of dysphagia., *Head and Neck Pathol.*, 7 (2013), 274–279.

[13] Makino, H., Miyashita, Masao., Nomura, T., Katsuta, M., Kashiwabara, M., Takahashi, K., Yamashita, K., Nakamizo, M., Yokoshima, K., Onda, M., Naito, Z., Tajiri, T., Solitary fibrous tumor of the cervical esophagus. *Dig. Dis. Sci.*, 52 (2007), 2195–2200.

[14] Gupte, A. R., Draganov, P. V. Eosinophilic esophagitis., *World J. Gastroenterol.*, 15 (2009), 17–24.

[15] Chehade, M., Lucendo, A. J., Achem, S. R., and Souza, R. F. Causes, evaluation, and consequences of eosinophilic esophagitis., *Ann. N.Y. Acad. Sci.*, 1300 (2013), 110–118.

[16] Philpott, H., Nandurkarb, S., Thienc, F., Gibsonb, P. R., Royced, S. G., Eosinophilic esophagitis: A clinicopathological review. *Pharmacol. Therapeut.*, 146 (2015), 12-22.

[17] Werneck-Silva, L. A., Prado, I. B., Role of upper endoscopy in diagnosing opportunistic infections in human immunodeficiency virus-infected patients. *World J. Gastroenterol*, 15 (2009), 1050–1056.

[18] Rosołowski, M., Kierzkiewicz, M. Etiology, diagnosis and treatment of infectious esophagitis., *Przegląd Gastroenterologiczny*, 8 (2013), 333–337.

[19] Cheng, H. T., Cheng, C. L., Cheng, H. L., Tang, J. H., Chu, Y. Y., Liu, N. J., Chen, P.C., Caustic ingestion in adults: The role of endoscopic classification in predicting outcome. *BMC Gastroenterol.*, 31 (2008), 1–7.

[20] Monjazeb, A. M., Blackstock, A. W., The Impact of multimodality therapy of distal esophageal and gastroesophageal junction adenocarcinomas on treatment-related toxicity and complications. *Semin. Radiat. Oncol.*, 23 (2013), 60–73.

[21] Kim, S. H., Jeong, J. B., Kim, J. W., Koh, S. J., Kim, B. G., Lee, K. L., Chang, M. S., Im, J. P., Kang, H. W., Shin, C. M., Clinical and endoscopic characteristics of drug-induced esophagitis., *World J. Gastroenterol.*, 20 (2014), 10994-10999.

[22] Felix, V. N., DeVault, K., Penagini, R., Elvevi, A., Swanstrom, L., Wassenaar, E., Crespin, O. M., Pellegrini, C. A., Wong, R. Causes and treatments of achalasia, and primary disorders of the esophageal body., *Ann. N.Y. Acad. Sci.*, 1300 (2013), 236–249.

[23] O'Neill, O. M., Johnston, B. T., Coleman, H. G., Achalasia: A review of clinical diagnosis, epidemiology, treatment and outcomes. *World J. Gastroenterol.*, 19 (2013), 5806–5812.

[24] Roman, S., Kahrilas, P.J., Management of spastic disorders of the esophagus., *Gastroenterol. Clin. North Am.*, 42 (2013), 27-43.

[25] Pietro, M. D. and Fitzgerald, R. C., Research advances in esophageal diseases: bench to bedside., *F1000 Prime Reports*. 44 (2013), 1–11.

[26] Falk, G. W., Fennerty, M. B., Rothstein, R. I., AGA Institute Technical Review on the use of endoscopic therapy for gastroesophageal reflux disease. *Gastroenterology*, 131 (2006), 1315–1336.

[27] Bell, R. C. W., Freeman, K. D., Clinical and pH-metric outcomes of transoral esophagogastric fundoplication for the treatment of gastroesophageal reflux disease., *Surg. Endosc.*, 25 (2011), 1975–1984.

[28] Diamantis, G., Scarpa, M., Bocus, P., Realdon, S., Castoro, C., Ancona, E., Battaglia, G., Quality of life in patients with esophageal stenting for the palliation of malignant dysphagia., *World J. Gastroenterol.*, 17 (2011), 144-150.

[29] Chuah, S. K, Chiu, C. H., Tai, W. C., Lee, J. H., Lu, H. I., Changchien, C. S., Tseng, P. H., Wu, K. L., Current status in the treatment options for esophageal achalasia., *World J. Gastroenterol.*, 19 (2013), 5421–5429.

[30] Ham, Y. H., Kim, G. H., Plastic and biodegradable stents for complex and refractory benign esophageal strictures. Clin Endosc., 47 (2014), 295–300.

Chapter 6

Is the Electrical Threshold of Sensation on the Soft Palate Indicative of the Recovery Process of the Swallowing Reflex Based on Functional Assessment?

Koichiro Ueda, Osamu Takahashi, Hisao Hiraba,
Masaru Yamaoka, Enri Nakayama, Kimiko Abe,
Mituyasu Sato, Hisako Ishiyama,
Akinari Hayashi and Kotomi Sakai

Additional information is available at the end of the chapter

http://dx.doi.org/10.5772/60771

1. Introduction

Patients with dysphasia have a variety of motor deficits in orofacial and pharyngeal movements. Disorders in the orofacial region, such as dysphasia developed, may be induced by cerebral vessel disease, cancer in the orofacial and neck region, and other conditions. Functional assessment of mastication and the deglutition is most likely to be performed using videoendoscopy (VE) and videofluoroscopy (VF), although electromyography (EMG), ultrasonography (US), and other modalities are also used. Although VE is the primary method for examination of swallowing, projection of VE during instantaneous variations in swallowing cannot be observed because of whiteout. On the other hand, although VF is the best choice for functional assessment of eating and swallowing, we cannot avoid a bombing experience. Therefore, we devised a new method to reduce the reliance on VF examination.

Electrical thresholds of the sensation of structures with primary disease in the orofacial region of patients with stroke, head and neck tumor, external injuries, and other conditions following orofacial treatments were examined. The results suggested a close relationship between the electrical threshold of sensation and the recovery process, because patients with various orofacial and neck diseases showed a lower threshold of electrical sensation associated with treatment. Thus, changes in the oral and pharyngeal phases using VF in patients with brain tumors, stroke, external injuries, amyotrophic lateral sclerosis and myasthenia gravis were investigated.

Many researchers have evaluated VF results based on the Videofluorographic Examination of Swallowing Worksheet developed by Logemann [8]. However, because the inspection items on this worksheet comprise many measurement items, numerous hospitals conduct their own modified VF assessments [2, 3, 5-7, 14]. Based on experiences in other hospitals, 11 key events were identified for the assessment of VF: bolus formation, tongue-to-palate contact, premature bolus loss, residue in the oral cavity, and oral transit time in the oral phase; and lift in the soft palate, triggering of the pharyngeal swallow, vallecula residue, pyriform sinus residue, pharyngeal transit time, and aspiration in the pharyngeal phase. Furthermore, these items were classified into three levels: grade 0 as normal, grade 1 as inadequate, and grade 2 as a true abnormality. The total scores for all items in the oral and pharyngeal phases separately are calculated and a higher sum in each phase represented a more serious condition is presumed. Electrical thresholds of sensation on the soft palate during the hospital visit were measured, too. Guidance regarding an accepted way of stretch training fitting various disorder parts, such as gum rubbing, the Mendelsohn maneuver, thermal tactile stimulation, the head lift exercise (Shaler exercise), the tongue holding maneuver and Sylvester maneuver. Trainings involved procedures suitable for each patient after obtaining first-person informed consent. For example, patients with the deglutition disorder were performed by thermal tactile stimulation during the hospital visit and Shaker exercise in the residence. Patients performed the training method best suited to their disease twice daily.

Finally, we examined the relationship between the total scores for all items in the oral and pharyngeal phases and the threshold of electrical sensation on the soft palate. We hypothesized that if electrical threshold measurement can be substituted for VF assessments, radiation exposure to patients can be reduced. Furthermore, electrical threshold stimuli on the soft palate and other areas are produced by an appeal of a loose press feeling in the stimulus area of subjects, not painful sensation.

2. Material and method

We aimed to elucidate the relationship between changes in the electrical threshold of sensations associated with various orofacial symptoms and the recovery processes of areas affected by orofacial disorders depending on the oral rehabilitation technique. Thus, we investigated the relationship between modified VF assessments and sensory electrical threshold evoked on the soft palate. In particular, electrical stimuli are appealed by a loose press feeling in the stimulus area of subjects, not painful sensation.

2.1. Subjects

First experiment: We examined 11 patients (8 males, 3 females; age range, 30-66 years) with various disorders in orofacial regions (facial muscles, n=4; lingual muscles, n=5; hypoesthesia of the soft palate, n=2) (Table 1). All medical treatments were performed over a long time period (range, 10-80 months). We compared the relationship between the degree of recovery following oral rehabilitation and the electrical threshold of sensation in the deficient orofacial regions.

The various disorders among the 11 patients were as follows: acoustic nerve tumor (n=1), diabetes (n=1), cerebral infarct (n=4), neck tumor (n=4), and facial nerve palsy (n=1) (Table 1). Guidance regarding an accepted way of stretch training fitting various disorder pats, such as gum rubbing, the Mendelsohn maneuver, thermal tactile stimulation, the head lift exercise (Shaker exercise), and the tongue holding maneuver were provided. Training involved procedures suitable for each patient after obtaining first-person informed consent. Patients performed the training method best suited to their disease twice daily. The thermal tactile stimulation was performed when the patients visited the hospital, and the relationships between the electrical threshold of sensation from one month to the next as well as the degree of recovery according to the training condition, including hearing investigation were examined.

Patient No.	Etiology	Location of disorder	Age	Sex	Time after onset
1	Accostic nerve tumor	unilateral tongue	55	F	60 months
2	Diabetes	unilateral tongue	59	F	120 months
3	Cerebral infarct	unilateral tongue	62	M	30 months
4	Neck tumor	unilateral tongue	30	M	48 months
5	Neck tumor	unilateral neck region	30	M	60 months
6	Neck tumor	unilateral mandibular part	43	F	36 months
7	Cerebral infarct	unilateral upper lip part	62	M	6 months
8	Neck tumor	unilateral neck region	30	M	50 months
9	Facial nerve palsy	unilateral tongue	35	M	3 months
10	Cerebral infarct	bilateral soft palate	66	M	36 months
11	Cerebral infarct	bilateral soft palate	62	M	6 months

Table 1. Patient characteristics in the first experiment. F: female, M: male.

Second experiment: Eight patients (six males, two females were evaluated; age range, 24-67 years) with glossopharyngeal nerve paralysis of the soft palatal lift. The duration of the patients' dysphasia symptoms ranged from 7 to 39 months before the investigation (Table 2). The eight patients exhibited various symptoms as follows: brain tumor (n=2), cerebral hemorrhage (n=2), cerebral contusion (n=2), amyotrophic lateral sclerosis (n=1), and myasthenia gravis (n=1) (Table 2). The degree of dysphagia was classified based on many VF assessments as described by Logemann [8] (underside of Modified VF worksheet, Table 3). The bolus formation, tongue-to-palate contact, premature bolus loss, and oral transit time were measured in the oral phase, while lift in the soft palate, triggering of pharyngeal swallow, epiglottic vallecula residue, pyriform sinus residue, pharyngeal transit time, and aspiration were measured in the pharyngeal phase. Thus, the analysis comprised the total assessments in the oral and pharyngeal phases. These items were divided into three levels: grade 0 as normal, grade 1 as inadequate, and grade 2 as a true abnormality.

Patient No.	Etiology	Location	Age	Sex	Time after onset	Status
1	Brain tumor	Brain stem	48	M	7 months	full oral
2	Brain tumor	Brain stem	54	M	9 months	NG
3	Cerebral hemorrhage	Multiple	67	M	7 months	NG
4	Cerebral hemorrhage	Middle cerebral artery territory	58	M	1 year 3months	full oral
5	Cerebral contusion	Multiple	19	M	10 months	NG
6	Cerebral contusion	Multiple	25	F	2 years 1 months	PEG
7	Amyotrophic lateral sclerosis	-	60	M	3 year 3 months	full oral
8	Myasthenia gravis	-	24	F	2 years 1 months	full oral

Table 2. Patient characteristics in the second experiment. NG: no symptoms, PEG: gastrostomy.

We utilized the total scores for all items in the oral and pharyngeal phases separately. In particular, we considered that a higher sum in each phase might indicate a more serious condition. All procedures were approved by the ethic committee at Nihon University School of Dentistry.

2.2. Threshold of electrical sensations

First experiment: A special electrode was designed for electrical stimulation of the tongue dorsum. This electrode consists of a button-like electrode with a central part (cathode, 0.5 mm across) and round wire (anode, 1.0 mm across) (Figure 1A). This electrode performed the local electrical stimulation. An electrode was applied to the facial skin as a skin patch (one side was the cathode and the other side was the anode) with a 25-mm distance between commercial electrodes (Figure 1B). The electrode applied to the soft palate was a circular disc cathode with a 1.0-cm diameter and circular disc anode with a 1.0-cm diameter made of stainless steel (Figures 1C and 1D). We categorized as "C" or "D" according to various oral conditions. The electrodes were separated according to their use in patients with natural teeth (Figure 1C) versus complete dentures (Figure 1D). The low electrode impedances were approximately 6.5-7.5 kΩ at 20 Hz as measured by Neuropack-μ, Nihon Koden Co.) and the stimulations were 0.2 msec in duration and 5 Hz in frequency.

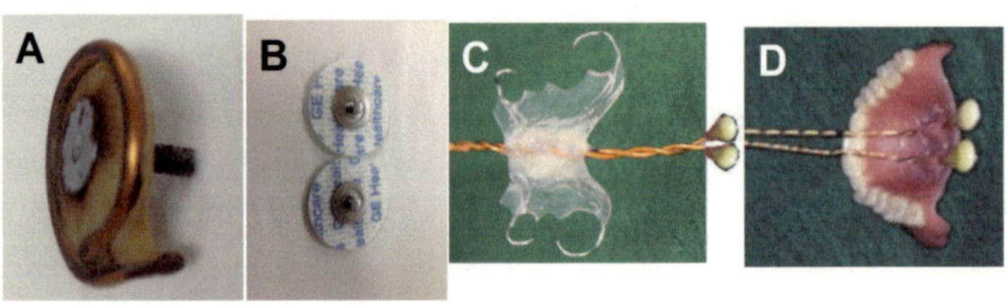

Figure 1. The electrode was used in various regions: (A) tongue dorsum, (B) facial skin, and (C,D) soft palate. (A) The special button-like electrode consists of a central part (cathode, 0.5 mm across) and round wire (anode, 1.0 mm across); this electrode is suitable for local stimulation. (B) Commercial-release electrodes were used for facial skin stimulation. (C, D) The electrodes were separated according to their use in patients with (C) natural teeth versus (D) complete dentures.

Second experiment: The electrodes for electrical stimulation were connected to thin acrylic maxillary splints or full dentures depending on their fit in the paralytic regions of each patient. The stimulus part for electrical stimulation were determined depending on exploration of the hypoesthesia on the soft plate. The electrode comprises a circular disc cathode and anode, both 1.0 cm in diameter, and is made of stainless steel. The electrode mounted at the top of the shielded elastic wire (braided wires) ensured good electrical contact with the moist nature of this part of the mouth. A silicon impression material (GC Co.) was used to cover the surfaces of the stimulating electrodes at low electrode impedances (approximately 6.5-7.5 kΩ at 20 Hz as measured by Neuropack-μ, Nihon Koden Co.). Stöhr and Petruch [12] and Stöhr et al. [13] reported that electrical stimulation in lips or gingival mucosa was appropriate in 0.1-0.2msec (duration) and 1-20 Hz (frequency). On the basis of these data, we decided to stimulate with 0.2msec in duration and 5 Hz in frequency. We employed the first sensation at the increased value with serial access from 0.2 mA. (depending on the mechanical mature).Measurements were performed three times, and the threshold value was averaged. We expected to determine the degree of recovery by the changes in the threshold of electrical sensations. We measured the threshold of electrical sensation in the soft palate with the use of Neuropack-μ every arrival at the hospital. The electrode was jointed with the dental resin on a palatal plate denture or full denture made from each patient, were always stimulated on the same point in every checks. We defined the electrical threshold as the patients were firstly sensed minimum values.

2.3. Modified VF worksheet

Although the VF worksheet proposed in Logemann's study [8] is used by many dentists and otolaryngologists, many medical institutions use a more concise version. We divided the dysphasia scale into the oral phase and pharyngeal phase. In the oral phase, we examined the bolus formation, tongue-to palate contact, premature bolus loss, residue in the oral cavity, and oral transit time. In the pharyngeal phase, we examined the lift in the soft palate, triggering of pharyngeal swallow, epiglottic vallecula, pyriform sinus residue, pharyngeal transit time, and aspiration.

For both the oral and pharyngeal phases, the bolus formation, tongue-to-palate contact, premature bolus loss, residue in the oral cavity, oral transit time, lift in the soft palate, and triggering of the pharyngeal swallow were categorized into three levels: grade 0 as normal, grade 1 as inadequate, and grade 2 as a true abnormality (Table 3). In particular, the amount of premature bolus loss, residue in the oral cavity, and epiglottic vallecula and pyriform sinus residue were divided into three levels: grade 0 indicated no residue, grade 1 indicated residue in <50% of the bolus, and grade 2 indicated residue in >50% of the bolus. Furthermore, aspiration was divided into three levels: grade 0 indicated no aspiration, grade 1 indicated supraglottic penetration and grade 2 indicated subglottic aspiration.

All oral and pharyngeal phase criteria were categorized into three levels, 0, 1 and 2. Based on the assortment of the three levels according to the standardized definition, wthat a more serious condition in the oral or pharyngeal phase would be indicated by a higher total for each criterion, as shown in the totals for the oral and pharyngeal phases in Table 3. We considered that assessments performed using these three simplified levels would provide consistency with respect to the criteria used during long-term evaluation (>2 months after symptom onset). The criterion for each phase (oral and pharyngeal) was employed by the total.

Parameter	Patient No.																							
	1			2			3			4			5			6			7			8		
	1st.	1 M	2 M	1st.	1M	2M	1st.	1M	2M	1st.	1M	2M	1st.	1M	2M	1st.	1M	2M	1st.	1M	2M	1st.	1M	2M
Oral phase																								
Bolus formation	0	0	0	2	2	2	1	1	1	1	1	1	2	1	1	2	2	2	1	1	2	1	1	1
Tongue-to-plate contact	0	0	0	1	1	1	0	0	0	0	0	0	2	1	1	2	2	2	2	2	2	0	0	0
Premature bolus loss	1	1	1	3	3	3	3	3	1	0	0	0	3	1	1	3	3	3	3	3	3	3	3	3
Residue in oral cavity	1	1	1	3	0	0	3	2	1	2	2	2	3	1	1	3	3	3	2	2	2	3	3	3
Oral transit time	1	0	0	1	1	1	1	0	0	0	0	0	1	2	1	1	1	1	1	1	1	1	1	1
Total in the Oral phase	3	2	2	10	7	7	8	6	3	3	3	3	11	6	5	11	11	11	9	9	10	8	8	8
Pharyngeal phase																								
Lift in the soft palate	2	2	2	2	0	0	2	2	1	2	2	2	2	1	1	2	1	1	2	2	2	2	2	2
Triggering of pharyngeal swallow	1	1	0	1	0	0	1	1	1	0	0	0	1	1	0	1	1	0	1	1	1	1	1	1
Vallecular residue	2	1	0	2	2	2	3	1	1	1	1	1	3	1	1	3	3	0	3	3	3	2	2	2
Pyriform sinus residue	2	2	1	3	2	2	3	1	1	1	1	1	3	1	1	3	2	1	1	2	2	0	0	0
Pharyngeal transit time	1	1	0	1	0	0	1	1	1	0	0	0	1	1	0	1	1	0	1	1	1	1	1	1
Aspiration	1	1	0	2	0	0	2	0	0	1	0	0	2	0	0	2	1	0	0	0	1	1	1	1
Total in the Pharyngeal phase	9	8	3	11	4	4	12	6	5	5	4	4	12	5	3	12	9	2	8	9	10	7	7	7
Threshold of sensation in a soft palate (mA)	8.6	5.6	2.2	8.0	2.2	1.6	7.3	3.4	2.9	5.6	2.2	2.1	6.8	5.5	2.1	7.0	6.1	3.1	2.8	3.3	2.8	3.3	3.0	3.2

1 st.: the first medical examination 1 M: the examination after one month 2 M: the examination after two month

Table 3. Measurements of videofluoroscopic dysphagia scale (VF assessments) and threshold of electrical sensation during the patients' hospital visits. Patients 1-6 had brain disease, and patients 7 and 8 had spinal cord disease and a muscular disorder, respectively..

3. Results

First experiment: We evaluated the recovery process of each patient as they performed routine exercises and gave an oral assessment of how they felt at each monthly hospital visit. The relationships between the recovery process and the electrical threshold of sensations are indicated by regression curves for each patient (Figures 1A, tongue dorsum; 1B, facial skin; and 1C, soft palate). The regression curves of the electrical threshold and time course showed ① y=-0.0442X+3.1564, r2=0.58404 (acoustic nerve tumor), ② y=-0.0105X+2.425, r2=0.0363 (diabetes), ③ y=-0.0269X+2.4865, r2=0.6517 (cerebral infarct) and ④ y=-0.0177X+4.2982, r2=0.02184 (neck tumor) on tongue dorsum stimulation, ⑤ y=-0.1669X+6.2984, r2=0.22006 (neck tumor), ⑥ y=-0.1605X+3.0904, r2=0.45346 (neck tumor), ⑦ y=-0.0159X+1.3826, r2=0.43144 (cerebral infarct), ⑧ y=-0.0237X+4.4219, r2=0.08506 (neck tumor), ⑨ y=0.0984X+4.1664, r2=0.5461 (facial nerve palsy) on facial skin stimulation, and ⑩ y=-0.0448X+12.404, r2=0.00864 (cerebral infarct), and ⑪ y=-0.0022X+3.5931, r2=3E-05 (cerebral infarct) on soft palate stimulation. These findings suggested that the electrical threshold stimulation decreased with the time course of the recovery process, because all "gradients" of these data were observed as negative values (Figure 2), although each r2 value (regression estimate of approximate curve) was indicated by divergence or convergence. In particular, although each disease showed a different slope, the recovery trend appeared to be unrelated to the onset of treatment.

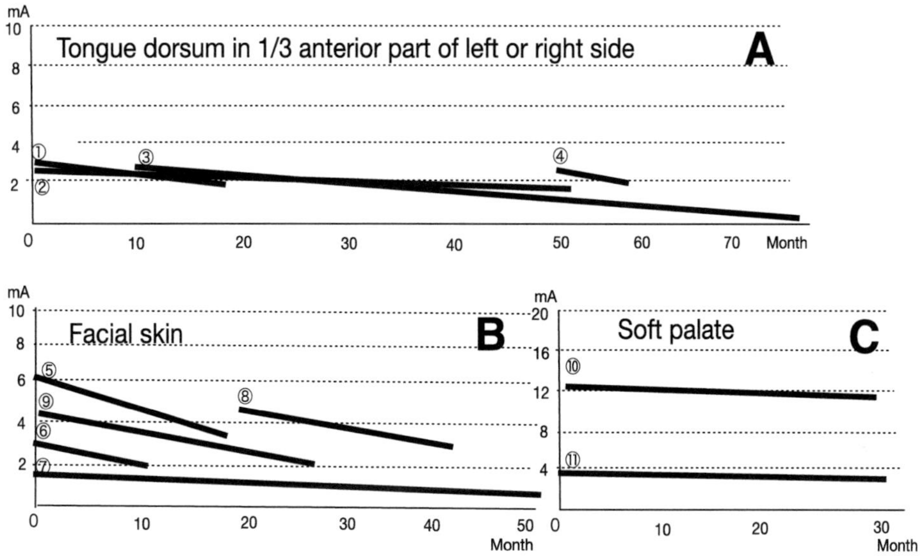

Figure 2. Changes in the recovery process of threshold electrical stimulation. Each start point indicated the start of treatment after onset of the disease.

Second experiment: All patients in the present study had severe swallowing dysfunctions as shown in Table 1. These disorders, which share characteristics in common with dysphasia, were divided into two types depending on the underlying cause. The location of the underlying cause was classified as either the brain (patients 1-6) or spinal cord (patients 7 and 8) (Table 2).

All criteria of the oral and pharyngeal phases were categorized into three levels: 0, 1 and 2 (Table 2). We investigated the relationship between the threshold of sensation and each value in the VF assessment of each patient's disease condition. These values were grouped into classes according to the data shown in Table 3. The total score of the VF assessments in the oral and pharyngeal phases and the threshold of sensation in each patient are shown in Figures 3Aa, 3Ab and 3B; the averages and standard deviations in each figure are indicated in Figures 3C and 3D. Almost all data showed a recovery trend (negative "gradient" of the regression curve) with the exception of amyotrophia lateral sclerosis and myasthenia gravis. Thus, amyotrophic lateral sclerosis and myasthenia gravis did not exert a curative influence on our treatment, because suggesting based on the VF and threshold that sensation did not recover (Figure 3: black lines, amyotrophic lateral sclerosis; red lines, myasthenia gravis). These results may suggest that such muscle diseases do not recovery with the type of training performed in this study. Although the average scores of the VF assessments and threshold electrical stimulation indicated a recovery trend for all diseases, separate analysis for each disease was importance to obtain more detailed data. Based on these findings, we believe that the electrical threshold of sensation on the soft plate may reflect the recovery process of swallowing reflex disorders.

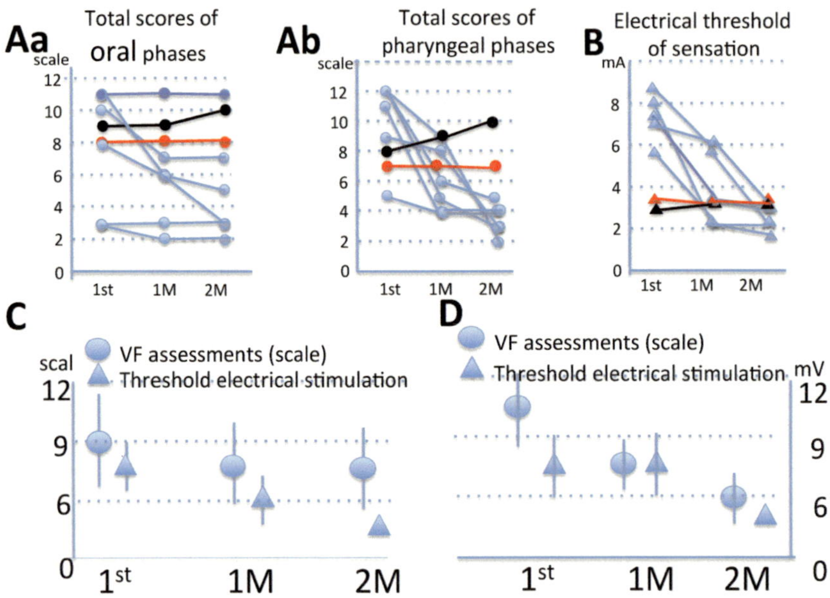

Figure 3. Relationship between total scores of VF assessments in (A) the oral phase and (D) the pharyngeal phase and the threshold of electrical sensation. (Aa) VF assessments in the oral phase. (Ab) VF assessments in the pharyngeal phase. (B) Electrical threshold of sensation. Black lines: amyotrophic lateral sclerosis. Red lines: myasthenia gravis. (C, D) Averages and standard deviations of VF assessments and electrical threshold of sensation.

4. Discussion

4.1. Total of VF assessments in the oral and pharyngeal phases and the threshold of electrical sensation

It was investigated that the relationship between the threshold of sensation and each value in the disease history of each patient. The relationship between the total in the oral phase and the threshold of sensation differed significantly (paired t-test, $P<0.05$). Furthermore, the relationship between the total in the pharyngeal phase and the threshold of sensation were statistically significant at $P<0.01$. The regression curves of each relationship were examined, too. The total scores of the VF assessments in the pharyngeal phase and the threshold of electrical sensation were strongly associated ($r2=0.75$). However, the total score of the VF assessments in the oral phase and the threshold of electrical sensation were not strongly associated (r2=0.13) (Figures 4A and 4B).

Because the total scores in the pharyngeal phase and the threshold of sensation showed a strong correlation, the decrease in electrical sensation might be related to recovery of the pharyngeal phase.

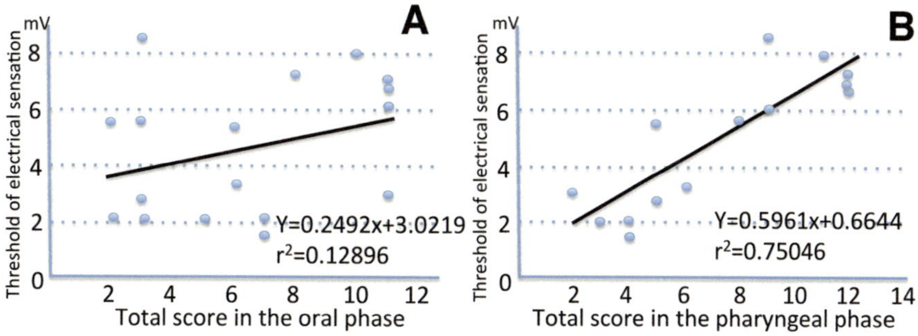

Figure 4. Relationship between (A) total score in the oral phase and threshold of sensation and (B) total score in the pharyngeal phase and threshold of sensation.

4.2. Relationship between VF assessments and electrical stimulations on the soft palate

We considered the presence of a relationship between the recovery process and electrical threshold of sensation, as shown in the first experiment. The results were assumed by a close relationship between the two. Why is there a relationship between a decrease in the threshold of electrical sensation and the recovery process? The well-known phenomenon of "active touch" or "haptic perception" is characterized by object perception through touch. It has been believed that sensory organs function by passive touch. However, Asanuma and Arissian [1] reported the functional role of peripheral input to the motor cortex during voluntary movements in the monkey. Specifically, they proposed that voluntary movements are induced by peripheral sensory inputs. Thus, we believe that measurements of the threshold of electrical sensation are necessary to measure recovery of voluntary movements.

Furthermore, our hypothesis involves the relationship between VF assessment parameters and electrical stimulation in patients with various disorders. VF assessments were divided into the oral and pharyngeal phases because the former is controlled by the first motor cortex of cerebral cortex (M1) and the latter is controlled by the brain stem. In particular, VF assessments of the oral phase are related to voluntary masticatory movements, while VF assessments of the pharyngeal phase are related to the swallowing reflex. We evaluated the relationship between VF assessment parameters and electrical stimulation in patients with various disorders using the swallowing worksheet proposed by Longemann [8], because we utilized measurements in the oral phase (related to masticatory processes) and pharyngeal phase (related to the swallowing reflex). In oral phase, we measured (1) bolus formation, (2) tongue-to-palate contact,

(3) premature bolus loss, (4) residue in oral cavity, and (5) oral transit time. On the other hand, measurements in the pharyngeal phase included (1) lift in the soft palate, (2) triggering of pharyngeal swallow, (3) epiglottic vallecula residue, (4) pyriform sinus residue, (5) pharyngeal transit time, and (6) aspiration. The relationship between total VF assessments in the oral phase and the threshold of electrical sensation showed a weak association with cerebral hemorrhage, cerebral contusion, amyotrophic lateral sclerosis and myasthenia gravis (Figure 4A). However, the relationship between total VF assessments in the pharyngeal phase and the threshold of electrical sensation had a strong association with these disorders (Figure 3B). On the other hand, a decrease in the electrical threshold of sensations following the treatment process was not observed in patients with amyotrophic lateral sclerosis or myasthenia gravis (black and red lines of Figures Aa, Ab and B).

In summary, the criteria for evaluating recovery of the swallowing reflex may be covered by the electrical threshold of sensation on the soft palate, and acceptance of the electrical stimulation will produce a reduction in the bombing experience. Why dose the threshold of electrical sensation reflect recovery of the swallowing reflex? The reflex arc progresses as follows: receptor organ, afferent fiber, central nerve for the reflex, efferent fiber and effector organ. In particular, initiation of the swallowing reflex starts from the regions that induce swallowing (primarily the soft palate, posterior part of tongue, and posterior wall of the pharynx). VF assessments of the pharyngeal phase exhibited the swallowing reflex, and this reflex was initiated by stimulation of the regions that induce swallowing. We consider that the stimulation of these regions involves perception by sensory organs, and the swallowing reflex is then evoked by the sensory stimulation.

4.3. Relationship between electrical sensation and voluntary movement or reflex

When we execute hand movements (especially during search behavior), we take notice of a keen sense in the fingers. Namely, our cutaneous sensation is excited before the execution of movements. This helps us to understand the inaccuracy and inadequacy of movements in patients with sensation disorders. In particular, when the patients with unilateral lingual nerve disease (e.g., secondary to sensory nerve damage during wisdom teeth extraction) are promoted to perform tongue protrusion, the tongue bends toward the diseased side. Furthermore, monkeys with tactile agnosia after blocking of the first somatosensory cortex (SI) exhibit poor performance in gripping an object (Hikosaka et al.) [4]. Nelson [9] reported somatosensory neuronal activity in the SI prior to movement. These results indicate that sensory information in the SI is necessary for the initiation and preparatory of the start of movements. Based on these findings, it is understandable that the somatosensory information obtained prior to movement excites the facial, intraoral, and pharyngeal regions. Sessle et al. [10]. Sessle [11], Stohr and Petruch [12] and Stohr et al. [13] reported that a close relationship between the facial motor and sensory cortices is needed during facial and tongue movements. We assumed the presence of a relationship between electrical sensation and the recovery process based on our findings in the orofacial region. However, two patients in the present study (nos. 7 and 8, Table 2) exhibited no change with electrical stimulation treatment. Both of these patients had muscular atrophy, a degenerative disease. These results may suggest that progressive deterioration of the muscle and spinal cord make reconstruction difficult. On the other hand, although a close relationship between VF assessment of the pharyngeal phase and electrical

http://dx.doi.org/10.5772/60771

stimulation on the soft palate was observed (cumulating tendency), there was a week relationship between VF assessment of the oral phase and electrical stimulation on the soft palate (scattering tendency) (Figures 4A and 4B). VF assessments of the oral phase involved stimulation of various regions of masticatory movements controlled by the M1. Because disorders of these regions become diffuse around the orofacial region, the electrical sensation of the soft palate cannot cover the entire disease region. However, VF assessments of the pharyngeal phase showed that the swallowing reflex was initiated by stimulation of the regions involved in induction of swallowing (primarily the soft palate, root of tongue, and posterior portion of wall of pharynx). We believe that this conclusion can be drawn from our experimental data: measurement of the electrical threshold can be performed as a substitute for VF assessment in the pharyngeal phase, and patients can undergo less radiation. Namely, the swallowing reflex, nasopharyngeal closure, elevation of hyoid bone and pharynx (laryngeal elevation), laryngeal closure (downward movement of the epiglottis), and esophageal sphincter relaxation are accomplished by serial processing after the initiation of sensory stimulation in the induced regions. We arrived at this conclusion from our experimental data.

Measurement of the electrical threshold can be performed as a substitute for VF assessment in the pharyngeal phase, and patients can undergo less radiation as a consequence.

5. Conclusion

Although VF (videofluoroscopic examination of swallowing) is the best choice for the functional assessment of eating (mastication) and swallowing, we cannot avoid a bombing experience. Therefore, we devised at new method to reduce the need for VF examination. The electrical threshold of sensation in centrally diseased sites of the orofacial region has long been examined in patients with stroke, head and neck tumor, external injury and other disorders following on the orofacial treatments. The results suggest a close relationship between the electrical threshold of sensation and the recovery process. Many researchers have evaluated the results of VF assessments based on the Videofluorographic Examination of Swallowing Worksheet developed by Logemann (1993). We selected 11 applicable items used by many hospitals: bolus formation, tongue-to-palate contact, premature bolus loss, residue in oral cavity, and oral transit time in the oral phase; and lift in the soft palate, triggering of pharyngeal swallow, vallecular residue, pyriform sinus residue, pharyngeal transit time, and aspiration in pharyngeal phase. In particular, we considered that a higher sum in each phase might indicate a more serious condition. We also measured the electrical threshold of sensation on the soft palate when patients visited the hospital. Why is the threshold of electrical sensation reflected by recovery of the swallowing reflex?

In particular, VF assessments in the oral phase are related to voluntary masticatory movement, while those in the pharyngeal phase are related to the swallowing reflex. Initiation of swallowing reflex starts from the regions that induce swallowing (primarily the soft palate, posterior part of tongue, and posterior wall of the pharynx). We propose that electrical thresholds in the soft plate can be assessable as the function of swallowing reflex.

Nomenclature

VE: videoendoscopic evaluation of swallowing. VF: videofluoroscopic examination of swallowing. SI: first somatosensory cortex. M1: first motor cortex.

Acknowledgements

This work was supported by Sato research grand and Sogoshigaku research grant of Nihon University School of Dentistry, by Grants-in-Aid for Scientific Research (21592539) and by a grant from the Ministry of Education, Culture, Sports, Science, and Technology to promote multi-disciplinary research projects.

Author details

Koichiro Ueda, Osamu Takahashi, Hisao Hiraba*, Masaru Yamaoka, Enri Nakayama, Kimiko Abe, Mituyasu Sato, Hisako Ishiyama, Akinari Hayashi and Kotomi Sakai

*Address all correspondence to: hiraba.hisao@nihon-u.ac.jp

Department of Dysphasia Rehabilitation, Physics, Nihon University School of Dentistry, Ichikawa Rehabilitation Hospital, Tokyo, Japan

References

[1] Asanuma H, Arissian K: Experiments on functional role of peripheral input to motor cortex during voluntary movements in the monkey. J Neurophysiol. 1984; 52:212–227.

[2] Baredes S, Shah CS, Kaufman R: The frequency of cricopharyngeal dysfunction on videofluoroscopic swallowing studies in patients with dysphagia. Am J Otolaryngol 1997; 18:185-189.

[3] Cook IJ1, Dodds WJ, Dantas RO, Massey B, Kern MK, Lang IM, Brasseur JG, Hogan WJ: Opening mechanism of the human upper esophageal sphincter. Am J Physiol 1989; 257: G748-G759.

[4] Hikosaka O, Tanaka M, Sakamoto M, Iwamura Y: Deficits in manipulation of objects; An analysis of behavioral changes induced by local injections of muscimol in the first somatosensory cortex of the conscious monkey. Brain Res 1985;325: 375-380.

[5] Jones B. The pharynx: disorders of function. Radiol Clin North Am 1994; 32: 1103-1115.

[6] Kahrilas PJ, Lin S, Rademaker AW, Logemann JA: Impaired deglutitive airway protection: a videofluoroscopic analysis of severity and mechanism. Gastroenterology 1997; 113: 1457-1464.

[7] Baijens LW, Speyer R, Roodenburg N, Manni JJ: The effect of neuromuscular electrical stimulation for dysphagia in opercular syndrome: a case study. Eur Arch Otorhinolaryngol 2008; 265: 825-830. DoI: 10.1007/s00405-007-0516-5.

[8] Logemann JA: Manual for the videofluorographic study of swallowing, 2nd edn. Austin: TX: Pro-Ed; 1993, p. 1-170.

[9] Nelson RJ: Set related and premovement related activity of promate primary somatosensory cortical neurons depends upon stimulus modality and subsequent movements. Brain Res Bull. 1988:21;411-424.

[10] Sessle BJ, Yao D, Nishiura H, Yoshino K, Lee J-C, Martin RE, Murray GM: Properties and plasticity of the primate somatosensory and motor cortex related to orofacial sensorimotor function. Clin Exp Pharmacol Physiol. 2005;32:109-114.

[11] Sessle BJ: Mechanisms of oral somatosensory and motor functions and their clinical correlates. J Oral Rehail. 2006;33: 243-264.

[12] Stöhr M, Petruch F: Somatosensory evoked potential following stiulation of the trigeminal nerve in man. J Neurol. 1979;220: 95-98.

[13] Stöhr M, Petruch F, Scheglmann K: Somatosensory evoked potentials following trigeminal nerve stimulation in trigeminal neuralgia. Ann Neurol. 1981;9: 63-66.

[14] Tachimura T: Nohara K, Wada T: Effect of Placement of a speech Appliance on Levotor veli palatini muscle activity during speech. Cleft Palate-Craniofacial J. 2000;37: 478-482.

Section 3

Management of Dysphagia

Chapter 7

Nutritional Support in Dysphagia

Vishal G. Shelat and Garvi J. Pandya

Additional information is available at the end of the chapter

http://dx.doi.org/10.5772/61243

1. Introduction

Dysphagia is defined as difficulty in swallowing. It is commonly caused due to neuromuscular (stroke, dementia, Parkinson's disease, myasthenia gravis, etc.), mechanical (oral cancer, oesophageal cancer, etc.), or other causes (radiotherapy treatment, gastroesophageal reflux disease, thrush, etc.). It risks aspiration and associated bronchopulmonary infections, fluid depletion, and under nutrition. It can alter nutritional equilibrium and can affect organ function and ultimately clinical outcome. To improve clinical outcomes, it is important to screen all at risk patients in order to identify patients at nutritional risk due to dysphagia [1–4]. Most dysphagia resolves within few weeks, but in some cases it may persist. This may affect the nutritional state of the individual who is already facing an illness or injury in first instance [5, 6]. Dysphagia and accompanying malnutrition is associated with excess morbidity and increased mortality rates [7, 8]. This chapter will focus on general principles of nutritional management in any patient including patients with dysphagia.

2. Nutritional screening and assessment

Up to 30% of all acute hospital admissions are malnourished and this is further deepened during hospitalisation [9]. Hence, all the patients should be screened for risk of malnutrition.

There are various scoring systems available to screen a patient at nutritional risk. Screening is based on history (weight loss, etc.) and physical examination (height, weight, and body mass index (BMI)).'Malnutrition universal screening tool' ('MUST') [Figure 1], rapid nutrition screen for hospitalised patients, nutrition risk index (NRI), Mini Nutritional Assessment-Short Form (MNA-SF), Short Nutritional Assessment Questionnaire (SNAQ©) (Table 1) and Nutrition Risk Screening (NRS-2002) are some of the commonly available and used composite tools in clinical practice [10–15]. An ideal screening tool should be easy to implement, accurate, reliable, inexpensive, and reproducible. NRS-2002 is the best instrument today because it is robust, simple, quick, validated, and based from an analysis of 128 controlled clinical trials. Patients with the risk criteria had a higher likelihood of a better clinical outcome from nutritional support than patients who did not fulfill the criteria [15]. NRS 2002 has also been used by nurses and dietitians in three hospitals of Denmark. Its reliability was validated by inter-observer variation between a nurse, a dietitian, and a physician with a k = 0.67. Its practicability was shown by the finding that 99% of 750 newly admitted patients could be screened [16]. Supplement 1 shows the 'TTSH Nutrition Screening Tool' (TTSH NST) used by the Nutrition and Dietetics department at Tan Tock Seng Hospital, Singapore. TTSH NST was developed from a cohort of younger hospitalised patients. This was later validated in a cohort of elderly patients using subjective global assessment (SGA) as a comparator. In 281 acute admissions to Tan Tock Seng Hospital with age range of 61–102 years, prevalence of malnutrition was 35% based on SGA. Risk of malnutrition as determined by TTSH NST with a cut-off of 4 had sensitivity, specificity, positive, and negative predictive values of 84%, 79%, 68%, and 90%, respectively, with area under the curve of 0.87. The optimal cut-off remained at 4 even for patients aged >85 years (AUC = 0.85). Risk of malnutrition was predictive of 6-month mortality (adjusted OR: 2.2, $P = 0.05$) and hospital length of stay ($P < 0.05$) [17].

Question	Score
Did you lose weight intentionally?	
• 6 Kg in past 6 months	3
• 3 Kg in the past month	2
Did you experience a decreased appetite over the past month?	1
Did you use supplemental drinks or tube feeding over the past month?	1

[a] Patients who scored 0 or 1 points were classified as well-nourished and did not receive intervention. Patients who scored 2 points were classified as moderately malnourished and received nutritional intervention. Patients who scored 3 points were classified as severely malnourished and received nutritional intervention and treatment by a dietician.

Reproduced from: *Am J Clin Nutr* 2005;82:1082-9. © 2005 American Society for Nutrition

Table 1. Short Nutritional Assessment Questionnaire [a]

Nutritional assessment is a more detailed process and is done in patients screened at risk or when metabolic or functional problems prevent a standard plan being carried out. There are few tools for evaluating the nutritional status of hospitalised patients. SGA, short nutritional assessment questionnaire, mini nutritional assessment (MNA), and corrected arm muscle area (CAMA) are tools used for nutritional assessment [18]. The assessment of nutritional status includes a nutritional history and physical examination in conjunction with appropriate laboratory studies [Figure 2]. Regurgitation, hoarse voice, coughing during or after swallowing, globus sensation, nasal regurgitation, recurrent chest infections, and frequent throat clearing symptoms may indicate dysphagia [19]. In all patients with dysphagia, a complete

http://dx.doi.org/10.5772/61243

evaluation of the cause of dysphagia must be performed and for the purpose of this chapter we will only discuss nutrition-related assessment.

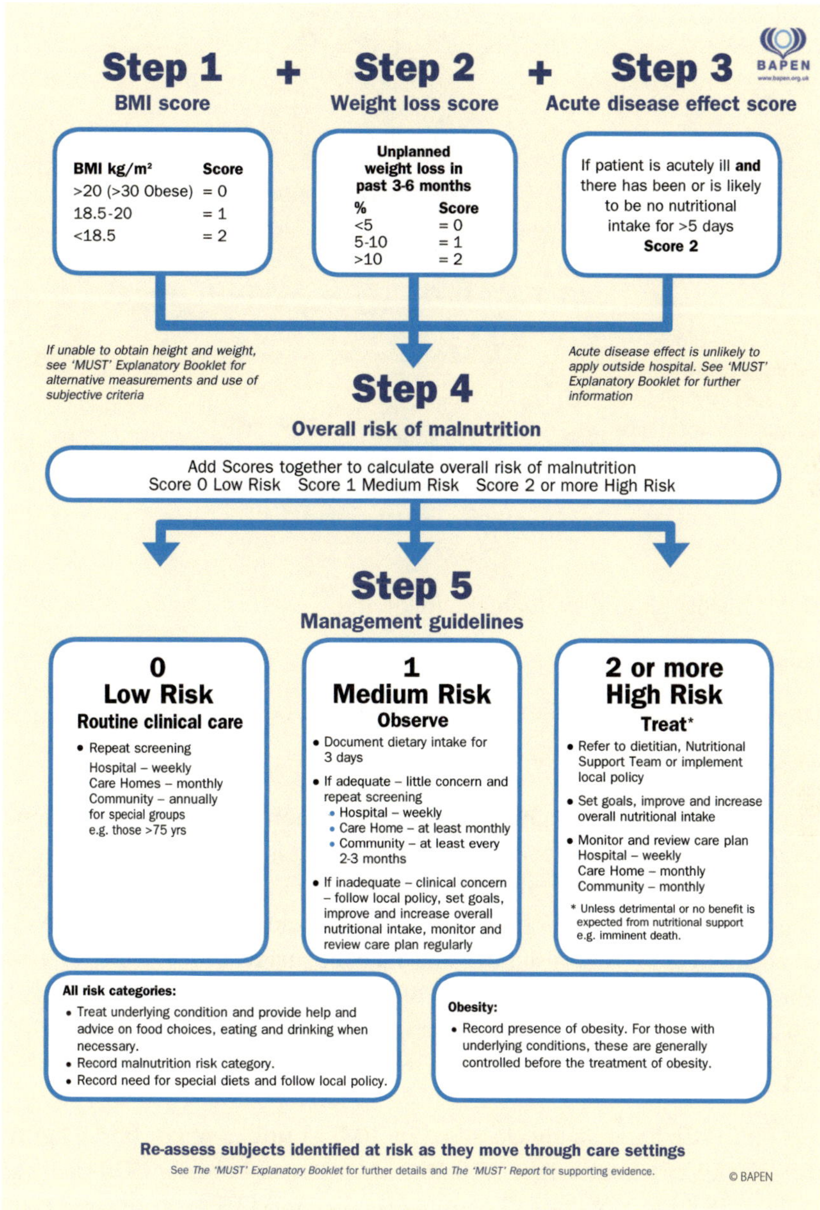

The 'Malnutrition Universal Screening Tool' ('MUST') is reproduced here with the kind permission of BAPEN (British Association for Parenteral and Enteral Nutrition). For further information on 'MUST' see www.bapen.org.uk Copyright © BAPEN 2012

Figure 1. 'MUST' flowchart

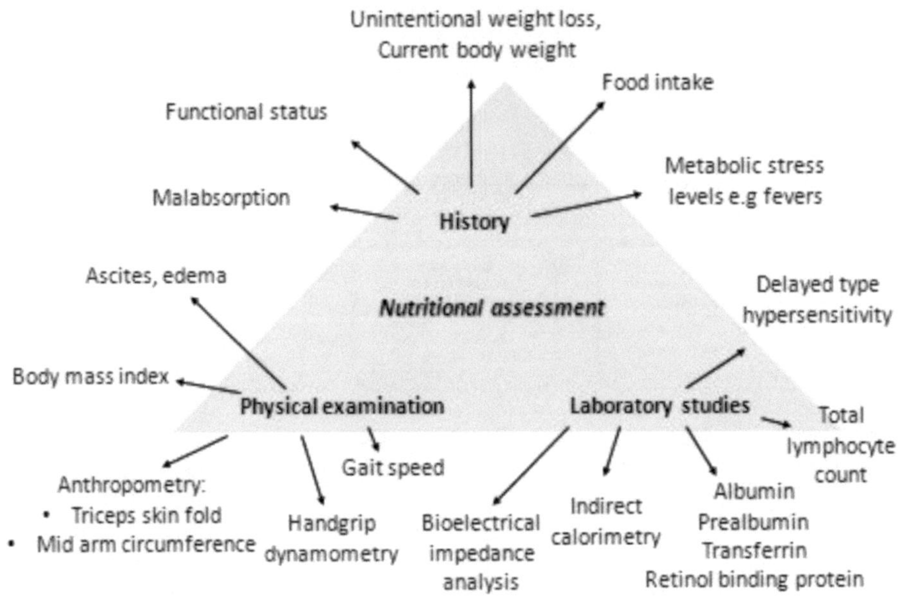

Figure 2. Nutritional assessment

The nutritional history should evaluate the following:

1. *Food intake*

A change in the dietary pattern due to dysphagia should be ascertained.

2. *Body weight*

The presence of unintentional weight loss over past six months should be ascertained. 10% or greater unintentional weight loss over the past six months is categorised as severe weight loss and is associated with a poor clinical outcome. In a study involving 3,047 patients enrolled in 12 chemotherapy protocols of Eastern Cooperative Oncology Group, Dewys WD, et al. has shown that chemotherapy response rates and median survival rates were lower in patients with weight loss [20]. The *functional status* of the patients (e.g., bedridden) and *metabolic stress* due to accompanied illness or injury also need to be ascertained.

3. *Physical examination*

Body mass index (BMI): Patients are classified by BMI as underweight (<18.5 kg/m^2), normal weight (18.5–24.9 kg/m^2), overweight (25.0–29.9 kg/m^2), class I obesity (30.0–34.9 kg/m^2), class II obesity (35.0–39.9 kg/m^2), or class III obesity (≥40.0 kg/m^2) [21].

Hand grip strength, gait speed, triceps skin fold thickness, mid-arm circumference, mucosal xerosis, and *edema* are some of the physical signs which could help establish malnutrition in patients with dysphagia. Handgrip strength reflects, in part, the association of muscle strength and lean body mass with malnutrition [22]. In a study conducted by the International Academy on

Nutrition and Aging (IANA) Task Force, gait speed at usual pace is found to be a consistent risk factor for disability, cognitive impairment, falls, institutionalisation, and/or mortality and at least as sensitive as composite tools [23].

4. *Laboratory studies*

Measurements of serum albumin, prealbumin, retinol-binding protein, transferrin, createnine height index, createnine extretion in urine and total lymphocyte count have been shown to correlate with clinical outcome. In a study involving 17 critically ill patients, Apelgren KN et al. have shown that a serum albumin <2.5 g/dL concentration is associated with an increased incidence of medical complications and death and it correctly separated 93% of patients in terms of survival prognosis [24]. Serum albumin levels are often used as a surrogate for preoperative nutritional assessment, but it is confounded by coexisting inflammation [25, 26]. Injury and inflammation decreases synthesis, increases degradation and transmembrane losses from the plasma compartment. In addition, albumin is also lost from open wounds (burns, etc.), peritonitis and through the gastrointestinal tract and/or kidneys in certain diseases. The association between hypoalbuminemia and poor clinical outcome is independent of both nutritional and inflammatory status [27]. Serum albumin is a good predictor of clinical outcomes but is a poor marker for nutritional assessment.

3. Nutritional pharmacology

If a patient is identified as at risk of malnutrition, appropriate intervention should be done to improve outcomes. Nutritional pharmacology is an emerging science over the last two decades. Nutrients such as arginine, glutamine, and long chain fatty acids (both omega 3 and omega 6) have been shown to improve clinical outcomes in diverse group of patients [28]. Arginine exhibits diverse effects including wound healing, protects against ischemia-reperfusion, improves macrophage function after injury, blocks adhesion molecules, inhibits lipid peroxidation, and improves cerebral and myocardial perfusion [28]. In a double blind randomised controlled trial involving 32 malnourished patients with head and neck cancer, Buijs N et al. concluded that perioperative arginine-enriched enteral nutrition improved long term overall survival and long term disease specific survival [29]. Glutamine is the most abundant amino acid and is a fuel of neutrophils, lymphocytes, and enterocytes. Glutamine is a conditionally essential amino acid in situations of stress. A recent Cochrane review including 4,671 patients with critical illness or elective major surgery concluded that glutamine supplementation reduced the infection rate and days on mechanical ventilation in critically ill or surgical patients [30]. Long chain fatty acids are important in function of cell membranes and act as intracellular messengers.

4. Enteral nutrition

Enteral route is physiologic and *'A functioning gastrointestinal system should be used to prevent its malfunction'*. Oral nutritional is ideal. Patients with dysphagia are at risk of aspiration pneumonia. Authors recommend a swallowing history and assessment prior to oral feeding. Until safety of oral feeding is established, tube feeding should be considered. Figure 3 outlines a simplistic approach in decision making for nutritional supplementation.

4.1. Formula feeds

There are various feeding formulas and selection should be based on fluid electrolyte and metabolic needs, digestion and absorption capacity, caloric and protein density of formula, physical characteristics of formula (osmolality, viscosity etc.), and cost. General purpose feeding formulas contain intact proteins and need an intact digestive and absorptive function of gastrointestinal system. Semi-elemental feeds contain free amino acids with minimal fat and are used in patients with compromised gastrointestinal function. There are also various disease-specific feeds available for patients with hepatic, renal, or pulmonary dysfunction. In addition, nutrient composition of the formulas can be altered to tailor individual patients need and such modular feeds require mixing by local pharmacy and are costly [31]. Once the feeding formula is decided and the nutritional requirement calculated, the rate and delivery of the feeding is established.

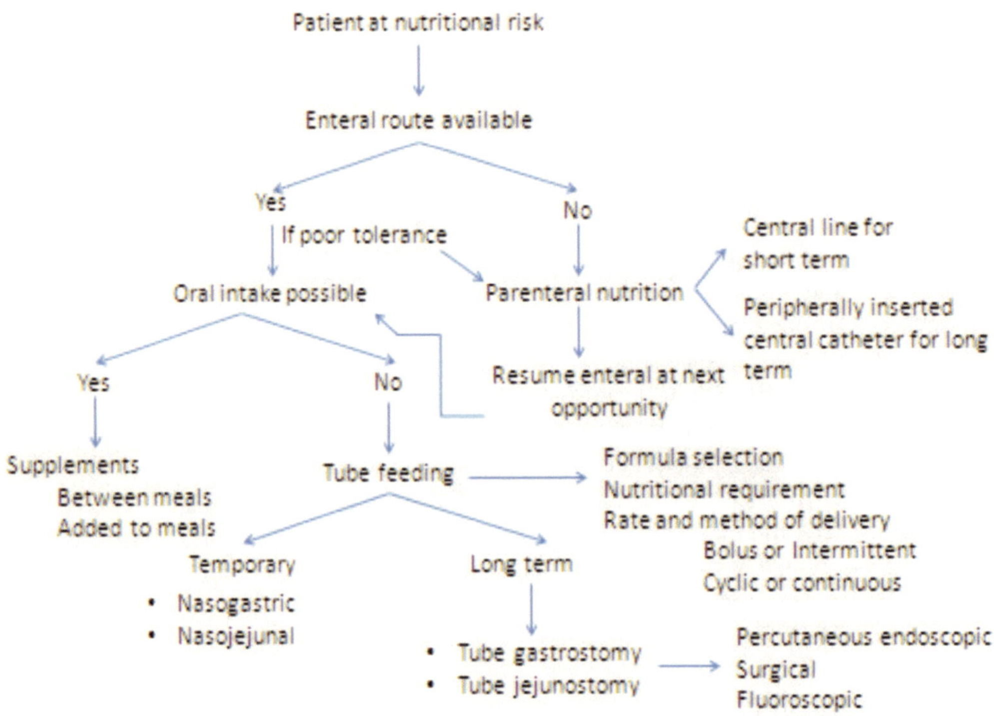

Figure 3. Algorithm of nutritional supplementation

4.2. Feed delivery

Intermittent bolus feeding is convenient to administer by nasogastric or percutaneous gastric tube and is suitable in ambulatory patients. Although there are no definitive studies, bolus feeding reduces lower esophageal sphincter pressure and may increase the chance for reflux and aspiration [32]. Intermittent cyclic feeding is indicated during weaning from tube feeding to oral feeding. It can be pump-assisted or gravity-assisted and feeding cycles of varying duration of period can be planned. This feeding is advantageous when an overnight tube feed is administered and the patient continues his normal oral intake during the day. Constant feeding infusion assisted by pump or gravity is indicated in bedridden patients with critical illness. Nasal tubes are associated with discomfort, excoriation and bleeding, and anosmia. Hence, when long-term feeding is required, percutaneous gastrostomy or jejunostomy tubes should be used. In a United Kingdom study involving 1,327 patients including 1,027 patients with gastrostomy tube insertion, Kurien M et al. has demonstrated that patients who undergo gastrostomy have significantly lower mortality than those who defer the procedure (11.2% vs. 35.5% at 30 days and 41.1% vs.74.3% at 1 year, $p<0.0001$) [33]. The most common indication of feeding gastrostomy remains inadequate swallowing as a result of a neurological event, oropharyngeal or esophageal cancer, or facial trauma [34]. Traditionally, tube feeding is delayed until the next day after the procedure. Authors' personal preference is to institute the feeding at the next opportunity. In a meta-analysis of six randomised controlled trials involving 467 patients, Bechtold ML et al. has shown that early feeding (defined as within 4 hrs) after percutaneous endoscopic gastrostomy placement was safe [35]. In patients with restricted mouth opening, oral cavity is inaccessible and a surgical gastrostomy needs to be created. Feeding gastrostomy is associated with the risk of aspiration and is not possible in patients with gastric outlet obstruction, gastroparesis, or gastric resection. In such patients, feeding jejunostomy is an alternative. Percutaneous feeding jejunostomy can also be inserted via the existing gastrostomy site. Percutaneous placement of feeding jejunostomy is technically difficult compared to gastrostomy. In a study involving 150 patients without a previous history of major abdominal surgery, Shike M et al. found that direct percutaneous endoscopic jejunostomy was successful in 129 procedures (86%) and aspiration occurred in 3% of patients [36]. Enteral nutrition preserves the gut integrity, reduces bacterial translocation, maintains the gut immune function, is easily administered and monitored, and cheaper compared to parenteral nutrition. However, it can also lead to complications.

4.3. Enteral nutrition: Common issues

Enteral nutrition causes mechanical problems with tube placement (migration, clogging etc.), metabolic problems (osmotic diarrhoea, overhydration, etc.), and is labour intensive (tube management, infusion pump device usage, etc.). In patients with tube feeding, prior to commencing feeding, a radiological confirmation of tube placement must be checked. Tube clogging could be prevented by using a wide tube, flushing the tube with water after medicine administration, minimising gastric aspirates to keep pH levels low, and using pancreatic enzymes mixed with bicarbonate [37]. Peristomal wound infections and leakage are also common problems associated with tube feeding and add to patient and family anxiety along with the nursing care burden [38]. In a Cochrane review with a pooled analysis of 1,271 patients from 12 randomised controlled trials, Lipp A et al. have shown that administration of prophylactic systemic antibiotics for percutaneous endoscopic gastrostomy tube placement reduces peristomal infection rates (OR 0.36, 95% CI: 0.26–0.50) [39]. Peristomal leakage can be reduced by appropriate fixation technique and antisecretory agents. In patients with persistent leakage, the tube should be withdrawn and replaced after few days or a new tube placed at the separate site, but no attempt should be made to control the leakage with a wider tube as it may exacerbate the leakage [40–42]. Diarrhoea remains the commonest gastrointestinal side effect of enteral tube feeding [43, 44]. Addition of fibre and probiotics has shown to reduce diarrhoea in enteral feeding. In a systematic review and meta-analysis including 51 studies, 43 randomised control trials and 1,762 subjects (1,591 patients and 171 healthy volunteers), Elia M et al. have shown that fibre supplementation was generally well tolerated and the incidence of diarrhoea reduced (OR 0.68, 95% CI: 0.48–0.96; 13 randomised control trials) [45]. In a randomised double blind placebo controlled trial involving 62 patients, Heimburger DC et al. have shown that most cases of diarrhoea in tube fed patients are caused by factors extraneous to tube feeding and lactobacillus treatment did not alter the risk of diarrhoea [46]. Patients on enteral feeding are also at risk of aspiration pneumonia. There are various strategies recommended to reduce the risk of aspiration namely head end of bed elevation, gastric residual volume measurement and postpyloric feeding. In a prospective randomized study involving 38 patients in medical and surgical intensive care units, endoscopically placed feeding jejunal tube-fed patients had a lower rate of pneumonia (nil vs. 10.5%) compared to patients fed by continuous gastric tube feeding [47]. In a literature review of 45 studies including patients with neurogenic oropharyngeal dysphagia over a period of 1978 to 1989, authors were not able to derive any meaningful conclusions with regard to superiority of postpyloric feeding due to limitations of individual studies with small sample size, inconsistent definitions of aspiration, varying feeding protocols, unspecified time frames, and heterogeneous populations [48]. Monitoring enteral nutrition involves fluid electrolyte balance, weight chart, serum electrolyte and glucose measurement, and stool charting. Refeeding syndrome is characterised by electrolyte depletion, fluid shifts, and glucose derangements that occur on reinstitution of nutrition in malnourished patients [49]. Chronically malnourished patients (e.g., patients with dysphagia) are at high risk of refeeding syndrome. In a study involving 321 patients with 92 patients at risk of refeeding hypophosphataemia, Zeki S et al. has shown that refeeding hypophosphataemia is more common in enteral-fed patients compared to parenteral nutrition [50]. Gradual introduction and progression of feeding over a few days with close monitoring of fluid and electrolytes can help in the prevention and early recognition of refeeding syndrome.

National Institute of Clinical Excellence (NICE) guidelines recommend that in an acute setting, if patients are unable to swallow safely or meet caloric needs orally, they should have an initial 2–4 week trial of nasogastric enteral tube feeding. Health care professionals with relevant skills and training in the diagnosis, assessment, and management of swallowing disorders should assess the prognosis and options for future nutrition support [19]. Before modifying nutritional support in a patient with dysphagia, level of alertness, need for feeding assistance, mobility, recurrent chest infections, metabolic needs, etc. should be considered [19].

http://dx.doi.org/10.5772/61243

5. Parenteral nutrition

In patients with short bowel or gastrointestinal intolerance, total parenteral nutrition is required. In general, parenteral nutrition should be considered if energy intake has been, or is anticipated to be, inadequate (<50% of daily requirements) for more than 7 days and enteral feeding is not feasible. Total parenteral nutrition requires labour-intensive monitoring for infection and haemodynamic stability. Metabolic complications, such as fluid overload, hypertriglyceridemia, hypercalcemia, hypoglycaemia, hyperglycaemia, and specific nutrient deficiencies, are usually caused by overzealous or inadequate nutrient administration. Catheter-related blood-borne infection is the most common life-threatening complication in patients who receive total parenteral nutrition and is commonly caused by *Staphylococcus epidermidis* or *Staphylococcus aureus* [51]. In a study involving 331 central venous catheters used for home parenteral nutrition with a median duration of 730 days, Buchman AL et al. have demonstrated increased rates of catheter-related blood-borne infections in patients receiving lipid emulsions, obtaining blood from catheter and administering medications via the catheter [52]. The incidence of most complications associated with the use of total parenteral nutrition is reduced with careful management and supervision, preferably by an experienced nutrition support team if available [53].

6. Nutrition support team

An interdisciplinary nutrition support team could include physicians, dieticians, pharmacists, and nurse clinicians. In a study involving 209 parenteral nutrition starts, Trujillo EB et al. have showed that non-indicated and preventable parenteral nutrition initiation, short-term (defined as less than 6 days) parenteral nutrition use and metabolic complications are less likely (34% vs. 66%, $p = 0.04$) when patients receive consultation by a multidisciplinary metabolic support service [54]. Nutritional support teams closely work with speech and swallowing assessment teams locally at Tan Tock Seng Hospital. In patients with non-obstructive dysphagia, video-fluoroscopy swallowing study is conducted prior to determining the route of feeding. It is possible that patients may be permitted oral feeds and in addition enteral tube feeding to ensure their caloric requirements are met.

7. Conclusion

Dysphagia patients are at risk of malnutrition. Malnutrition worsens during hospitalisation. Nutritional screening and assessment are paramount to improve outcomes. There are various tools to assist in nutritional screening and assessment and it is advisable to use the locally validated tool in clinical practise. Patients with dysphagia have special needs and this need to be considered during initiation and modification of nutrition therapy. Enteral nutrition is recommended wherever feasible. Nutrition support teams and swallowing therapy experts should be involved in all patients with dysphagia who require nutrition therapy.

Supplement

Tan Tock Seng HOSPITAL

Ward	Bed	Unit
Patient Details		

TTSH-Nutrition Screening Tool

Indicators *Refer to instructions overleaf*	**Scoring**	
Diagnosis nutritional risk level	Low	0
	Moderate	1
	High	2
Physical appearance	Normal	0
	Moderately underweight	1
	Severely underweight	2
Diet intake adequacy over past 5 days or more	Normal	0
	Reduced moderately	1
	Reduced severely	2
	Not available	--
Unintentional weight loss over past 6 months	No	0
	Unsure	1
	Yes, 0.5 – 3.0kg	2
	Yes, >3.0-7.0kg	3
	Yes, >7.0kg	4
	Yes, Unsure	2
Total Score*		

***IF SCORE IS 4 OR MORE, REFER TO THE DIETITIAN.**

Name /Sign ____________________

Date ____________________

Dietitian contacted ____________________

http://dx.doi.org/10.5772/61243

Tan Tock Seng
HOSPITAL

Instructions:. Score the patients for each criterion by referring to the tables below

<table>
<tr><td rowspan="2">Diagnosis
Nutritional
Risk Level</td><td colspan="2">High risk = 2</td><td colspan="2">Moderate risk = 1</td><td colspan="2">Low risk = 0</td></tr>
<tr><td colspan="2">AIDS
Burns, major
Cancer GI Tract/ Head & Neck
COPD- unstable
Dysphagia
Gastro- intestinal (GI) disease malabsorption/ maldigestion /Ileus GI obstruction /stricture/fistula
Hepatic Coma/encephalopathy
Infection -Prolonged/severe
Neurological severe deficits/coma
Skin Ulcers-pressure ulcers - stages III-IV
Pulmonary disease: Failure requiring ventilation
Radiation Therapy GI Tract
Renal Disease -ARF
Sepsis
SLE flare
Spinal Cord Injury- new
Surgery-GI major
Trauma-Head/Multi
Wounds, non healing</td><td colspan="2">Alzheimer' s disease /dementia
Cardiomyopathy
Chemotherapy
Congestive Heart Failure
Diabetes (Newly Diagnosed)
Diabetes (Uncontrolled)
Fractures, major
GI diseases all others
Infection with fever
Liver diseases-other
Nutritional anaemia
Pneumonia
Skin ulcers-diabetic, pressure ulcers - stage II
Psychological -Eating Disorders
Pulmonary Disease O2 dependant
Radiation Therapy H & N
Renal Disease- CRF
SLE stable
Substance abuse
Tuberculosis</td><td colspan="2">Angina
Cancer All others
Cardiac disease
COPD stable
DM (controlled)
Fractures, others
HIV +
Hypertension
Neurological no deficits
Peripheral vascular disease
Psychological-Others
Radiation Therapy: all others
Surgeries all not mentioned</td></tr>
<tr><td rowspan="2">Physical
Appearance</td><td colspan="2">Severely underweight = 2</td><td colspan="2">Moderately underweight =1</td><td colspan="2">Normal = 0</td></tr>
<tr><td colspan="2">• Severe loss of fat from triceps (minimal space between fingers)
• Hollowing, depression of temples, facial muscle wasting
• Protruding, prominent bones</td><td colspan="2">• Mild or moderate loss of fat from triceps and deltoid region
• Slight depression of temples, moderate facial muscle wasting
• Bones may show slightly</td><td colspan="2">At least normal muscle bulk and fat stores:
• Large space between fingers
• Rounded shoulders</td></tr>
<tr><td rowspan="2">Diet intake adequacy over past 5 days</td><td colspan="2">Reduced severely = 2</td><td colspan="2">Reduced moderately = 1</td><td colspan="2">Normal = 0</td></tr>
<tr><td colspan="2">• Takes less than ½ normal intake or has been NBM
• Does not take a diet supplement
• Less than 750 to 1000ml of a 1-calorie/ml formula per day via feeding tube or orally</td><td colspan="2">• Takes ½ -3/4 normal intake
• Occasionally takes a diet supplement
• 1000-1200ml of a 1-calorie /ml formula per day via feeding tube or orally</td><td colspan="2">• No change
• Takes formulas to supplement diet
• 1200-2000 ml of a 1-calorie/ml formula per day via feeding tube or orally</td></tr>
<tr><td rowspan="2">Unintentional weight loss</td><td>2</td><td>4</td><td>3</td><td>2</td><td>1</td><td>0</td></tr>
<tr><td>Yes, Unsure</td><td>Yes
> 7 kg</td><td>Yes
> 3- 7 kg</td><td>Yes
0.5 - 3kg</td><td>Unsure</td><td>No</td></tr>
</table>

Acknowledgements

We are grateful to the Department of Nutrition and Dietetics, Tan Tock Seng Hospital, Singapore, for permission to publish Tan Tock Seng Hospital Nutrition Screening Tool (TTSH NST).

Author details

Vishal G. Shelat[1*] and Garvi J. Pandya[2]

*Address all correspondence to: vgshelat@gmail.com

1 Tan Tock Seng Hospital, Singapore

2 Ministry of Health Holdings Pte Ltd, Singapore

References

[1] Martino R, Pron G, Diamant N. Screening for oropharyngeal dysphagia in stroke: Insufficient evidence for guidelines. Dysphagia 2000;15(1):19-30.

[2] Brown T, Findlay M, Von Dincklage J, Davidson W, Hill J, Isenring E, Talwar B,Bell K, Kiss N, Kurmis R, Loeliger J, Sandison A, Taylor K, Bauer J. Using a wiki platform to promote guidelines internationally and maintain their currency: Evidence-based guidelines for the nutritional management of adult patients with head and neck cancer. J Hum Nutr Diet 2013;26(2):182-190.

[3] Garg S, Yoo J, Winquist E. Nutritional support for head and neck cancer patients receiving radiotherapy: A systematic review. Support Care Cancer 2010;18(6):667-677.

[4] Beaver ME, Matheny KE, Roberts DB, Myers JN. Predictors of weight loss during radiation therapy. Otolaryngol Head Neck Surg 2001;125(6):645–648.

[5] Barer DH. The natural history and functional consequences of dysphagia after hemispheric stroke. J Neurol Neurosurg Psychiatry 1989;52(2):236-41.

[6] Teasell RW, Bach D, McRae M. Prevalence and recovery of aspiration post stroke: A retrospective analysis. Dysphagia 1994;9(1):35-9.

[7] Sala R, Munto MJ, de la Calle J, Preciado I, Miralles T, Cortes A, et al. Swallowing changes in cerebrovascular accidents: Incidence, natural history, and repercussions on the nutritional status, morbidity, and mortality. Rev Neurol 1998;27(159):759-66.

[8] Correia MI, Waitzberg DL. The impact of malnutrition on morbidity. Mortality, length of hospital stay and costs evaluated through a multivariate model analysis. Clin Nutr 2003;22(3): 235–239.

[9] Nutrition screening surveys in hospitals in the UK, 2007-2011. A report based on the amalgamated data from the four Nutrition Screening Week Surveys undertaken by BAPEN in 2007,2008, 2010 and 2011. Accessed http://www.bapen.org.uk/pdfs/nsw/bapen-nsw-uk.pdf on April 21, 2014.

[10] http://www.bapen.org.uk/must_tool.html. Accessed October 25, 2014.

[11] Kruizenga HM, van Tulder MW, Seidell JC, Thijs A, Ader HJ, van Bokhorst-de van der Schueren MA. Effectiveness and cost-effectivensss of early screening and treatment of malnourished patients. Am J Clin Nutr. 2005;82:1082-1089.

[12] Ferguson M, Capra S, Bauer J, Banks M. Development of a valid and reliable malnutrition screening tool for adult acute hospital patients. Nutrition 1999;15:458-64.

[13] Wolinsky FD, Coe RM, McIntosh WMA, et al. Progress in the development of a Nutritional Risk Index. J Nutr 1990;120:1549-1553.

[14] Reilly HM, Martineau JK, Moran A, Kennedy H. Nutritional screening—evaluation and implementation of a simple Nutrition Risk Score. Clinical Nutrition 1995;14:269-273.

[15] Kondrup J, Rasmussen HH, Hamberg O, et al. Nutritional Risk Screening (NRS 2002): A new method based on an analysis of controlled clinical trials. Clin Nutr 2003;22:321-336.

[16] Kondrup J, Johansen N, Plum LM, et al. Incidence of nutritional risk and causes of inadequate nutritional care in hospitals. Clin Nutr 2002;21:461-468.

[17] Lim YP, Lim WS, Tan TL, Daniels L. Evaluating the validity of a nutritional screening tool in hospitalized older adults. Ann Acad of Med Singapore. 2008;37(Suppl 11):S5.

[18] Detsky AS, McLaughlin JR, Baker JP, et al. What is subjective global assessment of nutritional status? J Parenter Enteral Nutr 1987;1(1):8-13.

[19] http://www.nice.org.uk/guidance/cg032/chapter/1-guidance#enteral-tube-feeding-in-hospital-and-the-community. Accessed October 25, 2014.

[20] Dewys WD, Begg C, Lavin PT, et al. Prognostic effect of weight loss prior to chemotherapy in cancer patients. Eastern Cooperative Oncology Group. Am J Med 1980;69(4):491-7.

[21] National Institutes of Health, National Heart, Lung, and Blood Institute. Clinical guidelines on the identification, evaluation, and treatment of overweight and obesity in adults—the evidence report. National Institutes of Health, National Heart, Lung, and Blood Institute. Obes Res. 1998;6(Suppl 2):S53-S54.

[22] Wang AY, Sea MM, Ho ZS, et al. Evaluation of handgrip strength as a nutritional marker and prognostic indicator in peritoneal dialysis patients. Am J Clin Nutr 2005;81(1):79-86.

[23] van Kan AG, Rolland Y, Andrieu S, et al. Gait speed at usual pace as a predictor of adverse outcomes in community-dwelling older people—an International Academy on Nutrition and Aging (IANA) Task Force. J Nutr Health Aging 2009;13(10):881-9.

[24] Apelgren KH, Rombeau JL, Twomey PL, Miller RA. Comparison of nutritional indices and outcome in critically ill patients. Crit Care Med 1982;10(5):305-7.

[25] Klein S. The myth of serum albumin as a measure of nutritional status. Gastroenterology 1990;99(6):1845–6.

[26] Don BR, Kaysen G. Serum albumin: Relationship to inflammation and nutrition. Semin Dial. 2004 Nov-Dec;17(6):432-7.

[27] Vincent JL, Dubois MJ, Navickis RJ, Wilkes MM. Hypoalbuminemia in acute illness: Is there a rationale for intervention? A meta-analysis of cohort studies and controlled trials. Ann Surg 2003;237(3):319-34.

[28] Alexander JW. Nutritional pharmacology in surgical patients. The American Journal of Surgery 2002;183:349–352.

[29] Buijs N, van Bokhorst-de van der Schueren MAE, Langius JAE, Leemans CR, Kuik DJ, Vermeulen M AR and van Leeuwen P AM. Perioperative arginine-supplemented nutrition in malnourished patients with head and neck cancer improves long-term survival. Am J Clin Nutr 2010;92(5):1151-6.

[30] Tao KM, Li XQ, Yang LQ, Yu WF, Lu ZJ, Sun YM, Wu FX. Glutamine supplementation for critically ill adults. Cochrane Database Syst Rev 2014 Sept 9;9:CD010050.

[31] Olree K, et al. Enteral formulations. In The ASPEN nutrition support practice manual, Silver Spring, Md, 1998, American Society for Parenteral and Enteral Nutrition.

[32] Metheny NA. Risk factors of aspiration. J Parenter Enteral Nutr 2002;26:S26-S31.

[33] Kurien M, Leeds JS, Delegge MH, Robson HE, Grant J, Lee FK, AcAlindon ME, Sanders DS. Mortality among patients who receive or defer gastrostomies. Clin Gastroenterol Hepatol 2013;11(11):1445-50.

[34] Itkin M, DeLegge MH, Fang JC, et al. Multidisciplinary practical guidelines for gastrointestinal access for enteral nutrition and decompression from the Society of Interventional Radiology and American Gastroenterological Association (AGA) Institute, with endorsement by Canadian Interventional Radiological Association (CIRA) and Cardiovascular and Interventional Radiological Society of Europe (CIRSE). Gastroenterology 2011;141:742-765.

[35] Bechtold ML, Matteson ML, Choudhary A, Puli SR, Jiang PP, Roy PK. Early versus delayed feeding after placement of a percutaneous endoscopic gastrostomy: A meta-analysis. Am J Gastroenterol 2008;103(11):2919-24.

[36] Shike M, Latkany L, Gerdes H, Bloch AS. Direct percutaneous endoscopic jejunostomies for enteral feeding. Gastrointest Endosc 1996;44(5):536-540.

[37] Sriram K, Jayanthi V, Lakshmi RG, George VS. Prophylactic locking of enteral feeding tubes with pancreatic enzymes. JPEN J Patenter Enteral Nutr 1997;21:353-356.

[38] Scharg SP, Sharma R, Jaik NP, Seamon MJ, et al. Complications related to percutaneous endoscopic gastrostomy (PEG) tubes. A comprehensive clinical review. J Gastrointestin Liver Dis 2007;16:407-418.

[39] Lipp A, Lusardi G. Systemic antimicrobial prophylaxis for percutaneous endoscopic gastrostomy. Cochrane Database Syst Rev. 2013;11:CD005571.

[40] Tsang TK, Eaton D, Falconio MA. Percutaneous ostomy dilatation: A technique for dilating the closed percutaneous endoscopic gastrostomy sites and reinserting gastrostomies. Gastrointest Endosc 1989;35(4):336-7.

[41] Schapiro GD, Edmundowicz SA. Complications of percutaneous endoscopic gastrostomy. Gastrointest Endosc Clin N Am 1996;6:409-422.

[42] Lynch CR, Fang JC. Prevention and management of complications of percutaneous endoscopic gastrostomy (PEG) tubes. Pract Gastroenterol 2004;28:66-76.

[43] Majid HA, Emery PW, Whelan K. Definitions, attitudes, and management practices in relation to diarrhea during enteral nutrition: A survey of patients, nurses, and dietitians. Nutr Clin Pract 2012;27:252-260.

[44] Whelan K, Schneider SM. Mechanisms, prevention, and management of diarrhea in enteral nutrition. Curr Opin Gastroenterol 2011;27:152-159.

[45] Elia M, Engfer MB, GreenCJ, Silk DB. Systematic review and meta-analysis: The clinical and physiological effects of fibre-containing enteral formulae. Aliment Pharmacol Ther 2008 27(2):120-45.

[46] Heimburger DC, Sockwell DG, Geels WJ. Diarrhea with enteral feeding: Prospective reappraisal of putative causes. Nutrition 1994;10(5):392-6.

[47] Montecalvo MA, Steger KA, Farber HW, et al. Nutritional outcome and pneumonia in critical care patients randomized to gastric versus jejunal tube feedings. The critical care research team. Crit Care Med 1992; 20(10):1377-87.

[48] Lazarus BA, Murphy JB, Culpepper L. Aspiration associated with long term gastric versus jejunal feeding: a critical analysis of the literature. Arch Phys Med Rehabil 1990;71(1):46-53.

[49] Marinella MA. The refeeding syndrome and hypophosphatemia. Nutr Rev 2003;61:320-323.

[50] Zeki S, Culkin A, Gabe SM, Nightingale JM. Refeeding hypophopphataemia is more common in enteral than parenteral feeding in adult patients. Clin Nutr 2011;30(3): 365-8.

[51] Dibb MJ, Abraham A, Chadwick PR, Shaffer JL, Teubner A, Carlson GL, Lal S. Central venous catheter salvage in home parenteral nutrition catheter-related blood stream infections: Long term safety and efficacy data. JPEN J Parenter Enteral Nutr. 2014 Sept 15. Pii: 0148607114549999 [Epub ahead of print].

[52] Buchman AL, Opilla M, Kwasny M, Zdiamantidis TG, Okamoto R. Risk factors for the development of catheter-related bloodstream infections in patients receiving home parenteral nutrition. JPEN J Parenter Enteral nutr 2013;38(6):744-9.

[53] Nehme AE. Nutritional support of the hospitalized patient. The team concept. JAMA 1980;243(19):1906-8.

[54] Trujillo EB, Young LS, Chertow GM, Randall S, Clemos T, Jacobs DO, Robinson MK. Metabolic and monetary costs of avoidable parenteral nutrition use. JPEN. J Parenter Enteral Nutr 1999;23(2):109-13.

Chapter 8

Decision Making for Enteral Nutrition in Adult Patients with Dysphagia – A Guide for Health Care Professionals

Nicoll Kenny and Shajila A. Singh

Additional information is available at the end of the chapter

http://dx.doi.org/10.5772/60987

1. Introduction

A review of current literature reveals high mortality rates post insertion of feeding tubes for the provision of long term enteral nutrition, most specifically post placement of a percutaneous endoscopic gastrostomy (PEG). The recommendation of enteral nutrition is often a complex decision, which requires the consideration of many aspects, including not only the medical need for nutritional support, but also the wishes of the patient and their families. The provision of artificial nutrition and hydration can be an emotional topic which leaves many health care professionals uncomfortable and unsure of what recommendations to make. This chapter aims to provide information about the different methods of enteral nutrition available and the indication for each one. It also hopes to present a number of factors that need to be considered by all health care professionals who are involved in the recommendation of enteral nutrition.

Enteral nutrition is the provision of sustenance into the stomach or small intestine and includes tube feedings as well as oral nutritional supplements [1]. The focus here is on enteral nutrition via tube feeding.

2. Indications for enteral nutrition

Optimal hydration and nutrition is required to meet the body's daily nutritional requirements. Patients with dysphagia may be unable to attain these minimum nutritional requirements with oral intake and require enteral nutrition [2-9]. These patients include those who are unable to swallow due to neurological damage or degeneration [4, 10-15], or those who have structural abnormalities that make oral nutrition impossible, as in the case of patients with advanced stage head and neck cancer or oesophageal cancer [16-18].

The most common indicator for long term enteral nutrition is a cerebral vascular accident (CVA) [3, 5, 10-12, 19-26]. Dysphagia with resulting malnutrition and/or dehydration is common in patients who have had a CVA, explaining the high need for enteral nutrition within this population [10, 13, 27-28]. Patients with other neurological deficits such as traumatic head injury or neuro-degenerative diseases, may also require short or long term enteral nutrition as a safe method of hydration and nutrition [7, 29-33].

Certain medical conditions are more likely to predispose patients to require enteral nutrition because of concomitant dysphagia and increased nutritional needs. Patients with head and neck cancer may develop dysphagia after radiation treatment as a result of tissue damage to the swallow mechanism [18] with a resultant need for prophylactic enteral nutrition [17]. Those patients who continue on oral intake may require enteral nutrition as a supplement to ensure sufficient intake of the daily nutritional requirements while receiving radiotherapy [18]. In cases of trauma to the body or after surgery, enteral nutrition is also recommended to aid sufficient caloric intake to minimise loss of body fat and to support recovery [15, 29, 31-32, 34-35].

3. Enteral nutrition routes

There are different enteral nutrition routes, and the route chosen is determined according to the length of time and the type of enteral support needed for a specific patient. The different types of enteral nutrition include nasogastric tubes (NGTs) and nasojejenal tubes (NJTs); surgically placed gastrostomy tubes (GTs) and jejenostomy tubes (JTs); and non-surgical placement methods include percutaneous endoscopic gastrostomy (PEG) or percutaneous endoscopic jejenostomy (PEJ).

Before the development of the PEG procedure by Gauderer and Ponsky in the early 1980s, a gastrostomy tube was placed under general anaesthetic. PEG has become the most popular method of tube placement because of the ease of insertion, minimal invasiveness and no requirement for a general anaesthetic [36-38]. A surgical gastrostomy may still be performed in cases where PEG is not possible due to obstruction which makes the passing of the scope down the gastrointestinal tract impossible [39].

4. Short term versus long-term enteral nutrition

The placement of NGTs are recommended for the delivery of early enteral nutrition in the acute stages of disease [2, 10, 13, 40]. The benefits of early enteral nutritional have been documented within various groups of patients [41-44]. NGTs are for short term use only and should not be in situ for periods longer than 4 to 6 weeks [2, 15], as they can cause serious complications including nasal ulceration, chronic sinusitis and increased risk of aspiration pneumonia [15, 39, 45].

http://dx.doi.org/10.5772/60987

NGTs are easy to insert and require no surgical procedure or administration of anaesthetics for placement [10, 14, 46]. However they are poorly tolerated by patients, and are often pulled out after insertion thereby reducing the nutritional advantage which was the aim of placement [47-49]. NGTs may be placed incorrectly by the professional inserting them, with incidences reported to range from 0.3 to 27% (cited by [50] in [51]). A misplaced NGT may result in aspiration pneumonia which can be fatal [51]. Patient positioning, with most hospitalized patients being in a sedated state or lying flat, during NGT feeding can also result in aspiration pneumonia [52-53]. An increase in reflux with NGT placement has been noted [39, 46] particularly in cases with pre-existing gastro-oesophageal reflux [54]. Similar negative effects have been noted with the use of PEGs [46].

If a patient requires enteral nutrition for a period longer than 4 to 6 weeks, and the prognosis justifies the intervention, placement of a gastrostomy or PEG tube for the provision of long term enteral nutrition could be considered [14, 19, 55, 56]. However, Maitines et al. (2009) suggest a longer period of at least 6 to 8 weeks with an NGT in situ, before considering a PEG to ensure a better outcome. Others [14] consider the prognosis and argue that a patient at the end stages of a disease should not be considered for PEG but should rather receive nutrition via NGT. No difference between NGT and PEG cohorts was found in the rate of complications [46], the rate of mortality post placement [45-46] or the occurrence of pneumonia post placement [46].

Higher complication rates for gastrostomies relative to PEG placements have been reported [57-58]. Complications include internal leakage, peritonitis, fistula, dislodgement, external leakage and skin infection. Higher mortality rates in surgical gastrostomy cases (29%, n=35) compared with PEG cases (17%, n=12) were not significantly different [58].

The reasons for high mortality rates include poor patient selection. Patients with risk factors for mortality have been recommended for a PEG resulting in poor outcomes that are being linked to the PEG procedure, when in fact these patients were at risk of death regardless of PEG placement [59-60]. There is strong evidence linking certain underlying medical conditions to higher mortality post PEG [5, 15, 36, 55-56, 59, 61-63]. The highest mortality rates occurred in patients who had CVA and malignancies [22, 62].

The timing of PEG placement [24, 64] is noted also to affect the outcome. It has been suggested that there be a 30 day delay in the placement of long term enteral nutrition to ensure a better chance of survival, leaving patients on short term enteral nutrition for a longer period [24, 64]. The notion of poor timing in the placement of PEG is linked to poor patient selection. If a patient has an underlying medical condition that places them at risk for mortality, it can be argued that they would have died regardless, and early PEG insertion, at a time when they are at risk of death due to an underlying medical condition, means that they die with a PEG in situ which makes their death a statistic of mortality post PEG placement. To counteract early PEG placement, it is suggested that if a patient has survived and still requires a PEG after their condition has stabilised, only then should it be considered. Abuksis et al. (2000) noted a lower mortality rate in patients who were deferred for the placement of a PEG until they were discharged from hospital and if it was still required at 30 days post discharge.

As an example, mortality in patients with CVAs usually occurs in the acute stage when a patient is still in the hospital [65]. Dysphagia is common following a CVA [65] and many CVA patients will regain their ability to swallow within two weeks post infarct [66]. A patient who receives a PEG at this stage is at high risk of dying due to the underlying medical condition of a CVA [65]. The high mortality will be reflected as a consequence of PEG placement in cases with a CVA. The timing for the placement of a PEG in a patient with a CVA is critical, and should only be considered if a patient has not regained their ability to swallow within four weeks [13, 67]. During the acute stages post CVA, an NGT is recommended for the provision of hydration and nutrition [13].

There are also a series of risk factors such as increased age, decreased body mass index, a higher number of co-morbidities, and decreased blood albumin levels have been identified as placing a patient at greater risk of mortality post PEG. Along with the primary medical condition and timing of placement, these factors also need to be considered when recommending a patient for a PEG to reduce the likelihood of poor outcomes. One such risk factor is increased age. Patients over the age of 60 were found to have the highest mortality rate at 30-days post insertion [20, 22-25, 55-56, 68-70]. Age together with diminished mental capacity, as with patients who have dementia, tripled mortality in the period after placement [22]. Such outcomes caution against PEG placement in older patients with dementia.

The positive outcomes of long term enteral nutrition should also guide decisions for such a recommendation. One such outcome post PEG placement is the ability to return to oral intake which can occur in patient populations with a range of medical conditions and depends on factors such as the presence of dysphagia, age, and the underlying medical condition that necessitated PEG placement [12, 17, 69]. Factors that determined a return to oral intake, were the ability to take some amount of nutrition orally at 3 and 6 months post PEG placement [12], regression of the tumour that had originally caused dysphagia post chemo/radiotherapy [12, 17] regaining of the swallow post CVA [12, 69], a younger age, the absence of dysphagia and intervention by a speech therapist to regain the swallow pre PEG placement [71].

The provision of nutrition into the stomach via NGT or gastrostomy/PEG is common [5, 21]. Gastrointestinal intolerance of tube feedings, identified by the presence of large gastric residual volumes, nausea and vomiting, ileus, abdominal distension, and diarrhoea [72], is a major factor limiting adequate enteral intake in patients. In cases such as these the stomach may be bypassed and nutrition delivered to a lower part of the gastro intestinal tract [4, 39, 73]. NJT/PEJ enteral nutrition has been noted to result in better energy intake due to improved absorption in the small bowel and a decreased risk of reflux related aspiration due to feeds being delivered into an area further away from the pharynx [74]. However, Davies et al. (2012) report no difference in energy intake and risk of aspiration between patients receiving enteral nutrition via NGT and NJT.

5. Decision making between the different routes of enteral nutrition

PEGs, GTs and NGTs have advantages and possible complications. The outcomes relate to mortality and improved nutrition. Adequate nutrition is linked to better medical outcomes and survival [35, 73]. PEG is noted to be superior to NGT with regard to improvement in general medical outcomes [46] with NGT candidates being statistically more prone to intervention failure, such as tube blockage or leakage, feed interruption and recurrent displacement, than patients who were fitted with PEG, regardless of the patient's underlying medical condition [46]. With better provision of feeds when a PEG is used, better medical outcomes may be expected as a patient is more likely to receive adequate hydration and nutrition.

When patients who had a CVA were considered as a separate group from other medical conditions, neither NGT nor PEG were superior in the delivery of nutrition. The presence of dysphagia was the key indicator for mortality rather than the type of enteral nutrition used [36].

There exists debate around which method of enteral intake is best suited for patients with head and neck cancer specifically. A large majority of patients with cancer are malnourished throughout the disease process and require enteral nutrition [75]. Determining the optimal mode of enteral nutrition in this patient population bears consideration of the benefits and drawbacks. Sobani et al. (2011) reported PEG as being superior to NGT in that it resulted in greater weight gain and lower mortality, but others [76] note a lower clinical risk of complications, and a greater chance of returning to full oral intake after a six month period, with patients left on NGT rather than fitted with a PEG. It was argued that a patient with an NGT would be more eager to feed orally in order to progress towards removal of the tube because of the visibility of an NGT, which can be unsightly to some. Beginning partial oral intake made muscle atrophy less likely and sped up the return to full oral intake, compared to those receiving nutrition exclusively via a PEG [76]. In patients with dysphagia and a range of medical conditions including neurological fallout and head and neck cancer, Gomes et al. (2012) noted no difference in mortality rates post PEG or NGT placement.

Mortality rates after PEG placement has been reported to be low as a direct result of the PEG procedure [11, 77]. However, Malmgren et al. (2011) suggest that the mortality rate in the first few weeks post PEG placement is 'high' and ranges between 10% and 36% depending on sample size and medical conditions [5, 22, 55-56, 69, 78-79). The greatest majority of patients died within a 30 day period post PEG placement and in patients with dementia, the mortality rate was as high as 54% [79]. The 30 day mortality rates were from both developed and developing countries where a variety of medical conditions were included in the sample.

Strong evidence links poor nutrition upon hospitalization with poor medical outcomes, such as greater incidence of morbidity and mortality [45, 73, 80]. Malnourishment is measured using the body mass index (BMI), with a BMI of <18.5 indicating malnutrition (WHO, 1995). Malnourishment can be as a result of the disease process or due to socioeconomic factors [81] and can be further exacerbated by hospitalization [13, 15, 35, 44, 48, 56, 73], because of interruptions in the provision of enteral nutrition, inadequate nutrition prescribed and the inability of a patient, who may be on oral intake, to physically eat independently [81]. Malnourishment at the time of PEG placement is a crucial factor noted to place a patient at risk for mortality [19, 45, 55-56, 70, 77].

Upon admission to hospital an NGT may be placed to improve nutrition before placement of a PEG [77]. But NGT feeds can result in minimal improvement in nutritional status because of interrupted feeds when the patient has a procedure, late placement and commencement of

30 day mortality rate (%)	Sample size (N)	Medical condition	Country	Researchers
15.8%	359	Head and neck cancer (n=97) CVA (n=73) Malignancy (n=61) Head injury (n=59) Cerebral palsy (n=38) Congenital anomaly (n=19) Motor neuron disease (n=7) Dementia (n=5)	Bosnia Herzegovina	Vanis, Saray, Gornjakovic & Mesihovic, 2012
22%	201	CVA (n=97) Malignant oesophageal obstruction (n=33) Dementia (n=16) Other neurologic disorders (n=13) Parkinsons (n=12) Other (n=23) Other malignancies (n=5)	Sweden	Malmgren et al., 2011
10%	77	Neurologic disorders (n=71) Head and neck cancer (n=6)	Turkey	Ermis et al., 2012
20%	128	CVA (n=34) Non neurologic cerebral hypoxia (n=30) Cranial tumour (n=23) Head and neck cancer (n=19) Motor neuron disease (n=13) Other (n=9)	Turkey	Gundogan et al., 2014
19%	83	CVA (n=83)	Norway	Ha & Hauge, 2003
22%	112	CVA (n=33) Head and neck cancer (n=27) Chronic neurological disorders (n=22) Other (n=30)	Britain	Longcroft-Wheaton et al., 2009
18.5%	187	Malignancy (n=187)	USA	Keung et al., 2012
36%	61	CVA (n=50) Dementia (n=21) Malignancy (n=9) Head and neck trauma (n=3)	Israel	Abuksis et al., 2004
28%	361	CVA (n=120) Dementia (n=103) Oropharyngeal malignancy (n=65) Other (n=73)	USA	Sanders et al., 2000

Table 1. International mortality rates 30 days post PEG placement

feeds or accidental removal of tubes [47-48, 72]. A nutritionally compromised patient would benefit from placement of a PEG with the aim of improving nutrition, based on evidence that PEG placement facilitates better improvement in nutrition [5, 75]. However PEG placement comes with a high risk of mortality due to the patient's initial poor nutritional status.

Based on the high mortality rate of malnourished patients, it is important to consider the nutritional status of individuals prior to PEG placement [19, 45, 55-56, 70, 77]. A review of the literature suggests that albumin levels may be used as a marker of a patient's nutritional status [82]. Albumin is a protein made by the liver, and is a measure of protein in the body. Albumin balances the amount of blood flowing through the body's arteries and veins and helps to transport calcium, progesterone, bilirubin and medications through the blood. A serum albumin test will measure the amount of protein in the blood and can be used as an indicator of the presence of liver or kidney disease [83] which can affect patient survival. Normal levels of albumin are considered to be in the range of 3.4-5.4 g/dL or 35-50 g/L, depending on how specific laboratories measure it. Blomberg et al., (2011) noted the link between low albumin levels pre-insertion of PEG and a high mortality rate post insertion. This link confirms that hypo- albuminaemia is a risk factor that should be considered in all patients being medically worked up for PEG placement [45, 56, 59, 77, 84]. Co morbidities like diabetes and cardiac disease were also noted to be significant risk factors for high mortality in patients post PEG placement [19, 56, 59, 70, 82].

6. The role of the speech language therapist (SLT)

Evidence exists to support the involvement of an SLT in the assessment and treatment of patients with dysphagia. Langmore et al. (2011) [108] suggested that it is important for an SLT to assess a patient with head and neck cancer and to determine the most optimal approach for each patient to be able to recover swallowing or to compensate for losses due to surgical or chemo-radiation intervention. The role of the SLT in the management of patients with dysphagia who may require enteral nutrition, is not to recommend the route of enteral nutrition, but rather to make a recommendation of whether or not the patient can eat orally and is safe to do so. All discussions and decisions relating to enteral nutrition, whether short or long term, should take place within an inter-professional team including the patient and caregivers.

Considering the multitude of risk factors that exist for poor outcomes post PEG insertion, it follows that a patient should be individually assessed for the presence of any risk factors before being recommended for the procedure [85-87]. A comprehensive assessment by the team needs to consider factors such as: 1) the potential benefits to the individual should they receive a PEG, 2) biochemical parameters, like blood albumin level, 3) multiple comorbidities, 4) prognosis, 5) and the presence of risk factors that may place a patient at risk of mortality post procedure, such as being over the age of 60 years and a low BMI [10, 19, 23, 25, 45, 56, 69, 87-89, 90].

Strong emphasis is placed upon a team approach when assessing patients who may be recommended for long term enteral nutrition [85-87]. A rigorous assessment, by a team, for each patient being considered for a PEG ought to be in place. The team needs to ensure that all risk factors which could affect outcome are considered and that an informed decision respects patient autonomy [60, 85-87]. A patient who is considered a high risk for mortality should not be considered a candidate for the procedure as it would be a futile intervention. Better patient selection would improve the outcome of patients who are recommended for and fitted with a PEG [91].

7. Ethical considerations

A patient may refuse a NGT or a PEG procedure and wish to begin/ continue oral intake, even if it means a shorter survival period. Patient's decisions need to be honoured and respected by health care professionals [92].

Where patients opt for enteral nutrition, despite the benefits that enteral nutrition can provide a patient, such as improved nutrition and a longer survival time, quality of life is affected [93]. Health care professionals should counsel patients on the effects that a PEG tube will have on their quality of life [94], by shifting the focus of management post PEG insertion to include social aspects and not only clinical needs [95].

The placement of a PEG for the provision of enteral nutrition is considered a life-saving procedure in some cases [93, 96] and many patients who have a PEG attest to this fact and the benefit that PEG feeding provides them [96-97]. One study noted particularly positive patient reports on their experiences living with a PEG tube, with 84% (N=51) noting a positive or neutral effect of the tube on their lives, 90% (N=51) expressing a view that the tube was worthwhile and 96% (N=51) noting that they would recommend it to another patient [97].

Negative experiences that a PEG has on patients' quality of life have been extensively reported. Common difficulties associated with having a PEG tube, which affect quality of life, include a high level of complication, like tube blockage, leakage and discomfort [94] interference with family life, social activities and hobbies [93-94, 98-99], interference with intimacy [94], negative reactions from others [95], a burden placed on family or caregivers [95] and a feeling of missing out on meal times and food [95]. Similar negative effects on quality of life are reported in patients who receive NGT feeds [98]. A study in Taiwan noted that the majority of patients are discharged home on NGT feeds because of a refusal to have a PEG placed [100]. Reasons included concern over leakage and infection following a PEG, a worry that the patient is too old and frail to undergo an operation and a cultural belief that the patient will not die "whole" if they have a PEG in situ [100].

In light of the high mortality rate post PEG placement, the concept of futility bears discussion. Futility refers to a medical intervention that would have no effect, or if there was an effect, it would not be one that the patient benefitted from [89]. Many patients receive long term enteral nutrition where no effect or benefit is proven in terms of nutritional improvement or survival

[56]. All aspects linked to possible mortality must be considered, and risks and benefits weighed before a recommendation for enteral nutrition is made. If a patient is considered to be a high risk for mortality, certain procedures that will cause further suffering and no benefit may be deemed futile [7], and should be avoided [21]. The decision to place a PEG should be based on the perceived benefit it will bring to the patient [89] and if no benefit is presumed, then the procedure should not be done. A patient who is identified as a high risk for mortality post PEG placement should not receive a PEG but rather they and their families should be counselled on the risks that exist and the reasons for deferred placement. A team can make a recommendation for enteral nutrition based on their knowledge but a cognitively intact patient must make the final decision after being fully informed about the benefits and risks involved in the proposed management plans [89].

The issue of futility in PEG placement is most particularly noted in the case of patients with advanced dementia being fitted with a tube for the provision of long term enteral nutrition [101-102]. In this population, the placement of a PEG has no benefit to the patient and can actually lead to decreased survival due to complications, such as aspiration, that result from the placement [89, 102]. The use of long term enteral nutrition in patients with malignancy, with the aim of nutritional gain, needs to be questioned as there is no real nutritional gain in these patients post placement [16, 62, 78].

Azzopardi and Ellul (2013) suggest that, in certain patient populations, the insertion of a PEG will only prolong a life which is of poor quality and it needs to be determined through discussion whether this decision is ethical. A consideration in South Africa particularly, is whether it would be appropriate to perform futile procedures in a resource constrained public hospital sector [103]. If PEGs are placed in cases where patients have poor prognosis and are considered high risk for mortality post PEG placement, an argument could be made that the scarce resources would be better directed to those patients with potentially better outcomes.

The use of protocols in patient care ensures adherence with best practice. They are important documents to which health care professionals should refer to guide practice that will result in the provision of the best possible care [104]. Protocols for the assessment and management of patients with dysphagia who require enteral nutrition exist [2, 38, 66, 105] but do not include considerations like assessment of risk factors to justify the PEG procedure. Further, adherence to protocols cannot be assumed. The presence of risk factors in patients do not always deter health professionals in making a recommendation for PEG placement, as is evident by the persistence of high mortality rates, despite the known effects of risk factors and their effect on mortality [56].

8. End of life and enteral nutrition

The decision to refer a patient for a PEG placement or not, includes holistic consideration of many factors to make a recommendation that is in the best interests of the patient.

The provision of hydration and nutrition at the end of life care is an area of debate and can become a highly emotional topic. Delegge et al. (2005) suggest that the decision to place a feeding tube consider the basic principles of professional ethics. Informed consent from an adult who is cognitively intact is imperative, and the benefits of the placement of enteral nutrition must outweigh the risk of the procedure, which should cause the patient no harm [89].

The concept of palliative care needs to be introduced as a real alternative for patients who are not considered candidates for PEG placement due to the presence of risk factors that place them at high risk for mortality. The World Health Organisation (2002) considers palliative care as "...an all-encompassing approach to care that begins months or years before death". PEG placement does not always benefit the patient, and although the actual PEG procedure does not harm the patient, the risk of mortality post placement is high, which in turn is harmful to the patient. The choice of refusing a PEG and remaining on oral intake as a form of palliative care should be made available to all patients and their caregivers, with provision of education and support for the decision they may make. The inclusion of a palliative care option for patients who do not wish to have a PEG placed would provide them with an alternative option, and it would also ensure that futile procedures are avoided which would uphold medical ethics.

The decisions around the recommendation of enteral nutrition, particularly in very ill patients who have a poor prognosis, are not easy for health care professionals to make. Clear guidelines that are based on evidence are crucial in order to help health care professionals navigate these difficult decisions that are often clouded with human emotion.

A role not often considered by SLTs is that of palliative care. The provision of artificial nutrition and hydration (ANH) to patients who are in the end stages of disease is debated, and can evoke emotional responses [106]. It is common for patients in the end stages of disease to have little or no oral intake [106]. Many practitioners may feel that depriving a patient of hydration and nutrition is unethical and can make health professionals uncomfortable [89,107]. A study of nurses' perceptions on ANH in palliative care yielded more clinical reasons for withholding of ANH than for providing it [106]. Reasons supporting provision of ANH were emotive, not based on clinical fact and were not in the best interests of the patient [106].

In practice, there comes a time, when a decision needs to be made about the hydration and nutrition needs of a patient in the end stages of disease. The SLT is often the professional who, based on the assessment of the patient's swallowing, is in a position to determine the feasibility of nutritional intake. It is important that the SLT and the inter-professional team are educated in the field of palliative care and ANH [106-107] to contribute to making an informed decision regarding a patient's options at end of life and reduce the number of inappropriate referrals for futile procedures with poor outcomes.

9. Conclusion

Based on a review of current literature some important points have been raised around the recommendation process for enteral nutrition in adult patients with dysphagia. The key focus in any decision making process for medical procedures should be on patient autonomy. If a patient consents to placement of a PEG for the provision of long term enteral nutrition, with a full understanding of the impact it will have on them, not only medically but socially and emotionally too, then a standard assessment procedure needs to follow. Assessment should be carried out by a team of health care professionals, including the SLT, and should include a consideration of the patients underlying medical condition, indication for PEG, prognosis of survival post procedure, age, nutritional status, the presence of co-morbidities and biochemical parameters. Based on the assessment findings, the team, in conjunction with the patient and their family, need to make a recommendation. If a patient is considered to be a high risk for mortality following PEG placement then alternate methods of intake need to be discussed with and recommended to the patient and their family, with education and counselling provided on the benefits and risks of oral intake as a form of palliation. A thorough assessment procedure will help to ensure that futile procedures are avoided and only patients who consent to and who will benefit from PEG placement are recommended for the procedure.

Author details

Nicoll Kenny[1*] and Shajila A. Singh[2]

*Address all correspondence to: nicollcbell@gmail.com

1 Chris Hani Baragwanath Academic Hospital, Speech Therapy and Audiology Department, Johannesburg, South Africa

2 University of Cape Town, Department of Communication Disorders, Cape Town, South Africa

References

[1] Lochs, H., Dejong, C., Hammarqvist, F., Hebuterne, X., Leon-Sanz, M., Schtz, T., van Gemert, W., van Gossum, A., Valentini, L., Lubke, H., Bischoff, S., Engelmann, N., & Thul, P. (2006). ESPEN Guidelines on Enteral Nutrition: Gastrosenterology. Clinical Nutrition, 25, 260-274. DOI:10.1016/j.clnu.2006.01.007.

[2] Bankhead, R., Boullata, J., Brantley, S., Corkins, M., Guenter, P., Krenitsky, J., Lyman, B., Metheny, N.A., Mueller, C., Robbins, S., & Wessel, J. (2009). A.S.P.E.N. Enteral Nutrition Practice Recommendations. Journal of Parenteral and Enteral Nutrition, 33, 122. DOI: 10.1177/0148607108330314.

[3] Blomberg, J., Lagergren, J., Martin, L., Mattsson, F., & Lagergren, P. (2012). Complications after percutaneous endoscopic gastrostomy in a prospective study. Scandinavian Journal of Gastroenterology, 47(6), 737-742. DOI:10.3109/00365521.2012.654404.

[4] DiBaise, J. K., & Scolapio, J. S. (2007). Home parenteral and enteral nutrition. Gastroenterology Clinics of North America, 36(1), 123. DOI:10.1016/j.gtc.2007.01.008.

[5] Erdil, A., Saka, M., Ates, Y., Tuzun, A., Bagci, S., Uygun, A., Yesilova, Z., Gulsen, M., Karaeren, N., & Dagalp, K. (2005). Enteral nutrition via percutaneous endoscopic gastrostomy and nutritional status of patients: Five-year prospective study. Journal of Gastroenterology & Hepatology, 20(7), 1002-1007. DOI:10.1111/j.1440-1746.2005.03892.

[6] Gundogan, K., Yurci, A., Coskun, R., Baskol, M., Gursoy, S., Hebbar, G., Ziegler, T. R. (2014). Outcomes of percutaneous endoscopic gastrostomy in hospitalized patients at a tertiary care center in turkey. European Journal of Clinical Nutrition, 68(4), 437-440. DOI:10.1038/ejcn.2014.11.

[7] Holmes, S. (2011). Importance of nutrition in palliative care of patients with chronic disease. Primary Health Care, 21(6), 31-39. Retrieved from http://web.b.ebscohost.com.ezproxy.uct.ac.za/ehost/pdfviewer/pdfviewer?sid=bbcd98c7-51e6-44f0-bbfa-91fbc7040303%40sessionmgr113&vid=1&hid=110.

[8] Sharp, H. M., & Shega, J. W. (2009). Feeding tube placement in patients with advanced dementia: The beliefs and practice patterns of speech-language pathologists. American Journal of Speech-Language Pathology, 18(3), 222-230. DOI: 10.1044/1058-0360(2008/08-0013.

[9] Vivanti, A. P., Campbell, K. L., Suter, M. S., Hannan-Jones, M., & Hulcombe, J. A. (2009). Contribution of thickened drinks, food and enteral and parenteral fluids to fluid intake in hospitalised patients with dysphagia. Journal of Human Nutrition and Dietetics: The Official Journal of the British Dietetic Association, 22(2), 148-155. DOI: 10.1111/j.1365-277X.2009.00944.

[10] Kobayashi, K., Cooper, G. S., Chak, A., Sivak Jr., M. V., & Wong, R. C. K. (2002). A prospective evaluation of outcome in patients referred for PEG placement. Gastrointestinal Endoscopy, 55(4), 500-506. DOI:10.1067/mge.2002.122577.

[11] Nicholson, F. B., Korman, M. G., & Richardson, M. A. (2000). Percutaneous endoscopic gastrostomy: A review of indications, complications and outcome. Journal of Gastroenterology & Hepatology, 15(1), 21-25. DOI:10.1046/j.1440-1746.2000.02004.

[12] Paramsothy, S., Papadopoulos, G., Mollison, L. C., & Leong, R. W. L. (2009). Resumption of oral intake following percutaneous endoscopic gastrostomy. Journal of Gastroenterology & Hepatology, 24(6), 1098-1101. DOI:10.1111/j.1440-1746.2009.05802.

[13] Prosser-Loose, E., & Paterson, P. G. (2006). The FOOD trial collaboration: Nutritional supplementation strategies and acute stroke outcome. Nutrition Reviews, 64(6), 289-294. DOI:10.1301/nr.2006.jun.289-294.

[14] Rio, A., Ellis, C., Shaw, C., Willey, E., Ampong, M., Wijesekera, L., Rittman, T., Nigel Leigh, P.,

[15] Stroud, M., Duncan, H., & Nightingale, J. (2003). Guidelines for enteral feeding in adult hospital patients. Gut, 52 (Suppl VII):vii1-vii12. DOI: 10.1136/gut.52.suppl_7.vii1.

[16] Baldwin, C., Spiro, A., McGough, C., Norman, A. R., Gillbanks, A., Thomas, K., Cunningham, D., O'Brien, M., & Andreyev, H. J. N. (2011). Simple nutritional intervention in patients with advanced cancers of the gastrointestinal tract, non-small cell lung cancers or mesothelioma and weight loss receiving chemotherapy: A randomised controlled trial. Journal of Human Nutrition & Dietetics, 24(5), 431-440. DOI: 10.1111/j.1365-277X.2011.01189.

[17] Nguyen, N. P., North, D., Smith, H. J., Dutta, S., Alfieri, A., Karlsson, U., Lee, H., Martinez, T., Lemanski, C., Nguyen, L. M., Ludin, A., & Sallah, S. (2006). Safety and effectiveness of prophylactic gastrostomy tubes for head and neck cancer patients undergoing chemoradiation. Surgical Oncology, 15(4), 199-203. DOI:http://dx.doi.org.ezproxy.uct.ac.za/10.1016/j.suronc.2006.12.002.

[18] Wermker, K., Jung, S., Huppmeier, L., Joos, U., & Kleinheinz, J. (2012). Prediction model forearly percutaneous endoscopic gastrostomy (PEG) in head and neck cancer treatment. Oral Oncology, 48, 355-360. DOI:10.1016/j.oraloncology.2011.11.005.

[19] Longcroft-Wheaton, G., Marden, P., Colleypriest, B., Gavin, D., Taylor, G., & Farrant, M. (2009). Understanding Why Patients Die After Gastrostomy Tube Insertion: A Retrospective Analysis of Mortality. Journal of Parenteral and Enteral Nutrition, 33 (4), 375-379. DOI: 10.1177/0148607108327156.

[20] Kirchgatterer, A., Bunte, C., Aschl, G., Fritz, E., Hubner, D., Kranewitter, W., Fleischer, M., Hinterreiter, M., Stadler, B., & Knoflach, P. (2007). Long-term outcome following placement of percutaneous endoscopic gastrostomy in younger and older patients. Scandinavian Journal of Gastroenterology, 42(2), 271-276. DOI: 10.1080/00365520600880864.

[21] Lee, C., Im, J., Kim, J., Kim, S., Ryu, D., Cha, J.M., E.Y., Kim, E.R., & Chang, D. (2013). Risk factors for complications and mortality of percutaneous endoscopic gastrostomy: A multicenter, retrospective study. Surgical Endoscopy, 27(10), 3806-3815. DOI: 10.1007/s00464-013-2979-3.

[22] Malmgren, A., Hede, G. W., Karlström, B., Cederholm, T., Lundquist, P., Wirén, M., & Faxén-Irving, G. (2011). Indications for percutaneous endoscopic gastrostomy and survival in old adults. Food & Nutrition Research, 55, 1-6. DOI:10.3402/fnr.v55i0.6037.

[23] Richter-Schrag, H-J., Richter, S., Ruthmann, O., Olschewski, M., Hopt, UT., & Fischer, A. (2011). Risk factors and complications following percutaneous endoscopic gastrostomy: A case series of 1041 patients. Canadian Journal of Gastroenterology, 25(4), 201-206. Retrieved from http://www-ncbi-nlm-nih-gov.ezproxy.uct.ac.za/pmc/articles/PMC3088695/pdf/cjg25201.pdf.

[24] Smith, B., Perring, P., Engoren, M., & Sferra, J. J. (2008). Hospital and long-term outcome after percutaneous endoscopic gastrostomy. Surgical Endoscopy, 22(1), 74-80. DOI:10.1007/s00464-007-9372-z.

[25] Smoliner, C., Volkert, D., Wittrich, A., Sieber, C. C., & Wirth, R. (2012). Basic geriatric assessment does not predict in-hospital mortality after PEG placement. BMC Geriatrics, 12, 52-52. DOI:10.1186/1471-2318-12-52.

[26] Thomson, M. A., Carver, A. D., & Sloan, R. L. (2002). Percutaneous endoscopic gastrostomy feeding in a district rehabilitation service. Clinical Rehabilitation, 16(2), 215-220. DOI:10.1191/0269215502cr476oa.

[27] Crary, M. A., Humphrey, J. L., Carnaby-Mann, G., Sambandam, R., Miller, L., & Silliman, S. (2012). Dysphagia, nutrition, and hydration in ischemic stroke patients at admission and discharge from acute care. Dysphagia 28(1), 69-7. DOI:10.1007/s00455-012-9414-0.

[28] Sura, L., Madhavan, A., Carnaby, G., & Crary, M. A. (2012). Dysphagia in the elderly: Management and nutritional considerations. Clinical Interventions in Aging, 7, 287-298. DOI:10.2147/CIA.S23404.

[29] Darbar, A. (2001). Nutritional Requirements in Severe Head Injury. Nutrition, 17, 71-72. PII S0899-9007(00)00476-7.

[30] Denes, Z. (2004). The influence of severe malnutrition on rehabilitation in patients with severe head injury. Disability and Rehabilitation, 26(19), 1163-1165. DOI: 10.1080/09638280412331270380.

[31] Hartl, R., Gerber, L.M., Quanhong, N., & Ghajar, J. (2008). Journal of Neurosurgery, 109, 50-59. DOI: 10.3171/JNS/2008/109/7/0050.

[32] Vizzini, A., & Aranda-Michel, J. (2011). Nutritional support in head injury. Nutrition, 27(2), 129-132. DOI:10.1016/j.nut.2010.05.004.

[33] Zhang, L., Sanders, L., & Fraser, R. J. L. (2012). Nutritional support teams increase percutaneous endoscopic gastrostomy uptake in motor neuron disease. World Journal of Gastroenterology: WJG, 18(44), 6461. DOI:10.3748/wjg.v18.i44.6461.

[34] de Aguilar-Nascimento, J. E., Bicudo-Salomao, A., & Portari-Filho, P. (2012). Optimal timing for the initiation of enteral and parenteral nutrition in critical medical and surgical conditions, Nutrition, 28(9), 840-843. DOI:10.1016/j.nut.2012.01.013.

[35] Vassilyadi, F., Panteliadou, AK., & Panteliadis, C. (2013). Hallmarks in the History of Enteral and Parenteral Nutrition : From Antiquity to the 20th Century. Nutrition in Clinical Practice, 28: 209. DOI: 10.1177/0884533612468602.

[36] Laskaratos, F., Walker, M., Walker, M., Gowribalan, J., Gkotsi, D., Wojciechowska, V.,... Jenkins, A. (2013). Predictive factors for early mortality after percutaneous en-

doscopic and radiologically-inserted gastrostomy. Digestive Diseases and Sciences. DOI 10.1007/s10620-013-2829-0.

[37] Swaminath, A., Longstreth, G.F., Runnman, E.M., Yang, S.J. (2010). Effect of Physician Education and Patient Counseling on Inpatient Nonsurgical Percutaneous Feeding Tube Placement Rate, Indications, and Outcome. Southern Medical Journal, 103 (2), 126-130. DOI: 10.1097/SMJ.0b013e3181c9800f.

[38] Wilhelm, S.M., Ortega, K.A., Stellato, T.A. (2010). Guidelines for identification and management of outpatient percutaneous endoscopic gastrostomy tube placement. The American Journal of Surgery, 199, 396-400.

[39] McClave, S. A., & Chang, W. (2003). Complications of enteral access. Gastrointestinal Endoscopy, 58(5), 739-751. DOI:http://dx.doi.org.ezproxy.uct.ac.za/10.1016/S0016-5107(03)02147-3.

[40] Maitines, G., Ugenti, I., Memeo, R., Clemente, N., & Lambrenghi, O.C. (2009). Endoscopic gastrostomy for enteral nutrition in neurogenic dysphagia: Application of a nasogastric tube or percutaneous endoscopic gastrostomy. Chirurgia Italiana Journal 61(1), 33-38. Retrieved from http://europepmc.org/abstract/med/19391337.

[41] Davies, A. R., Morrison, S. S., Bailey, M. J., Bellomo, R., Cooper, D. J., Doig, G. S., Finfer, S.R., & Heyland, D. K. (2012). A multicenter, randomized controlled trial comparing early nasojejunal with nasogastric nutrition in critical illness. Critical Care Medicine, 40(8), 2342-2348. DOI: 10.1097/CCM.0b013e318255d87e.

[42] Doig, G. S., Heighes, P. T., Simpson, F., & Sweetman, E. A. (2011). Early enteral nutrition reduces mortality in trauma patients requiring intensive care: A meta-analysis of randomized controlled trials. Injury, 42, 50-56. DOI:10.1016/j.injury.2010.06.008.

[43] Lu, G., Huang, J., Yu, J., Zhu, Y., Cai, L., Gu, Z., & Su, Q. (2011). Influence of early post-burn enteral nutrition on clinical outcomes of patients with extensive burns. Journal of Clinical Biochemistry and Nutrition, 48(3), 222-225. DOI:10.3164/jcbn.10-91.

[44] Silva, M.A., dos Santos, S.G.F., Tomasi, C. D., da Luz, G., Paula, M.M., Dal Pizzol, F., & Ritter, C. (2013). Enteral nutrition discontinuation and outcomes in general critically ill patients. Clinics (São Paulo, Brazil), 68(2), 173-178. DOI: 10.6061/clinics/2013(02)OA09.

[45] Azzopardi, N., & Ellul, P. (2013). Pneumonia and mortality after percutaneous endoscopic gastrostomy insertion. The Turkish Journal of Gastroenterology: The Official Journal of Turkish Society of Gastroenterology, 24(2), 109-116. DOI: 10.4318/tjg.2013.0512.

[46] Gomes, C.A.R., Lustosa, S. A. S., Matos, D., Andriolo, R., Waisberg, D. R., & Waisberg, J. (2012). Percutaneous endoscopic gastrostomy versus nasogastric tube feeding

for adults with swallowing disturbances. Cochrane Database of Systematic Reviews, 3, 1-50. DOI:10.1002/14651858.CD008096.pub3.

[47] Beavan, J., Conroy, S. P., Harwood, R., Gladman, J. R. F., Leonardi-Bees, J., Sach, T., Bowling, T., Sunman, W., & Gaynor, C. (2010). Does looped nasogastric tube feeding improve nutritional delivery for patients with dysphagia after acute stroke? A randomised controlled trial. Age and Ageing, 39, 624-630. DOI: 10.1093/ageing/afq088.

[48] Kim, H., Stotts, N. A., Froelicher, E. S., Engler, M. M., Porter, C., & Kwak, H. (2012). Adequacy of early enteral nutrition in adult patients in the intensive care unit. Journal of Clinical Nursing, 21, 2860-2869. DOI:10.1111/j.1365-2702.2012.04218.

[49] Roy, P., Person, B., Souday, V., Kerkeni, N., Dib, N., & Asfar, P. (2005). Percutaneous radiologic gastrostomy versus nasogastric tube in critically ill patients. Clinical Nutrition, 24(2), 321-325. DOI:10.1016/j.clnu.2004.11.006.

[50] Wu, P.Y., Kang, T.J., Hui, C.K., Hung, M.H., Sun, W.Z., & Chan, W.H. (2006). Fatal massive hemorrhage caused by nasogastric tube misplacement in a patient with mediastinitis. Journal of Formosan Medical Association, 105, pp. 80-85

[51] Hegde, H., V., & Rao, P. R. (2010). A near miss; malpositioned nasogastric tube in the left bronchus of a spontaneously breathing critically-ill patient. Current Anaesthesia & Critical Care, 21, 94-96. DOI:10.1016/j.cacc.2009.12.002.

[52] Dziewas, R., Ritter, M., Schilling, M., Konrad, C., Oelenberg, S., G., Nabavi, D., Stogbauer, F., Ringelstein, E.B., & Lüdemann, P. (2004). Pneumonia in acute stroke patients fed by nasogastric tube. Journal of Neurology, Neurosurgery & Psychiatry, 75(6), 852-856. DOI:10.1136/jnnp.2003.019075.

[53] Mizock, B.A. (2007). Risk of Aspiration in Patients on Enteral Nutrition: Frequency, Relevance, Relation to Pneumonia, Risk Factors, and Strategies for Risk Reduction. Current Gastroenterology Reports, 9, 338-344. Retrieved from http://link.springer.com.ezproxy.uct.ac.za/journal/11894/9/4/page/1.

[54] Jung, S.H., Dong, S. H., Lee, J.Y., Kim, N.H., Jang, J.Y., Kim, H.J., Kim, B.H., Chang, Y.W., & Chang, R. (2011). Percutaneous Endoscopic Gastrostomy Prevents Gastroesophageal Re?ux in Patients with Nasogastric Tube Feeding: A Prospective Study with 24- Hour pH Monitoring. Gut and Liver, 5(3), 288-292. DOI.org/10.5009/gnl.2011.5.3.28.

[55] Abuksis, G., Mor, M., Plaut, S., Fraser, G., & Niv, Y. (2004). Outcome of percutaneous endoscopic gastrostomy (PEG): Comparison of two policies in a 4-year experience. Clinical Nutrition (Edinburgh, Scotland), 23(3), 341-346. DOI:10.1016/j.clnu.2003.08.001.

[56] Johnston, S. D., Tham, T. C. K., & Mason, M. (2008). Death after PEG: Results of the national confidential enquiry into patient outcome and death. Gastrointestinal Endoscopy, 68(2), 223-227. DOI:10.1016/j.gie.2007.10.019.

[57] Dwyer, K.M., Watts, D.D., Thurber, J.S., Benoit, R.S., & Fakhry, S.M. (2002). Percutaneous endoscopic gastrostomy: The preferred method of elective feeding tube placement in trauma patients. Trauma, 52, 26-32. Retrieved from http://journals.lww.com/jtrauma/Abstract/2002/01000/Percutaneous_Endoscopic_Gastrostomy__The_Preferred.7.aspx.

[58] Moller, P., Lindberg., C-G., & Zilling, T. (1999). Gastrostomy by various techniques: Evaluation of indications, outcome, and complications. Scandanavian Journal of Gastroenterology,34, 1050-1054.

[59] Kurien, M., Leeds, J. S., Robson, H. E., James, G., Hoeroldt, B., Dear, K., Kapur, K., Grant, J., McAlindon, M.E., & Sanders, D. S. (2011). Survival following gastrostomy insertion: Are there differences in mortality according to referral indication? Gut, 60,A18-A19. DOI: 10.1136/gut.2011.239301.37.

[60] Richards, D., Tanikella, R., Arora, G., Guha, S., & Dekovich, A. (2013). Percutaneous endoscopic gastrostomy in cancer patients: Predictors of 30-day complications, 30-day mortality, and overall mortality. Digestive Diseases & Sciences, 58(3), 768-776. DOI:10.1007/s10620-012-2397-8.

[61] Grant, D. G., Bradley, P. T., Pothier, D. D., Bailey, D., Caldera, S., Baldwin, D. L., & Birchall, M. A. (2009). Complications following gastrostomy tube insertion in patients with head and neck cancer: A prospective multi-institution study, systematic review and meta-analysis. Clinical Otolaryngology, 34(2), 103-112. DOI:10.1111/j.1749-4486.2009.01889.

[62] Poulose, B., Kaiser, J., Beck, W., Jackson, P., Nealon, W., Sharp, K., & Holzman, M. (2013). Disease-based mortality after percutaneous endoscopic gastrostomy: Utility of the enterprise data warehouse. Surgical Endoscopy, 27(11), 4119-4123. DOI: 10.1007/s00464-013-3077-2.

[63] Schettler, A., Momma, M., Markowski, A., Schaper, R., Klamt, S., Vaezpour, R., & Schneider, A. (2013). Pp215-mon complication rate and mortality after percutaneous endoscopic gastrostomy are low and depend on the indication. Clinical Nutrition, 32, S202-S202. DOI:10.1016/S0261-5614(13)60525-7.

[64] Abuksis, G., Mor, M., Segal, N., Shemesh, I., Plout, S., Sulkes, J., Fraser, G.M., & Niv, Y. (2000). Percutaneous endoscopic gastrostomy: High mortality rates in hospitalized patients. The American Journal of Gastroenterology, 95(1), 128-132. DOI:10.1111/j.1572-0241.2000.01672.x.

[65] Cowey, E. (2012). End of life care for patients following acute stroke. Nursing Standard, 26(27), 42-46. Retrieved from http://web.b.ebscohost.com.ezproxy.uct.ac.za/ehost/pdfviewer/pdfviewer?sid=be9f53c3-a7f3-4c75-a392-ffef3e0bcec7%40sessionmgr198&vid=1&hid=110.

[66] Westaby, D., Young, A., O'Toole, P., Smith, G., & Sanders, D.S. (2010). The provision of a percutaenously placed enteral tube feeding service. Gut, 59, 1592-1605. DOI: 10.1136/gut.2009.204982.

[67] Kumar, S., Langmore, S., Goddeau, R., J., Alhazzani, A., Selim, M., Caplan, L. R., Zhu, L.,

[68] Grant, M. D., Rudberg, M. A., & Brody, J. A. (1998). Gastrotomy placement and mortality among hospitalized medicare beneficiaries. JAMA: The Journal of the American Medical Association, 279(24), 1973-1976. Retrieved from http://jama.jamanetwork.com.

[69] Ha, L., & Hauge, T. (2003). Percutaneous endoscopic gastrostomy (PEG) for enteral nutrition in patients with stroke. Scandinavian Journal of Gastroenterology, 38(9), 962. DOI 10.1080/00365520310005190.

[70] Zopf, Y., Maiss, J., Konturek, P., Rabe, C., Hahn, E. G., & Schwab, D. (2011). Predictive factors of mortality after PEG insertion: Guidance for clinical practice. JPEN.Journal of Parenteral and Enteral Nutrition, 35(1), 50-55. DOI: 10.1177/0148607110376197.

[71] Yokohama, S., Aoshima, M., Koyama, S., Hayashi, K., Shindo, J., & Maruyama, J. (2010). Possibility of oral feeding after induction of percutaneous endoscopic gastrostomy. Journal of Gastroenterology & Hepatology, 25(7), 1227-1231. DOI:10.1111/j. 1440-1746.2009.06190.

[72] MacDougall, C. (2010). SASPEN Case Study: Nutrition in the ICU and multi-organ failure. South African Journal of Clinical Nutrition, 23(3):157-159. Retrieved from http://www.ajol.info/index.php/sajcn/article/view/59893.

[73] Codner, P. A. (2012). Enteral nutrition in the critically ill patient. Surgical Clinics of North America, 92(6), 1485-1501. DOI:10.1016/j.suc.2012.08.005.

[74] Heyland, D.K., Drover, J.W., Dhaliwal, R., & Greenwood, J. (2002). Optimizing the benefits and minimizing the risks of enteral nutrition in the critically ill: Role of small bowel feeding. Journal of Parenteral and Enteral Nutrition, 26(6), 51-57. DOI: 10.1177/014860710202600608

[75] Sobani, Z., Ghaffar, S., & Ahmed, B. N. (2011). Comparison of outcomes of enteral feeding via nasogastric versus gastrostomy tubes in post operative patients with a principle diagnosis of squamous cell carcinoma of the oral cavity. Journal of the Pakistan Medical Association, 61(10), 1042-1045. Retrieved from http://ecommons.aku.edu/pakistan_fhs_mc_surg_otolaryngol_head_neck/12.

[76] Sheth C.H., Sharp S. & Walters E.R. (2013) Enteral feeding in head and neck cancer patients at a UK cancer centre. Journal of Human Nutrition and Dietetics, 26(5), 421-428. DOI:10.1111/jhn.12029

[77] Blomberg, J., Lagergren, P., Martin, L., Mattsson, F., & Lagergren, J. (2011). Albumin and C-reactive protein levels predict short-term mortality after percutaneous endo-

scopic gastrostomy in a prospective cohort study. Gastrointestinal Endoscopy, 73(1), 29-36. DOI:10.1016/j.gie.2010.09.012.

[78] Keung, E. Z., Liu, X., Nuzhad, A., Rabinowits, G., & Patel, V. (2012). In-hospital and long-term outcomes after percutaneous endoscopic gastrostomy in patients with malignancy. Journal of the American College of Surgeons, 215(6), 777-786. DOI:10.1016/j.jamcollsurg.2012.08.013.

[79] Sanders, D.S., Carter, M.J., D'Silva, J., James, G., Bolton, R.P., & Bardhan, K.D. (2000). Survival Analysis in Percutaneous Endoscopic Gastrostomy Feeding: A Worse Outcome in Patients with Dementia. The American Journal of Gastroenterology, 95(6), 1472-1475. DOI: 10.1016/S0002-9270(00)00871-6.

[80] Koretz, R. L., Avenell, A., Lipman, T. O., Braunschweig, C. L., & Milne, A. C. (2007). Does enteral nutrition affect clinical outcome? A systematic review of the randomized trials. American Journal of Gastroenterology, 102(2), 412-429. DOI:10.1111/j.1572-0241.2006.01024.

[81] Norman, K., Pitchard, C., Lochs, H., & Pirlich, M. (2008) Prognostic impact of disease-related malnutrition. Clinical Nutrition, 27, 5-15. DOI:10.1016/j.clnu.2007.10.007.

[82] Pear, S.M. (2007). Patient Risk Factors and Best Practices for Surgical Site Infection Prevention. Managing Infection Control. Accessed electronically from http://www.kchealthcare.com/media/1515/patient_risk_factors_best_practices_ssi.pdf on 07 July 2014

[83] Pratt, D.S. (2010). Liver chemistry and function tests. In: Feldman M, Friedman LS, Brandt LJ, eds. Sleisenger and Fordtran's Gastrointestinal and Liver Disease. 9th ed. Philadelphia: Saunders Elsevier, chapter 73. Retrieved from: http://www.nlm.nih.gov/medlineplus/ency/article/003480.htm

[84] Nair, R., Hertan, H., & Pitchumoni, C. S. (2000). Hypoalbuminemia is a poor predictor of survival after percutaneous endoscopic gastrostomy in elderly patients with dementia. The American Journal of Gastroenterology, 95 (1), 133-136. DOI:10.1111/j.1572-0241.2000.01673.x.

[85] O'Mahony, S. (2012). Dif?culties with percutaneous endoscopic gastrostomy (PEG): a practical guide for the endoscopist. Irish Journal of Medical Science, 182, 25-28. DOI 10.1007/s11845-012-0845-2.

[86] Playford, D. (2010). Oral feeding dif?culties and dilemmas: a guide to practical care particularly towards the end of life. Advances in Clinical Neuroscience and Rehabilitation, 10 (3), 39-40.

[87] Tanswell, I., Barrett, D., Emm, C., Lycett, W., Charles, C., Evans, K., & Hearing, S. D. (2007). Assessment by a multidisciplinary clinical nutrition team before percutaneous endoscopic gastrostomy placement reduces early postprocedure mortality..Journal of Parenteral and Enteral Nutrition, 31(3), 205-211. DOI: 10.1177/0148607107031003205.

[88] Buscaglia, J.M. (2006). Common issues in PEG tubes- what every fellow should know. Gastrointestinal Endoscopy, 64 (6), 970-972. DOI:10.1016/j.gie.2006.07.042.

[89] DeLegge, M. H., McClave, S. A., DiSario, J. A., Baskin, W. N., Brown, R. D., Fang, J. C., & Ginsberg, G. G. (2005). Ethical and medicolegal aspects of PEG-tube placement and provision of artificial nutritional therapy. Gastrointestinal Endoscopy, 62(6), 952-959. DOI:http://dx.doi.org.ezproxy.uct.ac.za/10.1016/j.gie.2005.08.024.

[90] Kurien, M., McAlindon, M. E., Westaby, D., & Sanders, D. S. (2010). Percutaneous endoscopic gastrostomy (PEG) feeding. BMJ: British Medical Journal (Overseas & Retired Doctors Edition), 340(7756), 1074-1078. DOI:10.1136/bmj.c2414.

[91] Daniel, K., Rhodes, R., Vitale, C., & Shega, J. (2014). American Geriatrics Society Feeding Tubes in Advanced Dementia Position Statement. Journal of the American Geriatrics Society, 62, 1590-1593. DOI: 10.1111/jgs.12924.

[92] Jordan, S., Philpin, S., Warring, J., Cheung, W.Y., & Williams, J. (2006). Percutaneous endoscopic gastrostomies: the burden of treatment from a patient perspective. Journal of Advanced Nursing, 56(3), 270-281. DOI: 10.1111/j.1365-2648.2006.04006.x.

[93] Rogers, S.N., Thomson, R., O'Toole, P., & Lowe, D. (2007). Patients experience with long-term percutaneous endoscopic gastrostomy feeding following primary surgery for oral and oropharyngeal cancer. Oral Oncology, 43(5), 499-507. DOI:10.1016/j.oraloncology.2006.05.002.

[94] Brotherton, A., Abbott, J., & Aggett, P. (2006). The impact of percutaneous endoscopic gastrostomy feeding upon daily life in adults. Journal of Human Nutrition and Diet, 19, 355-367. Retrieved from http://web.b.ebscohost.com.ezproxy.uct.ac.za/ehost/pdfviewer/pdfviewer?sid=1395252e-c7c2-4cb1-821d-ca78e8e674dd%40sessionmgr112&vid=0&hid=109.

[95] Anis, M.K., Abid, S., Jafri, W., Abbas, Z., Shah, H.A., Hamid, S., & Wasaya, R. (2006). Acceptability and outcomes of the Percutaneous Endoscopic Gastrostomy (PEG) tube placement- patients' and care givers' perspectives. Biomed Central Gastroenterology, 6(37). DOI:10.1186/1471-230X-6-37.

[96] Osborne, J.B., Collin, L.A., Posluns, E.C., Stokes, E.J., & Vandenbussche, K.A. (2012). The experience of head and neck cancer patients with a percutaneous endoscopic gastrostomy tube at a Canadian cancer center. Nutrition in Clinical Practice, 27(5), 661-668. DOI: 10.1177/0884533612457181.

[97] Brotherton, A., & Judd, P.A. (2007). Quality of life in adult enteral tube feeding patients. Journal of Human Nutrition and Diet, 20, 513-522. Retrieved from http://web.b.ebscohost.com.ezproxy.uct.ac.za/ehost/pdfviewer/pdfviewer?sid=9fef6b68-b6a0-46a2-bf7f-9231ce6fcf3b%40sessionmgr198&vid=1&hid=109.

[98] Martin, L., Blomberg, J., & Lagergren, P. (2012). Patients' perspectives of living with a percutaneous endoscopic gastrostomy (PEG). Biomed Central Gastroenterology, 12, 126-134. Retrieved from http://web.b.ebscohost.com.ezproxy.uct.ac.za/ehost/

pdfviewer/pdfviewer?sid=e8e849fd-2b09-4ae2-bfc8-8900217edf23%40ses-sionmgr198&vid=0&hid=109

[99] Lin, L.C., Li, M.H., & Watson, A. (2011). A survey of the reasons patients do not chose percutaneous endoscopic gastrostomy/jejunostomy (PEG/PEJ) as a route for long-term feeding. Journal of Clinical Nursing, 20, 802-810. doi: 10.1111/j.1365-2702.2010.03541.x.

[100] Goldberg, L.S., & Altman, K.W. (2014). The role of gastrostomy tube placement in advanced dementia with dysphagia: a critical review. Clinical Intervention in Aging, 9, 1733-1739. DOI.org/10.2147/CIA.S53153.

[101] Sampson, E.L., Candy, B., & Jones, L. (2009). Enteral tube feeding for older people with advanced dementia. Cochrane Database of Systematic Reviews,2. DOI: 10.1002/14651858.CD007209.pub2.

[102] Naidoo, S. (2012). The South African national health insurance: a revolution in health-care delivery. Journal of Public Health, 34(1), pp. 149-150. DOI:10.1093/pubmed/fds008.

[103] Heyland, D.K., Cahill, N.E., Dhaliwal, R., Sun, X., Day, A.G., & McClave, A. (2010). Impact of Enteral Feeding Protocols on Enteral Nutrition Delivery: Results of a Multicenter Observational Study. Journal of Parenteral and Enteral Nutrition, 34, 675-684. DOI: 10.1177/014607110364843.

[104] Loser, C., Aschi, G., Hebuterne, X., MArthus-Vliegen, E.M.H., Muscaritoli, M., Niv, Y., Rollins, H., Singer, P., & Skelly, R.H. (2005). ESPEN guidelines on artificial enteral nutrition - Percutaneous endoscopic gastrostomy (PEG). Clinical Nutrition, 24, 848-861. DOI: 10.1016/j.clnu.2005.06.013.

[105] Dev, R., Dalal, S., & Bruera, E. (2012). Is there a role for parenteral nutrition or hydration at the end of life? Current Opinion in Supportive and Palliative Care, 6(3), 365-370. DOI: 10.1097/SPC.0b013e328356ab4a.

[106] Stiles, E. (2013). Providing artificial nutrition and hydration in palliative care. Nursing Standard, 27(20), 35-42. Retrieved from http://web.a.ebscohost.com.ezproxy.uct.ac.za/ehost/pdfviewer/pdfviewer?sid=db9450ad-a4f4-45ad-8e1d-81850172d273%40sessionmgr4002&vid=0&hid=4206

[107] Byron, E., de Casterle, D., & Gastmans, C. (2012). 'Because we see them naked" - Nurses experiences in caring for hospitalised patients with dementia: Considering artificial nutrition and hydration (ANH). Bioethics, 26(6), 285-295. DOI:10.1111/j.1467-8519.2010.01875.

[108] Langmore, S., Krisciunas, G.P., Miloro, K.V., Evans, S. R., & Cheng, D.M. (2011). Does PEG Use Cause Dysphagia in Head and Neck Cancer Patients? Dysphagia, 27, 251-259. DOI 10.1007/s00455-011-9360-2.

Chapter 9

Dysphagia and the Family

Rebecca L. Nund, Nerina A. Scarinci,
Bena Cartmill and Elizabeth C. Ward

Additional information is available at the end of the chapter

http://dx.doi.org/10.5772/60856

1. Introduction

The medical effects of dysphagia, including dehydration, malnutrition, and aspiration, that lead to pneumonia are well documented throughout the literature, as are the negative consequences of dysphagia on an individual's functioning and quality of life. What is less known, however, is how the family members of people with dysphagia are impacted by this condition. Understanding the issues faced by individuals who support and care for family members with dysphagia, and exploring how health professionals can best support the needs of the entire family is an important and emerging area of both research and clinical practice.

2. The biopsychosocial effects of dysphagia

Dysphagia is traditionally defined as a difficulty or abnormality in swallowing. In adulthood, it is predominantly an acquired condition and may result from a wide variety of etiologies. It can also result from changes associated with the effects of normal aging [1]. Over the past four decades, the bulk of research conducted in the field of dysphagia and its management has focused on understanding this condition at an impairment level. Through this historical body of work, swallowing is now understood to be a complex physiological process that involves precision timing and coordination of multiple structures within the neuromuscular system. Oropharyngeal dysphagia can be associated with a range of physiological impairments, which may lead to difficulty in oral preparation of the bolus, moving the bolus posteriorly toward the pharynx, triggering and coordinating the pharyngeal swallow, clearing the bolus into the upper esophagus, and protecting the airway from food and fluid entry [2]. Depending on the etiology of the condition causing dysphagia, individuals may also be affected by associated impairments such as xerostomia (dry mouth), taste changes, or excessive secretions that may further impact capacity, motivation, and desire to eat. The associated medical effects resulting from difficulty in swallowing may include dehydration, malnutrition [3], and respiratory dysfunction (including pneumonia) [4], and ultimately can lead to death in severe cases [5].

The traditional management approaches that have evolved in parallel with our understanding of the process of normal swallowing have also been predominantly based on impairment. Interventions including postural strategies, swallowing techniques, and modification of food and fluid textures are used as first-line treatment options to compensate for specific physiological impairments and to improve the efficiency and safety of oropharyngeal swallowing function. Active rehabilitation programs, which are typically implemented in parallel to compensatory measures, are developed following a combination of clinical and objective assessments (videofluoroscopy or fiber-optic endoscopic evaluation of swallowing) and involve behavioral and medical interventions designed to improve swallowing physiology for long-term gain.

While management services for adult-acquired dysphagia remain predominantly focused on remediating physiological impairments, in particular, the need to consider the wider psychosocial impacts of dysphagia has been highlighted in the past decade. It is now recognized that health professionals must consider dysphagia and its effects more broadly, and that dysphagia is, in fact, a multifaceted condition. In addition to its impact on the medical condition of the individual, dysphagia has also been demonstrated to effect functioning in daily life and overall quality of life [6]. Eating and drinking is a source of human pleasure. Dysphagia can make this process and the activities surrounding it laborious, uncomfortable, and difficult [7]. Irrespective of the cause, dysphagia has been found to have a significant negative impact on the quality of life both immediately and months or years following its onset [5, 6, 8]. In the geriatric population, reduced quality of life has been associated with self-perceived swallowing difficulties, a condition that older people did not necessarily associate with normal aging [9].

Recent studies have also demonstrated the impact of dysphagia on psychosocial health. In a population-based study, dysphagia was reported by 16% of those surveyed, with intermittent dysphagia associated with anxiety and progressive dysphagia associated with depression [10]. Anxiety and depression are also significantly worse in head and neck cancer survivors with dysphagia than those without dysphagia, irrespective of treatment type [8, 11]. For people with dysphagia, difficulty in swallowing has been found to affect socialization, eating out, family rituals, cooking, and shopping [12-14]. As such, the concept of dysphagia needs to be reconsidered. Dysphagia is more than simply a physical difficulty. Rather it represents a complex and multilayered condition that may impact on a person's physical, emotional, and social life and carries significant burden surrounding functioning in everyday activities.

In order to embrace a wider view of dysphagia, a new conceptual framework is required. The International Classification of Functioning, Disability and Health (ICF) [15] (Figure 1) has been both proposed [16] and used [17-21] as a consistent and universal taxonomy to report research outcomes regarding dysphagia. The ICF is a conceptual framework that provides a biopsychosocial perspective of functioning, and uses an internationally recognized language [15]. It has the potential to describe the far-reaching complexities of dysphagia through the consideration of functioning from the perspective of the body, the individual, and society in two

http://dx.doi.org/10.5772/60856

parts: (1) functioning and disability and (2) contextual factors [15]. Functioning and disability comprises (a) the body functions and body structures and (b) activities and participation. The contextual factors are comprised of (a) environmental factors and (b) personal factors (WHO, 2001) (Figure 1).

Each of the components of the ICF consists of various domains and categories that are referred to as the units of classification. Therefore, the functioning of an individual with a health condition can be documented using the appropriate category code and then adding qualifiers, which are numeric codes that specify the magnitude of the individual's functioning or disability within that category [15]. An alphanumeric coding system is used for coding health conditions in the ICF. The letters *b, s, d,* and *e* represent body functions, body structures, activities and participation, and environmental factors respectively. A numeric code then follows these letters, which denotes the domain (or chapter number), followed by additional sublevels of coding, and then the qualifiers (WHO, 2001). For example, changes to taste would be linked to the code b250 - taste function where *b* represents the body functions domain and the numbers (i.e., 250) represent the various levels of classification.

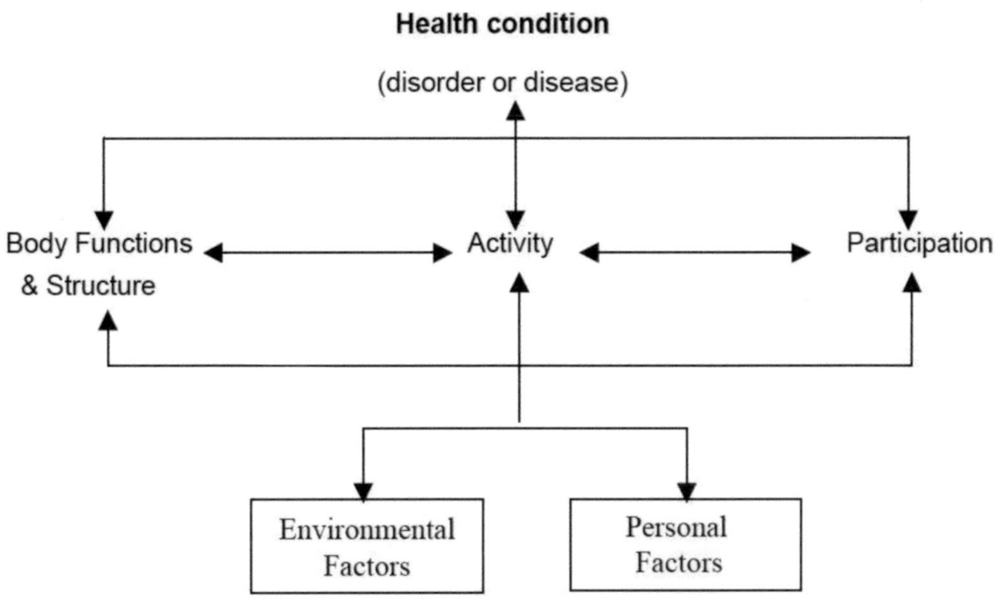

Figure 1. International Classification of Functioning, Disability and Health (ICF) [15]

Recently, a study examining the consumer's perspective of living with dysphagia following management for head and neck cancer utilized the ICF to classify patients' physical, emotional, and psychosocial concerns relating to their dysphagia [20]. The results demonstrated that dysphagia impacted on body functions, activities and participation, and environmental factors almost equally, with changes to body structures rarely mentioned by people with dysphagia. Therefore when dysphagia is examined more broadly, using a framework such as the ICF, it clearly has far-reaching life effects beyond the physiological changes to the swallow and the medical implications of dysphagia.

3. The effects of dysphagia on the family

Mealtimes, eating, and drinking are profoundly social activities that sustain not only our physiological needs but also our social and emotional life [22]. The meanings we attach to food, and the processes of eating and swallowing are deeply connected to our most valued activities and experiences, and are integral to how we see ourselves as individuals and in relation to others [23]. As such the negative effects of dysphagia are recognized to influence more than just the life of the person with the condition.

In a recent study that mapped the experiences of living with dysphagia following nonsurgical head and neck cancer management to the ICF, a number of environmental factors were identified to influence the functioning (and disability) of the individuals with dysphagia [20]. In particular, family members were identified as important sources of support for people with dysphagia throughout the trajectory of care, particularly in regards to meal preparation and the encouragement to keep eating [20]. In addition to playing an important support role, there is emerging evidence to indicate that families also experience negative effects as a result of living with and supporting individuals with dysphagia [24-26]. For the purposes of this chapter, family is defined as any individual who plays a significant role in the life of the person with dysphagia. This definition encompasses a broad concept of family, and is consistent with other literature, whereby family is described as being two or more people who are related in any way, including through a continuing biological, legal, or emotional relationship [27].

Recent research has demonstrated the pervasive effects of dysphagia on family members following a number of different etiologies including head and neck cancer treatment [24, 26, 28, 29], stroke [25], traumatic brain injury [25], and motor neuron disease [30]. This body of evidence has revealed that families are important members of the support team for people with dysphagia as they provide valuable practical and emotional support. The high levels of burden experienced by family members in relation to food and meal preparation may hinder their ability to function effectively as a support system for the individual with dysphagia [24, 26, 31]. It can also affect their physical and psychological health, and quality of life [24, 25, 32].

Verdonck de Leeuw et al. [32] found that the presence of a gastrostomy tube, a surrogate indicator of dysphagia, in people with head and neck cancer was the only significant predictor of distress in family carers. Supporting this, the family members of people with head and neck cancer and dysphagia have been shown to experience a reduced quality of life both before cancer treatment and in the early acute phase, with significant improvements shown between 3 and 12 months post-treatment [24]. Evidence supports that the family member's quality of life was found to significantly correlate with the functioning of their family member with dysphagia [24]. Therefore, the presence of dysphagia has the potential to have significant effects, not only on the life of the person with dysphagia but also on their family. Despite differing etiologies, family members of people with dysphagia consistently report negative effects on their everyday lives as a result of the dysphagia particularly in relation to: managing modified diets/fluids, and providing appropriate meals; negative influences of dysphagia on family dynamics and social activities; and the emotional impacts of dysphagia [24-26, 28-30].

3.1. Managing modified diets and fluids and providing appropriate meals

A number of studies have noted that family members of people with dysphagia report experiencing distress associated with food preparation and mealtime activities [24-26, 31]. Consistently across multiple studies, family members reported changes to their meal preparation, noting a need for more conscious and intentional thought and planning, and the need to cook two separate meals [24-26]. Preparing food and meals is one of the most significant ways of providing care, and demonstrating love and concern for others [22, 24, 33]. Though often discounted as trivial, there are a number of important skills involved in the work of "feeding the family" [22]. These skills include: planning meals, learning the food preferences of others, learning about food and preparation techniques, provisioning and shopping for food, preparing meals, serving meals, feeding, and cleaning up from meals.

Meals have been described as fundamental to our daily thinking and acting and are core component to how we organize our days [34]. It is has been estimated that the average person makes over 260 decisions a day regarding eating and that more than 200 of these choices are made subconsciously [35]. When it comes to preparing meals for an individual with dysphagia, decisions regarding eating and drinking are likely to increase and will likely no longer be subconscious. Putting a meal together requires more than cooking as it takes "thoughtful foresight, simultaneous attention to several different aspects of a project, and a continuing openness to ongoing events and interactions" (p. 55) [22]. When a family member has dysphagia, putting a meal together becomes a more intense and time-consuming process [26].

3.2. Influence of dysphagia on family dynamics and social activities

Dysphagia has a recognized influence on family dynamics [24-26, 30, 31]. Many families report the need to accommodate the needs of their family member with dysphagia and consistently find a disruption to family mealtimes [26]. For a number of families, their meals are now dictated by what their family member with dysphagia can eat and some families also eat textured modified diets [26]. In addition, several families have commented that they no longer ate meals together as they did not want to eat in front of their family member with dysphagia [26, 30]. Those that did reported changes to the meaning and experiences of family meals [24-26]. In some studies family members reported leaving the dinner table because they could not cope with their family member's dysphagia [25, 26]. Family mealtimes are often acknowledged as an important get-together time to enrich family life and "eating together means staying together" (p. 11) [34]. When one member of the family can no longer fully engage in the mealtime experience because of dysphagia, the effects are felt by the entire family unit as there is a loss in the social bonds of food and meals [24-26, 30, 31].

The effects of dysphagia, on family members at mealtimes, are not limited to the home. Numerous studies have documented the negative effects of dysphagia on family member's social lives including eating out at restaurants and attending significant events such as weddings and holidays leading to further feelings of frustration and isolation [24-26]. Some family members reported looking for opportunities to eat foods that their family member could no longer eat when their family member with dysphagia was not present [26]. Despite the disruptions to family meals and social engagements, the family members in one study reported that they believed the dysphagia did not have a significant impact on their relationship, but had in fact brought them closer together, indicating that family members learn to adapt and adjust to the dysphagia [26].

3.3. Emotional impacts of dysphagia

Numerous emotional impacts of dysphagia on family members have been discussed in the current literature. These emotional impacts have been expressed around a variety of areas. Johansson and Johansson [25] noted that family members of people with dysphagia following stroke or traumatic brain injury expressed concern about their family member's health and well-being, particularly regarding nutrition, weight maintenance, and the need to pay special attention to texture-modified diets. These findings are similar to those found in family members of people with dysphagia following head and neck cancer. Both Patterson et al. [24] and Nund et al. [26] discussed feelings of fear, guilt, frustration, anger, stress, and helplessness over the enforced changes to meal preparation [24,26]. In addition, family members expressed feelings of insecurity, uncertainty, loneliness, and frustration [24-26] when leaving the care of the hospital services. Family members in these studies reported feeling ill-prepared and anxious regarding the increased responsibilities for their family member's food and eating [25-27]. These findings across studies highlight the need for specific interventions for family members to build capacity and provide support in the multiple roles they undertake in caring for their family member with dysphagia [26].

4. Third-party disability in dysphagia

The impact of dysphagia on an individual's family is increasingly being acknowledged as an important consequence of dysphagia [24-26]. The effects of a health condition, such as dysphagia, on the functioning (and disability) of family has been termed "third-party disability" and identified as an area for future work by the WHO [15]. The concept of third-party disability is raised in the situation where the family member may not have a health condition; however, they may experience activity limitations and participation restrictions as a result of their family member's dysphagia.

Although the concept of third-party disability is still under some conceptual debate, to date the ICF has been used successfully to describe the third-party disability of spouses of older people with hearing impairment [36]; close family members of people with aphasia [37]; and more recently, family members of people with dysphagia following head and neck cancer [38].

A model extending the ICF to explain third-party disability has been proposed [36] and an adapted version of this model, specifically relating to dysphagia, is shown in Figure 2. This adapted model demonstrates how the functioning and disability of an individual with dysphagia acts as an environmental factor for the family member, influencing their functioning (and disability).

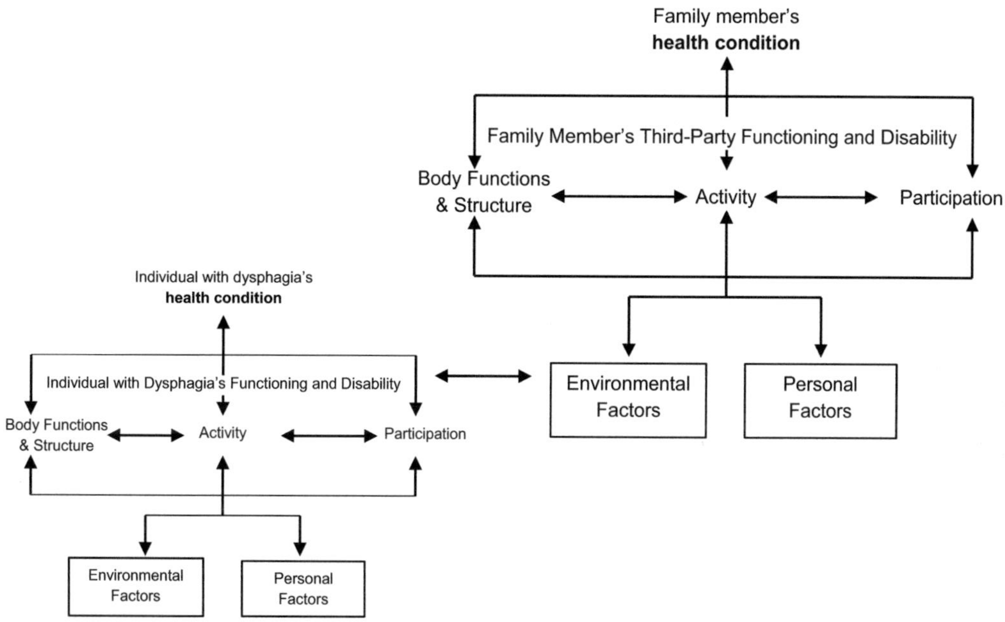

Figure 2. Application of the ICF to family members of people with dysphagia (adapted from Scarinci et al. [36])

In a recent study that mapped family members ' experience of dysphagia following head and neck cancer to the ICF, Nund et al. [38] found that the majority of their concerns were linked to the activities and participation component of the ICF (e.g., difficulties or changes to meal preparation were linked to the activities and participation component). It should be noted, however, that these difficulties were generally determined to be performance problems rather than capacity limitations [38]. The difficulties experienced by family members regarding meal preparation were not related to impairments in their body functions, or even in their capacity to prepare a meal. Rather, family members reported experiencing difficulties preparing meals because their family member with dysphagia had specific requirements regarding food and fluids [38].

This finding is consistent with the definition of third-party disability whereby although the family member does not have a health condition, they experience activity limitations and participation restrictions as a result of their partner's health condition (i.e., as a result of their partner's dysphagia) [14]. In this mapping process, it was observed that the most relevant domains of the activities and participation component of the ICF were those of interpersonal interactions and relationships, domestic life, general tasks and demands, learning and applying knowledge, self-care, major life areas, and community, social and civic life [38]. The number of relevant activity and participation domains highlights the pervasive effects of dysphagia on the life of the carer and demonstrates that food and meals underpin a number of life areas for family members of head and neck cancer survivors with dysphagia. This study confirmed that ICF terminology can be used successfully to describe the multifaceted and complex effects of dysphagia on family members of people treated nonsurigcally for head and neck cancer.

5. Strategies used by family members to cope with dysphagia

In reponse to the pervasive effects of dysphagia, studies reported to date have identified a number of strategies and processes family members adopt to adjust and cope with their family member's dysphagia and the associated impacts on their life [24-26]. A predominant theme across studies is the acceptance of a new normal. That is accepting that meal preparation, mealtimes, and social occassions may never be the same. In order to reach this point, family members across studies noted the need to negotiate changing roles in regards to their family members dysphagia and the need to take on more roles within the household [24-26].

Other strategies reported by family members include maintaining a positive attitude; looking for opportunities to eat foods that their partner could not eat when they were not present; and using trial and error strategies to learn what foods their family member could and could not eat. Each of these strategies and adjustment processes were often made without the support of health professionals and family members across studies have consistently reported the need for further education, training, and support from health professionals to help them adapt and adjust to their family member's dysphagia regardless of etiology or severity of dysphagia [25, 26, 29].

6. Role of family-centered care in dysphagia management

Given the emerging evidence supporting the important role of family members in the provision of informal care for people with dysphagia, and the potential for third-party disability in family members of people with dysphagia, active involvement of family members in all aspects of dysphagia assessment and intervention is clearly indicated. This could be achieved in dysphagia management by shifting from a patient-focused, impairment-based model of intervention, to providing a more holistic, family-centered approach. The Institute for Patient- and Family-Centered Care [39] define family-centered care (FCC) as "... an approach to the planning, delivery, and evaluation of healthcare that is governed by mutually beneficial partnerships between healthcare providers, patients and families." Although traditionally used in pediatrics, FCC can be applied to people of all ages, and used in any health care setting [39, 40].

http://dx.doi.org/10.5772/60856

The term "family-centered care" is sometimes used synonymously with patient-centered care and client-centered care. However, an important distinction between FCC and the other forms of centeredness is that FCC seeks to explicitly assist families in ways that are important to family members [41, 42]. As such, FCC ensures that care is planned around the whole family; and importantly, the entire family is recognized as receivers of care, not just the individual with dysphagia [43, 44]. In the context of third-party disability, FCC is the most relevant type of centeredness in health care because it emphasizes the importance of health care that is mutually beneficial to all [45].

The principles of FCC originated in the field of psychology, and specifically, family-systems theory. According to family-systems theory, the behavior of any individual should be viewed in the context of their family's social system [46]. This consideration is supported by empirical evidence showing that family relationships affect biological systems, psychological well-being, and health behavior [47]. Therefore, consideration of the contribution of family relationships to health outcomes is an important consideration for any health service. Family-systems theory also supports the notion that family members play an important role in promoting ongoing change and development in an individual's functioning, and these changes have the potential to affect the entire family unit.

Given FCC has its roots in theories from psychology, there is a body of evidence in the field of psychology supporting the efficacy of involving family members in interventions. The range of psychological disorders for which involvement of family members has been investigated has been diverse, but includes such conditions as obsessive compulsive disorder and problem-gambling [48-57]. This body of research has shown that interventions that include family members are more effective than individual treatment [52, 54]. Research has also demonstrated that the inclusion of family members in intervention increases opportunities for the family to improve their communication [53, 57]. Involvement of family members also allows professionals to obtain a more holistic view of the true impact of the problem as well as the role of family dynamics [56].

Research in pediatric health care has long demonstrated the benefits of FCC for children with a variety of health conditions. A recent systematic review highlighted the benefits for both patients and family members in terms of improvements in the health condition, improved efficiencies and access to health care services, and improved communication between health care professionals and families [58]. In terms of family functioning, a meta-analysis by Dunst et al. [59] also showed improved family behavior and functioning as a result of FCC. More recently, the application of FCC to adult health care services has been discussed in the literature [40], with a number of documented benefits. Studies have shown that active engagement of family members in medical consultations for patients with chronic conditions results in greater patient engagement in decision making [60], improved recall of information [61], improved satisfaction with care and health-related quality of life [62, 63], increased compliance with medical treatments [64], decreased depression rates, and overall better family dynamics for patients and family members [65, 66]. These benefits have been shown to be especially strong for families of patients with physical health conditions due to the physical assistance provided by these family members on a daily basis [67-69]. In the case of dysphagia, it is expected that due to the chronic nature of this condition and the ongoing supports required by family members in mealtime preparation and assistance, the application of FCC for this population would yield similar benefits.

The Institute for Patient- and Family-Centered Care [39] describes four key components for applying FCC, which could be implemented in dysphagia management: (1) respect and dignity for patients and family members, such that health care professionals listen to and honor the perspectives and choices of patients and family members; (2) the provision of complete and unbiased information to patients and family members such that they can participate effectively in the decision-making process; (3) participation of patients and family members in all aspects of care and decision making; and (4) collaboration with patients and family members in all levels of health care, including policy and program development, implementation and evaluation, facility design, professional education, and in the delivery of care.

In listening and honoring the perspective and choices of people with dysphagia and their family members, clinicians should follow the recommendations outlined by Laidsaar-Powell et al. [70] in order to optimize family member involvement. These include: encouraging, welcoming and involving family members in all aspects of the consultation; and determining the reason for the presence of family members from the perspective of both the patient and family member. Although family members of people with dysphagia may attend consultations with the patient, their role may traditionally be viewed by the health professional as that of "support person" for the individual with dysphagia. However, a recent systematic review of family member involvement in physician consultations highlighted that family members may play a number of roles in supporting patients, ranging from being a memory aide and transcriber to providing emotional support and serving as an advocate and interpreter [70].

A narrow perception of these roles by health professionals may serve to prevent full and active participation in the management plan, with a recent study indicating that health professionals may miss valuable opportunities for engaging family members in designing chronic care management plans, and failing to facilitate participation of family members in consultations [71]. Thus, in order to facilitate FCC in dysphagia management, clinicians should not only be mindful of highlighting helpful behaviors from family members; but also clarifying and agreeing on the role of the family member in the initial stages of the consultation. Laidsaar-Powell et al. [70], however, highlight the importance of respecting patient preferences for family member involvement, ensuring that patients consent to and support the involvement of their family member.

In dysphagia management, the provision of health information that is complete and unbiased is especially important given the health-related quality of life implications of dysphagia [2, 5]. Both people with dysphagia and their family members report the need for more personalized and practical information regarding dysphagia management [13, 26, 28-31]. Johnson [72] further emphasizes the importance of providing complete and unbiased information on a continuous basis. This, of course, is especially important for people with dysphagia who may not understand or have difficulty following recommendations due to associated cognitive impairments [73], and require their family member to take full responsibility for the decision-making process. In dysphagia management, health information must be both family-centered and holistic in nature, to ensure that the full consequences of dysphagia on the everyday lives of people with dysphagia and their family members are discussed. Previous research has documented the desire of both people with dysphagia and their families to receive more information regarding the potential everyday impacts of dysphagia and how these impacts can be managed [14, 26]. In addition to providing information about the everyday impacts of dysphagia, in order to provide effective FCC, health professionals should also provide information about the role of family members in the management process [74], including issues relating to meal preparation, shopping for textured modified foods, household organization, nutrition, and encouraging their family member with dysphagia to keep eating [26], and importantly, discussion of strategies and resources that may aid them in this role.

Another consideration for clinicians is how this information provided to people with dysphagia and their family members could most effectively inform shared decision making. Shared decision-making is one of the key principles of FCC and involves active participation of both the patient and family in the decision-making process. Kaizer et al. [73] described a shared decision-making model that was used with people with dysphagia and their family members in a rehabilitation hospital setting. Kaizer et al. [73] acknowledged that the use of a family-centered shared decision-making model was important in the management of dysphagia as the success of dysphagia recommendations required considerable cooperation and participation of both people with dysphagia and their family members. Engagement of people with dysphagia and their family in the decision-making process is especially important to ensure that they understand and agree with the recommendations being made. In situations when patients and families feel "forced" to follow a management plan they do not agree with, divisions may develop between family members, hampering positive relations between the patient and family and the health care team [73].

It is clear that in order to promote the best possible outcomes for people with dysphagia, and minimize the third-party disability experienced by family members of people with dysphagia, the provision of more holistic, family-centered approach to dysphagia management is recommended. This chapter has provided some key evidence supporting the use of FCC in other areas of health care, which could readily be applied to services for people with the dysphagia and their families. Some important considerations for the successful implementation of FCC have also been discussed, with concepts from other fields of health care applied to dysphagia rehabilitation.

7. Conclusion

Current research has documented both the medical, psychosocial, and health-related quality of life impacts of dysphagia. In addition, emerging research is also demonstrating the pervasive nature of dysphagia on family members. Though the physiological impacts of dysphagia are generally well recognized and managed, people with dysphagia and their families may also experience significant negative effects on their daily lives including impacts on meal preparation, family dynamics and family mealtimes, social occasions, and psychological effects. Though clinicians generally recognize the importance of family members, many focus their attention on the individual with dysphagia and therefore the effect of dysphagia on family members is rarely assessed or managed. Providing a more holistic and family-centered approach to dysphagia assessment and management, using a framework such as the ICF, may not only assist the family, but may also result in more positive long-term outcomes for people with dysphagia. In the next decade, further research is required to document the effects of dysphagia on the family and to develop new and innovative treatments for family-centered care in dysphagia management.

Author details

Rebecca L. Nund[1,2*], Nerina A. Scarinci[1], Bena Cartmill[2,3] and Elizabeth C. Ward[1,2]

*Address all correspondence to: r.nund@uq.edu.au

1 School of Health and Rehabilitation Sciences, The University of Queensland, St Lucia Campus, Brisbane, Australia

2 Centre for Functioning and Health Research, Metro South Hospital and Health Services, Brisbane, Australia

3 Speech Pathology Department, Princess Alexandra Hospital, Brisbane, Australia

References

[1] Sura, L., et al., Dysphagia in the elderly: management and nutritional considerations. Clin Interv Aging, 2012. 7(1): 287-98.

[2] Logemann, J.A., Evaluation and treatment of swallowing disorders. 2nd ed. 1998, Austin, TX: PRO-ED.

[3] Foley, N.C., et al., A review of the relationship between dysphagia and malnutrition following stroke. Journal of Rehabilitation Medicine, 2009. 41(9): 707-713.

[4] Perry, L. and C.P. Love, Screening for dysphagia and aspiration in acute stroke: A systematic review. Dysphagia, 2001. 16(1): 7-18.

[5] Leow, L.P., et al., The impact of dysphagia on quality of life in ageing and Parkinson's disease as measured by the swallowing quality of life (SWAL-QOL) questionnaire. Dysphagia, 2010. 25(3): 216-220.

[6] Davis, L.A., Quality of life issues related to dysphagia. Topics in Geriatric Rehabilitation, 2007. 23(4): 352-365.

[7] Vesey, S., Dysphagia and quality of life. British Journal of Community Nursing, 2013. 18(Sup5): S14-S19.

[8] García-Peris, P., et al., Long-term prevalence of oropharyngeal dysphagia in head and neck cancer patients: impact on quality of life. Clinical Nutrition, 2007. 26(6): 710-717.

[9] Chen, P.-H., et al., Prevalence of perceived dysphagia and quality-of-life impairment in a geriatric population. Dysphagia, 2009. 24(1): 1-6.

[10] Eslick, G.D. and N. Talley, Dysphagia: epidemiology, risk factors and impact on quality of life-a population-based study. Alimentary pharmacology & therapeutics, 2008. 27(10): 971-979.

[11] Nguyen, N.P., et al., Impact of dysphagia on quality of life after treatment of head-and-neck cancer. International Journal of Radiation Oncology Biology Physics, 2005. 61(3): 772-778.

[12] Regnard, C., et al., Gastrostomies in dementia: Bad practice or bad evidence? Age and Ageing, 2010. 39(3): 282-284.

[13] Nund, R.L., et al., The lived experience of dysphagia following non-surgical treatment for head and neck cancer. International Journal of Speech-Language Pathology, 2014. 16(3): 282-289.

[14] Nund, R.L., et al., Survivors' experiences of dysphagia-related services following head and neck cancer: Implications for clinical practice. International Journal of Language & Communication Disorders, 2014. 49(3): 354-363.

[15] World Health Organization, International Classification of Functioning, Disability and Health. 2001, Geneva: World Health Organization.

[16] Threats, T.T., Use of the ICF in dysphagia management. Seminars in Speech and Language, 2007. 28(4): 323-333.

[17] Cartmill, B., et al., Long-term functional outcomes and patient perspective following altered fractionation radiotherapy with concomitant boost for oropharyngeal cancer. Dysphagia, 2012. 27(4): 481-490.

[18] Frowen, J.J. and A.R. Perry, Swallowing outcomes after radiotherapy for head and neck cancer: a systematic review. Head & Neck, 2006. 28(10): 932-944.

[19] Hutcheson, K.A. and J.S. Lewin, Functional outcomes after chemoradiotherapy of laryngeal and pharyngeal cancers. Current Oncology Reports, 2012. 14(2): 158-165.

[20] Nund, R.L., et al., Application of the International Classification of Functioning, Disability and Health (ICF) to people with dysphagia following non-surgical head and neck cancer management. Dysphagia, 1.-12. 2014. 29:692-703.

[21] Roe, J.W.G., et al., Swallowing outcomes following intensity modulated radiation therapy (IMRT) for head & neck cancer: A systematic review. Oral Oncology, 2010. 46(10): 727-733.

[22] DeVault, M.L., Feeding the family: The social organization of caring as gendered work. 1991, Chicago, IL: University of Chicago Press.

[23] DeRenzo, E.G., Ethical considerations in dysphagia treatment and research: Secular and sacred, in Dysphagia: A continuum of care, B.C. Sonies, Editor. 1997, Aspen Publishers: Gaithersburg, MD. 91-106.

[24] Patterson, J.M., et al., Head and neck cancer and dysphagia; caring for carers. Psycho-Oncology, 2013. 22(8): 1815-1820.

[25] Johansson, A.E.M. and U. Johansson, Relatives' experiences of family members' eating difficulties. Scandinavian Journal of Occupational Therapy, 2009. 16(1): 25-32.

[26] Nund, R.L., et al., Carers' experiences of dysphagia in people treated for head and neck cancer: A qualitative study. Dysphagia, 2014. 29(4): 450-458.

[27] Kilmer, R.P., J.R. Cook, and E. Munsell, Moving from principles to practice: Recommended policy changes to promote family-centered care. American Journal of Community Psychology, 2010. 46(3-4): 332-341.

[28] Mayre-Chilton, K.M., B.P. Talwar, and L.M. Goff, Different experiences and perspectives between head and neck cancer patients and their care-givers on their daily impact of a gastrostomy tube. Journal of Human Nutrition and Dietetics, 2011. 24(5): 449-459.

[29] Penner, J.L., et al., Family members experiences caring for patients with advanced head and neck cancer receiving tube feeding: A descriptive phenomenological study. Journal of Pain and Symptom Management, 2012. 44(4): 563-571.

[30] Stavroulakis, T., et al., The impact of gastrostomy in motor neurone disease: Challenges and benefits from a patient and carer perspective. BMJ Supportive & Palliative Care, 2014.

[31] Locher, J.L., et al., Disruptions in the organization of meal preparation and consumption among older cancer patients and their family caregivers. Psycho-Oncology, 2010. 19(9): 967-974.

[32] Verdonck-de Leeuw, I.M., et al., Distress in spouses and patients after treatment for head and neck cancer. The Laryngoscope, 2007. 117(2): 238-241.

[33] Reid, J., et al., The experience of cancer cachexia: A qualitative study of advanced cancer patients and their family members. International Journal of Nursing Studies, 2009. 46(5): 606-616.

[34] Meiselman, H.L., Dimensions of the meal. Journal of Foodservice, 2008. 19(1): 13-21.

[35] Wansink, B., Mindless eating: Why we eat more than we think. 2010, New York: Bantam.

[36] Scarinci, N.A., L. Worrall, and L. Hickson, The ICF and third-party disability: Its application to spouses of older people with hearing impairment. Disability & Rehabilitation, 2009. 31(25): 2088-2100.

[37] Grawburg, M., et al., Describing the impact of aphasia on close family members using the ICF framework. Disability & Rehabilitation, 2013. 36: 1184-95.

[38] Nund, R.L., et al., Third-party disability in carers of people with dysphagia following non-surgical management for head and neck cancer. Disability & Rehabilitation, 2015.

[39] Institute for Patient- and Family-Centered Care. Frequently asked questions. 2010. September 15, 2014.

[40] Bamm, E.L. and P. Rosenbaum, Family-centered theory: Origins, development, barriers, and supports to implementation in rehabilitation medicine. Archives of Physical Medicine and Rehabilitation 2008. 89(8): 1618-24.

[41] Crais, E.R., V.Roy, and K. Free, Parents' and professionals' perceptions of the implementation of family-centered practices in child assessments. American Journal of Speech-Language Pathology, 2006. 15(4): 365-377.

[42] Dempsey, I. and D. Keen, A review of processes and outcomes in family-centered services for children with a disability. Topics in Early Childhood Special Education, 2008. 28(1): 42-52.

[43] Dunst, C.J., Family-centered practices: Birth through high school. The Journal of Special Education, 2002. 36(3): 141-149.

[44] Shields, L., J. Pratt, and J. Hunter, Family centred care: A review of qualitative studies. Journal of Clinical Nursing, 2006. 15(10): 1317-1323.

[45] Johnson, B.H., Family-centered care: Facing the new millennium. Interview by Elizabeth Ahmann. Pediatric Nursing, 2000. 26(1): 87-90.

[46] Goldenberg, H. and I. Goldenberg, Family therapy: An overview. 8th ed. 2013, Belmont, CA: Brooks/Cole.

[47] Martine, L.M. and R. Schultz, Involving family in psychosocial interventions for chronic illness: Are there added benefits to patients and family members? Current Directions in Psychological Science, 2007. 16: 90-94.

[48] Black, D.R., L.J. Gleser, and K.J. Kooyers, A meta-analytic evaluation of couples weight-loss programs. Health Psychology, 1990. 9(3): 330-347.

[49] Edwards, M.E. and Steinglass, Family therapy treatment outcomes for alcoholism. Journal of Marital and Family Therapy, 1995. 21(4): 475-509.

[50] Eisler, I., The empirical and theoretical base of family therapy and multiple family day therapy for adolescent anorexia nervosa. Journal of Family Therapy, 2005. 27(2): 104-131.

[51] Eisler, I., et al., Family therapy for adolescent anorexia nervosa: The results of a controlled comparison of two family interventions. Journal of Child Psychology and Psychiatry, 2000. 41(6): 727-736.

[52] Emmelkamp, P.M.G. and I. De Lange, Spouse involvement in the treatment of obsessive-compulsive patients. Behaviour Research and Therapy, 1983. 21(4): 341-346.

[53] Kalischuk, R.G., et al., Problem gambling and its impact on families: A literature review. International Gambling Studies, 2006. 6(1): 31-60.

[54] Mehta, M., A comparative study of family-based and patient-based behavioural management in obsessive-compulsive disorder. The British Journal of Psychiatry, 1990. 157(1): 133-135.

[55] Renshaw, K.D., G. Steketee, and D.L. Chambless, Involving family members in the treatment of OCD. Cognitive Behaviour Therapy, 2005. 34(3): 164-175.

[56] Steinberg, M.A., Couples treatment issues for recovering male compulsive gamblers and their partners. Journal of Gambling Studies, 1993. 9(2): 153-167.

[57] Tepperman, J.H., The effectiveness of short-term group therapy upon the pathological gambler and wife. Journal of Gambling Behavior, 1985. 1(2): 119-130.

[58] Kuhlthau, K.A., et al., Evidence for family-centered care for children with special health care needs: A systematic review. Academic Pediatrics, 2011. 11(2): 136-143..

[59] Dunst, C.J., C.M. Trivette, and D.W. Hamby, Meta-analysis of family-centered help-giving practices research. Mental Retardation and Developmental Disabilities Research Reviews, 2007. 13(4): 370-378.

[60] Clayman, M.L., et al., Autonomy-related behaviors of patient companions and their effect on decision-making activity in geriatric primary care visits. Social Science & Medicine, 2005. 60(7): 1583-1591.

[61] Jansen, J., et al., The role of companions in aiding older cancer patients to recall medical information. Psycho-Oncology, 2010. 19(2): 170-179.

[62] Street, R.L. and H.S. Gordon, Companion participation in cancer consultations. Psycho-Oncology, 2008. 17(3): 244-251.

[63] Wolff, J.L. and D.L. Roter, Hidden in plain sight: Medical visit companions as a resource for vulnerable older adults. Archives of Internal Medicine, 2008. 168(13): 1409-1415.

[64] DiMatteo, M.R., Social support and patient adherence to medical treatment: A meta-analysis. Health Psychology, 2004. 23(2): 207-218.

http://dx.doi.org/10.5772/60856

[65] Visser-Meily, A., et al., Intervention studies for caregivers of stroke survivors: A critical review. Patient Education and Counseling, 2005. 56(3): 257-267.

[66] Van Horn, E., J. Fleury, and S. Moore, Family interventions during the trajectory of recovery from cardiac event: An integrative literature review. Heart & Lung, 2002. 31(3): 186-198.

[67] Martire, L.M., The "relative" efficacy of involving family in psychosocial interventions for chronic illness: Are there added benefits to patients and family members? Families, Systems, & Health, 2005. 23(3): 312-328.

[68] Nezu, A.M., et al., Project Genesis: Assessing the efficacy of problem-solving therapy for distressed adult cancer patients. Journal of Consulting and Clinical Psychology, 2003. 71(6): 1036-1048.

[69] Martire, L.M., et al., Feasibility of a dyadic intervention for management of osteoarthritis: A pilot study with older patients and their spousal caregivers. Aging & Mental Health, 2003. 7(1): 53-60.

[70] Laidsaar-Powell, R.C., et al., Physician-patient-companion communication and decision-making: A systematic review of triadic medical consultations. Patient Education and Counseling, 2013. 91(1): 3-13.

[71] Boehmer, K.R., et al., Missed opportunity? Caregiver participation in the clinical encounter. A videographic analysis. Patient Education and Counseling, 2014. 96(3): 302-307.

[72] Johnson, B.H., The changing role of families in health care. Children's Health Care, 1990. 19(4): 234-241.

[73] Kaizer, F., A.M. Spiridigliozzi, and M.R. Hunt, Promoting shared decision-making in rehabilitation: Development of a framework for situations when patients with dysphagia refuse diet modification recommended by the treating team. Dysphagia, 2012. 27(1): 81-87.

[74] Wolff, J.L., et al., Going it together: Persistence of older adults' accompaniment to physician visits by a family companion. Journal of the American Geriatrics Society, 2012. 60(1): 106-112.

Section 4

Dysphagia in Specific Populations

Chapter 10

Dysphagia in Parkinson's Disease

Rosane Sampaio Santos,
Carlos Henrique Ferreira Camargo,
Edna Márcia da Silva Abdulmassih and
Hélio Afonso Ghizoni Teive

Additional information is available at the end of the chapter

http://dx.doi.org/10.5772/60983

1. Introduction

Parkinson's disease (PD) is the second most common neurodegenerative disorder among the elderly after Alzheimer's disease. It affects around 1% of the population over 65 years of age and has a prevalence of 4% or more among individuals over the age of 85 years [1]. The condition is primarily the result of a progressive, chronic loss of dopaminergic neurons in the substantia nigra and striatum and presents with or without intracytoplasmic Lewy body deposits [1-3]. A monogenic etiology is found in only around 5% of cases. In cases that do not have a monogenic etiology, the condition is known as sporadic or idiopathic PD and occurs as a result of interaction between a series of hereditary and environmental factors [3].

Bradykinesia, tremors, rigidity, and postural instability are the main motor signs of PD [4]. PD also presents with a series of non-motor manifestations, including changes in behavior, cognition, learning, and the autonomic nervous system. Dysautonomias are major complications of PD and include orthostatic (postural) hypotension (OH), constipation, anhydrosis, erectile dysfunction, sialorrhea, dysphagia, esophageal dysmotility, gastroparesis, irritable bladder symptoms, and nocturia [5-7].

Dysphagia is a problematic and sometimes dangerous feature of PD. Oropharyngeal dysphagia can have a negative impact on quality of life [8,9] and increases the risk of aspiration pneumonia, which is often a cause of death in PD [10,11]. Subjective dysphagia occurs in one third of PD patients. Objectively measured dysphagia rates are much higher, with four out of five patients being affected. The prevalence of dysphagia in four studies was between 72% and 87%, with a pooled prevalence estimate of 82% (95% CI 77%–87%), suggesting that while the condition is common in PD, patients do not always report swallowing difficulties unless asked. This under-reporting calls for a proactive clinical approach to dysphagia, particularly in light of the serious clinical consequences of the condition [12].

The aim of this chapter is to show dysphagia as a symptom/sign and an important cause of disability in patients with PD.

2. Definition and classification of Parkinsonism and PD

PD is a progressive parkinsonism of undetermined cause without features suggestive of an alternative diagnosis. It responds to dopaminergic treatment and is associated with depletion of dopaminergic neurons and the presence of Lewy body inclusions in some of the remaining nerve cells [13-15].

The diagnosis of PD is based on clinical criteria as there is no definitive laboratory test to diagnose the disorder. Pathological confirmation of Lewy bodies on autopsy, a hallmark of PD, has historically been considered the standard criterion for diagnosis [13]. In clinical practice, diagnosis is usually based on the presence of a number of cardinal motor features, response to levodopa, associated symptoms, and the exclusion of other disorders [15]. When patients have a classical presentation, diagnosis of PD is relatively simple. However, differentiating PD from other forms of parkinsonism in the early stages of the disease, when signs and symptoms overlap with other syndromes, can be difficult [16]. Criteria for diagnosis of PD were developed by the UK Parkinson's Disease Society Brain Bank (Table 1) and the National Institute of Neurological Disorders and Stroke (NINDS) [7,14]. When standard clinical criteria such as the UK Parkinson's disease brain bank criteria are used, significantly more accurate clinical diagnosis of the disease is possible; however, as many as 10% of patients diagnosed with the disease in life will still need to be reclassified at post-mortem examination [17]. These criteria have been estimated to have a diagnostic specificity and sensitivity of 98.6% and 91.1%, respectively [18].

Parkinsonian disorders can be classified into four categories: primary (idiopathic) parkinsonism, secondary (acquired, symptomatic) parkinsonism, heredodegenerative parkinsonism, and multiple system degeneration (parkinsonism plus syndromes). A number of features, including tremor, early gait abnormality (e.g., freezing), postural instability, pyramidal tract signs, and response to levodopa, can be used to distinguish PD from other parkinsonian disorders. While differences in the density of postsynaptic dopamine receptors in PD patients or patients with atypical parkinsonian disorders have been used to account for the poor response to levodopa therapy in the latter group, other explanations may also be possible [19].

http://dx.doi.org/10.5772/60983

UK Parkinson's Disease Society Brain Bank
Step 1
Bradykinesia
At least one of the following criteria:
Muscular Rigidity
4–6 Hz rest tremor
Postural instability not caused by primary visual, vestibular, cerebellar, or proprioceptive dysfunction
Step 2
Exclude other causes of parkinsonism
Step 3
At least three of the following supportive (prospective) criteria:
Unilateral onset
Rest tremor
Progressive disorder
Persistent asymmetry affecting the side of onset most
Excellent response (70%–100%) to levodopa
Severe levodopa-induced chorea (dyskinesia)
Levodopa response for 5 years or more
Clinical course of 10 years or more

Table 1. Diagnostic criteria for Parkinson's disease (PD) [7,14]

3. Non-motor symptoms in Parkinson's disease

In his "Essay on the Shaking Palsy," James Parkinson did not consider PD to be just a motor disorder, and in 1817 he described the presence of sleep disturbance, constipation, dysarthria, dysphonia, dysphagia, sialorrhea, urinary incontinence, and constant sleepiness with slight delirium [20]. What has been well established is that in PD patients, non-motor symptoms (NMS) occur in more than 90% of individuals in all stages of the disorder and include a variety of symptoms from neuropsychiatric and autonomic dysfunction to sleep disturbances and little-understood and little-reported sensory symptoms such as pain and impaired vision [21]. These NMS frequently occur throughout the course of PD and may occur concurrently with motor symptoms or precede their onset by several years [22]. In advanced PD, NMS have been recognized as important factors associated with impaired quality of life [23] and impose a considerable economic burden on patients' families and society [24].

In contrast to the motor symptoms of PD, NMS are often under-recognized during routine clinical visits and poorly managed in clinical practice [21,25]. Indeed, they have only recently been considered sufficiently important to warrant study by clinicians and researchers. In a prospective study of 101 PD patients, neurologists failed to identify the presence of depression, anxiety, and fatigue in over 50% of patients and the presence of sleep disturbance in 40% [26].

4. Clinical features and diagnosis of dysphagia in Parkinson's disease

Oropharyngeal dysphagia in PD may limit or preclude safe oral feeding, reducing the patient's full capacity in society and resulting in social, psychological, and economic problems for the individual [27].

One of the first reports of parkinsonian dysphagia was in 1817 by James Parkinson, who described a typical case of PD with weight loss, difficulty in swallowing solids and liquids, sialorrhea, and reduced tongue movements [21].

In 1983, Longemann proposed the videofluoroscopic swallowing study (VFSS) as a means of assessing the dynamics of swallowing. Parkinsonian VFSS [27] can show specific impairments, such as those in the oral pharyngeal and esophageal phases. In the oral phase, these include orofacial tremor, difficulty forming a cohesive food bolus, prolonged swallowing time, limited tongue and mandibular excursion during mastication, and the presence of repetitive antero-posterior movements of the tongue during bolus propulsion (lingual festination). Pharyngeal phase impairments include delayed pharyngeal response with consequent stasis in the valleculae and piriform sinuses, with the risk of laryngeal penetration and aspiration, and impairment of pharyngeal muscle contraction and cricopharyngeal function [28]. Impairments in the esophageal phase of swallowing include reduced peristalsis and reduced transit time. All of these disturbances occur together with the traditional motor symptoms of PD (bradykinesia and rigidity) as a result of degeneration of the autonomic nerve system and voluntary muscle system [29, 30].

The incidence of swallowing disorders in PD varies from 50% to 100% of patients. Another characteristic reported in studies of dysphagia in PD is that it may be present without symptoms, making it difficult to identify the condition early and, consequently, to plan a more efficient therapeutic approach [27].

Interestingly, many patients who do not complain of feeding difficulties report having eliminated certain types of food that caused them swallowing difficulties, often restricting themselves to food with a purée consistency. Some patients report weight loss associated with swallowing disorders.

As a result of swallowing disturbances, parkinsonian patients may present with tracheal aspiration (entry of material into the airway), which is generally asymptomatic and known as silent aspiration. Tracheal aspiration related to swallowing is a major cause of morbidity and mortality in PD, suggesting a reduction in voluntary mechanisms that protect the upper airways [31].

http://dx.doi.org/10.5772/60983

5. Management of dysphagia in patients with Parkinson's disease

Treatment of PD has traditionally been pharmacologic and was revolutionized by the discovery that levodopa is able to penetrate the blood--brain barrier and be converted to dopamine in the central nervous system. However, the effect of pharmacologic treatment on oral communication and swallowing is still controversial.

Drug treatment appears to have little effect on speech and swallowing disturbances compared with the major effect it has on motor symptoms in the trunk and limbs. In a study on voice and swallowing, when patients were asked about the effects of medication, all reported clear improvements in general physical symptoms, but only three out of twenty-four patients reported improvements in oral communication and swallowing symptoms. This suggests that both dysarthrophonia and dysphagia are related to dysfunction of nondopaminergic neuronal pathways [27].

Although the subject of much controversy in the past, the value of speech therapy has been confirmed in several objective studies [29-31]. The effects of speech therapy on voice and swallowing were analyzed in a study, which showed that there was a 100% improvement in symptoms after therapy, particularly increased sphincteric action of the larynx [27].

Speech therapy for parkinsonian dysphagia includes exercises to increase mobility of oropharyngeal and laryngopharyngeal structures involved in mastication and swallowing, specific techniques to improve formation and propulsion of the bolus, and maneuvers that increase airway protection during swallowing. In cases of severe dysphagia, speech language pathologists work with compensatory strategies such as modifications in bolus consistency and viscosity and postural maneuvers [31].

In 1987, Lorraine Olson Raming and Carolyn Mead developed an effective treatment program for individuals with PD voice tremor. The technique is known as LSVT (Lee Silverman Voice Treatment) and was named after the first patient who received the treatment (Lee Silverman). The basic principle used in this approach involves increasing vocal effort to enable patients to speak louder. An important study reported significant improvements in swallowing in patients who received LSVT treatment. Temporal measurements such as oral and pharyngeal transport time, duration of contact between the base of the tongue and the pharynx and duration of velopharyngeal closure and laryngeal elevation were taken. There was a 51% improvement in dysphagia after LSVT [32].

Biofeedback is a technique that uses visual or auditory references and electromyography, mirrors or other tools to show physiological events to the patient. It is used to enhance learning by means of exteroceptive systems, which replace inadequate proprioceptive signals, to improve voluntary motor control, to provide more specific, faster sensory information and to facilitate motor relearning. Visual information can compensate for sensorimotor loss by allowing individuals to assimilate lost or altered information and reduce body asymmetry by reestablishing a central motor program that takes into account position and movement [32,33].

Doppler sonar has been investigated as a method for assessing swallowing [34]. The feasibility of using this method as an aid to the assessment of swallowing and the benefits it brings have been confirmed in recent studies. The use of Doppler sonar to provide biofeedback of swallowing in PD patients not only helps them understand the swallowing process and how they can influence it, but also enables them to derive satisfaction from performing an activity over which they previously seemed to have no control.

6. Conclusion

Oropharyngeal dysphagia is a common symptom in PD and can develop at any time during the course of the disease. In fact, some authors have suggested that dysphagia may be one of the initial symptoms of PD.

Treatment of dysphagia in PD requires specialized rehabilitation combining treatment strategies that maximize social functioning, minimize the swallowing burden on the patient, and improve mental health [35].

Author details

Rosane Sampaio Santos[1], Carlos Henrique Ferreira Camargo[2*],
Edna Márcia da Silva Abdulmassih[3] and Hélio Afonso Ghizoni Teive[3]

*Address all correspondence to: chcamargo@uol.com.br

1 Tuiuti University of Paraná, Brazil

2 Hospital Universitário dos Campos Gerais, Department of Medicine, State University of Ponta Grossa, Brazil

3 Hospital de Clínicas, Federal University of Paraná, Brazil

References

[1] Diedrich M, Kitada T, Nebrich G, Koppelstaetter A, Shen J, Zabel C, et al. Brain region specific mitophagy capacity could contribute to selective neuronal vulnerability in Parkinson's disease. Proteome Sci. 2011;9(59):1-18.

[2] Moore S, Dilda V, Hakim B, Macdougall HG. Validation of 24-hour ambulatory gait assessment in Parkinson's disease with simultaneous video observation. Biomed Eng Online. 2011 Sep 21;10:82.

[3] Klein C, Westenberger A. Genetics of Parkinson's disease. Cold Spring Harb Perspect Med. 2012 Jan;2(1):1-15.

[4] Rodriguez-Oroz MC, Jahanshahi M, Krack P, Litvan I, Macias R, Bezard E, et al. Initial clinical manifestations of Parkinson's disease: features and pathophysiological mechanisms. Lancet Neurol. 2009 Dec;8(12):1128-1139.

[5] Oka H, Masayuki Y, Onouchi K, Morita M, Mochio S, Suzuki M, et al. Characteristics of orthostatic hypotension in Parkinson's disease. Brain. 2007;130:2425-2432.

[6] Varanese S, Birnbaum Z, Rossi R, Di Rocco A. Treatment of advanced Parkinson`s disease. Parkinsons Dis. 2011 Feb 7;2010:480260. doi: 10.4061/2010/480260.

[7] Hughes AJ, Daniel SE, Kilford L, Lees AJ. Accuracy of clinical diagnosis of idiopathic Parkinson's disease: a clinicopathologic study of 100 cases of Parkinson's disease. J Neurol Neurosurg Psychiatry. 1992 Mar;55(3):181-184.

[8] Plowman-Prine EK, Sapienza CM, Okun MS, Pollock SL, Jacobson C, Wu SS, et al. The relationship between quality of life and swallowing in Parkinson's disease. Mov Disord. 2009;24:1352-1358.

[9] Han M, Ohnishi H, Nonaka M, Yamauchi R, Hozuki T, Hayashi T, et al. Relationship between dysphagia and depressive states in patients with Parkinson's disease. Parkinsonism Relat Disord. 2011;17:437-439.

[10] Beyer MK, Herlofson K, Arsland D, Larsen JP. Causes of death in a community-based study of Parkinson's disease. Acta Neurol Scand. 2001;103:7-11.

[11] Mehanna R, Jankovic J. Respiratory problems in neurologic movement disorders. Parkinsonism Relat Disord. 2010;16:628-638.

[12] Kalf JG, de Swart BJ, Bloem BR, Munneke M. Prevalence of oropharyngeal dysphagia in Parkinson's disease: a meta-analysis. Parkinsonism Relat Disord. 2012 May;18(4): 311-315.

[13] Gibb WR, Lees AJ. The relevance of the Lewy body to the pathogenesis of idiopathic Parkinson's disease. J Neurol Neurosurg Psychiatry. 1988;51:745-752.

[14] Gelb DJ, Oliver E, Gilman S. Diagnostic criteria for Parkinson disease. Arch Neurol. 1999;56:33-39.

[15] Tolosa E, Wenning G, Poewe W. The diagnosis of Parkinson's disease. Lancet Neurol. 2006;5:75-86.

[16] Rao G, Fisch L, Srinivasan S, et al. Does this patient have Parkinson disease? JAMA. 2003;289:347-353.

[17] Hughes AJ, Daniel SE, Lees AJ. Improved accuracy of clinical diagnosis of Lewy body Parkinson's disease. Neurology. 2001;57:1497-1499.

[18] Hughes AJ, Daniel SE, Ben-Shlomo Y, Lees AJ. The accuracy of diagnosis of parkinsonian syndromes in a specialist movement disorder service. Brain. 2002;125(part 4): 861-870.

[19] Jankovic J. Parkinson's disease: clinical features and diagnosis. J Neurol Neurosurg Psychiatry. 2008;79:368-376.

[20] Teive HA. Charcot's contribution to Parkinson's disease. Arq Neuropsiquiatr. 1998 Mar;56(1):141-145.

[21] Chaudhuri KR, Odin P, Antonini A, Martinez-Martin P. Parkinson's disease: the non-motor issues. Parkinsonism Relat Disord. 2011 Dec;17(10):717-723.

[22] Tolosa E, Gaig C, Santamaria J, Compta Y. Diagnosis and the premotor phase of Parkinson disease. Neurology. 2009;72:S12-S20.

[23] Li H, Zhang M, Chen L, Zhang J, Pei Z, Hu A, et al. Nonmotor symptoms are independently associated with impaired health-related quality of life in Chinese patients with Parkinson's disease. Mov Disord. 2010;25:2740-2746.

[24] Wang G, Cheng Q, Zheng R, Tan YY, Sun XK, Zhou HY, et al. Economic burden of Parkinson's disease in a developing country: a retrospective cost analysis in Shanghai, China. Mov Disord. 2006;21:1439-1443.

[25] Chen W, Xu ZM, Wang G, Chen SD. Non-motor symptoms of Parkinson's disease in China: a review of the literature. Parkinsonism Relat Disord. 2012 Jun;18(5):446-452.

[26] Shulman LM, Taback RL, Rabinstein AA, Weiner WJ. Non-recognition of depression and other non-motor symptoms in Parkinson's disease. Parkinsonism Relat Disord. 2002;8:193-197.

[27] Carrara-Angelis E. Voz e deglutição. In: Andrade LAF, Barbosa RE, Cardoso F, Teive HAG. Doença de Parkinson: estratégias atuais de tratamento. 2. ed. São Paulo: Segmento Farma, 2006. pp. 197-207.

[28] Troche MS, Sapienza CM, Rosenbek JC, et al. Effects of bolus consistency on timing and safety of swallow in patients with Parkinson's disease. Dysphagia. 2008;23:26-32.

[29] Potulska A, Friedman AA, Królicki L, et al. Swallowing disorders in Parkinson's disease. Parkinsonism Relat Disord. 2003;9:349-353.

[30] Gross RD, Atwood CW Jr, Ross SB, Eichhorn KA, Olszewski JW, Doyle PJ. The coordination of breathing and swallowing in Parkinson's disease. Dysphagia. 2008;23:136-145.

[31] Jost WH. Gastrointestinal dysfunction in Parkinson's Disease. J Neurol Sci. 2010;289(1-2):69-73.

[32] Carrara-Angelis E, Moura LF, Ferraz HB. Effect of voice rehabilitation on oral communication of Parkinson's disease patients. Acta Neurol Scand. 1997;96:199-250.

[33] Perez-Lloret S, Nègre-Pagès L, Ojero-Senard A, Damier P, Destée A, Tison F, Merello M, Rascol O, COPARK Study Group. Oro-buccal symptoms (dysphagia, dysarthria,

http://dx.doi.org/10.5772/60983

and sialorrhea) in patients with Parkinson's disease: preliminary analysis from the French COPARK cohort. Eur J Neurol. 2012;19:28-37.

[34] Santos RS, Abdulmassi EM, Zeigeilboim BS, Teive HAG. Analysis of Swallowing sounds through sonar doppler in patients with Parkinsons disease. Parkinsonism Relat Disord. 2012;18:S20.

[35] Leow LP, Huckabee ML, Anderson T, Beckert L. The Impact of dysphagia on quality of life in ageing and Parkinson's disease as measured by the swallowing quality of life (SWAL-QOL) questionnaire. Dysphagia. 2009;25(3):216-220.

Chapter 11

Dysphagia in Dystonia

Carlos Henrique Ferreira Camargo, Edna Márcia da Silva Abdulmassih, Rosane Sampaio Santos and Hélio Afonso Ghizoni Teive

Additional information is available at the end of the chapter

http://dx.doi.org/10.5772/60765

1. Introduction

The word *dystonia* comes from the modern Latin *dys-* and the Greek *tonos* [1,2]. It is defined as a state of disordered tonicity, especially of muscle tissue. The word tone itself has musical connotations. It derives from the thirteeth-century old French *ton*, of the voice. The Latin word *tonus* meant a stretching, quality of sound, tone, or accent and in turn is derived from the Greek *tonos*, similarly translated as stretching, tension and raising of the voice and pitch. In modern usage, the word dystonic is applied to abnormal tension resulting in abnormal postures present in many disorders [2]. The definition of dystonia was recently revisited. In 2013, an international consensus committee proposed the following revised definition: *Dystonia is a movement disorder characterized by sustained or intermittent muscle contractions causing abnormal, often repetitive, movements, postures, or both. Dystonic movements are typically patterned, twisting, and may be tremulous. Dystonia is often initiated or worsened by voluntary action and associated with overflow muscle activation* [3].

The condition affects most voluntary muscles and is known as cervical dystonia (CD) when the neck muscles are affected. The term spasmodic torticollis was previously used for this syndrome, but it does not stress the dystonic nature of the disease [4]. Oromandibular dystonia (OMD) spasms of the masticatory, facial and lingual muscles result in repetitive and sometimes sustained jaw opening, closure, deviation or any combination of these, as well as abnormal tongue movements [5].

Various studies have shown that before treatment is started, some focal craniocervical dystonias such as spasmodic dysphonia and CD can be accompanied by a range of swallowing difficulties [6-15]. The incidence of dysphagia varies between 22 and 100 % of CD patients and is usually over 50 %. It increases significantly after botulinum toxin (BoNT) injection [8,11,12]. Dysphagia is suspected in 36 % of patients with CD on the basis of clinical assessment, and the incidence increases to 72 % on electrophysiological evaluation of oropharyngeal swallowing and after selective rhizotomy [8,9]. Similarly, dysphagia in patients with spasmodic dysphonia has been reported before and after treatment of this condition [13-15]. Because of the anatomical distribution of the affected muscles, OMD and co-existing oral-buccal-lingual (OBL) dyskinesias are associated with abnormal perioral, oral and lingual movements that can interfere with tasks such as chewing, swallowing and speaking, leading to social embarrassment and even eating disorders and weight loss. Eating dysfunction has been reported in 15.6 % of OMD cases [16]. Pharyngeal OMD often affects the pharyngeal constrictor muscles and can occur with spasmodic dysphonia. Choking and difficulty in swallowing are common complaints. After treatment of spasmodic dysphonia, there may be an unexpected improvement in pharyngeal dystonia. Treatment for pharyngeal constriction muscle dysfunction is nearly always associated with dysphagia [17].

Although new radiologic changes were observed in 50 % of CD patients following BoNT-A treatment, clinically only 33 % of the patients reported new dysphagia symptoms. The severity of the new dysphagia symptoms correlated strongly with the severity of new radiologic pharyngeal abnormalities [8].

In this chapter the role of dysphagia as a clinical symptom of cranio-cervical dystonia is discussed and the occurrence of dysphagia as a common adverse effect of treatment for dystonias is described.

2. Classification of dystonias

If defining dystonia is difficult and controversial, classifying the various forms of dystonias is a much more complex task, primarily because the term dystonia can mean not only a disease but also a symptom that can be part of many disorders with a wide range of causes. In an attempt to clarify the term, three "surnames" for dystonia were proposed: "symptom", "movement" and "disorder". A patient may complain of dystonia if, for example, he has a twisted neck. The patient has a dystonia symptom (dystonia^{Sx}). On examination, the signs of dystonia may be confirmed. This patient then has a dystonia movement (dystonia^{Mov}). Finally, dystonia as a disorder (dystonia^{Dx}) requires a clinicopathologic understanding of the etiology of the disease, i.e., whether it is genetic, late-onset, post-traumatic, or has other etiologies [18]. These new definitions led to the replacement of the 1998 dystonia classification [3] by a new one in 2013. The dystonias are now subdivided according to whether they are the result of pathological changes or structural damage, have acquired causes or are hereditary. If there is no clearly defined etiology, the dystonia can be classified as idiopathic familial or idiopathic sporadic [3].

Recent years have seen significant progress being made in our understanding of the genetics of dystonias as new loci and genes have been identified. For generalized dystonias, the genetic mechanisms are better understood, while for focal dystonias, the genes and genetic susceptibility to the disorder are not yet well identified. Hereditary dystonias (dystonia^{Dx}) are clinically and genetically heterogeneous. The known genetic forms include all monogenic inheritance

http://dx.doi.org/10.5772/60765

patterns (autosomal recessive, autosomal dominant, and X-linked). Table 1 shows the hereditary dystonias grouped according to their similarities. They are divided according to their clinical features (axis I) and etiology (axis II) in line with the new 2013 classification.

3. Phenomenology and clinical features of cranio-cervical dystonias

3.1. Blepharospasm

Blepharospasm (BSP) is a form of focal dystonia characterized clinically by involuntary periocular spasms resulting in forceful eye closure [20,21,22]. BSP is characterized by tonic, phasic or combined involuntary tonic-phasic contractions of the orbicularis oculi muscles, producing repeated and frequent blinking and persistent forceful closure of the eyelids with various degrees of functional blindness. The characteristic features of BSP include sensory tricks that patients use to relieve their symptoms (geste antagoniste) and a high frequency of ocular symptoms starting before or at the onset of the spasm [20,21,22]. BSP may be associated with inhibition of the levator palpebrae muscle (apraxia of eyelid opening) or involuntary movements in the lower face or jaw muscles [20,21,22]. Apraxia of eyelid opening may in turn be associated with other neurological conditions, such as progressive supranuclear palsy and corticobasal degeneration [21,22].

3.2. Oromandibular dystonia

OMD refers to involuntary spasms of masticatory, lingual, and pharyngeal muscles that result in jaw closing (JC), jaw opening (JO), jaw deviation (JD), or a combination of these abnormal movements [22,23]. When OMD is associated with blepharospasm, the combination is referred to as "cranial dystonia" or, less appropriately, as "Meige's syndrome" [24]. Because of the anatomical distribution of the affected muscles, OMD and co-existing OBL dyskinesias are associated with abnormal perioral, oral and lingual movements that can interfere with chewing, swallowing and speaking, leading to social embarrassment [25] and even eating disorders and weight loss [26]. Examination may reveal a variety of antagonistic maneuvers, or sensory tricks, including touching the lips or chin, chewing gum, or biting on a toothpick [21]. Even using these sensory tricks, patients often feel socially embarrassed by the spasms, which give them a disfigured appearance [22].

3.3. Lingual dystonia

Dystonic involvement of the tongue is a well-recognized feature of tardive dystonia as well as OMD, both primary and secondary, although primary focal lingual dystonia (PFLD) has only rarely been described. PFLD presents as an action dystonia during speech or in paroxysmal episodic lingual dystonic spasms [27]. A rare disorder, it can be severe enough to affect speech, swallowing and breathing. Tardive lingual dystonia secondary to dopamine-receptor-blocking drugs may manifest as a relatively isolated problem. Although severe tongue protrusion, particularly during eating, is characteristic of neuroacanthocytosis, it can also be seen in other rare forms of symptomatic dystonias such as pantothenate kinase-associated neurodegeneration and Lesch–Nyhan syndrome [21].

3.4. Laryngeal dystonia

Laryngeal dystonia (spasmodic dysphonia) is a neurological voice disorder with low prevalence. It is characterized by involuntary adductor (toward the midline) or abductor (away from the midline) vocal fold spasms during phonation that cause phonatory breaks [20,22]. Some patients also present with a mixed type of this disorder. Onset of laryngeal dystonia frequently occurs late in life and presents in mild to severely disabling forms that lead to long-lasting impaired verbal communication. Adductor spasmodic dysphonia (SD) is undoubtedly the most common form [22]. Both forms rarely occur in the same individual. Around one-third of SD sufferers also present with voice tremor, which makes the pitch and loudness of the voice waver at 5 Hz during vowels and is most apparent when the sound "/a/" (as in "all") is produced for at least 5 s [28].

3.5. Cervical dystonia

CD is characterized by involuntary posturing of the head as a result of involuntary spasms, jerks, or tremors (or a combination of all three) and is often associated with neck pain. Clinical classification is based on the position of the head and type of movement. The most common form is rotational torticollis (>50 %). Other relatively frequent forms include laterocollis and retrocollis, while anterocollis and complex forms of CD (in which there is no predominant component) are less common. Patients frequently present with a combination of abnormal patterns, even when it is possible to identify a predominant component [29]. A number of sensory tricks, including touching the contralateral side of the face as well as ipsilateral to the direction of head rotation, can produce a temporary improvement in involuntary neck movements. As with other forms of focal dystonia, the symptoms of CD are exacerbated by stress and improved by relaxation [20,29].

Clinical category	Designation	Clinical characteristics	Locus	Gene	Inheritance pattern
Isolated dystonias					
Persistent dystonias					
Childhood- or adolescent-onset dystonias	DYT1	Early-onset primary generalized dystonia	9q	*TOR1-A or DYT1*	AD
	DYT2	Autosomal recessive idiopathic dystonia	-	-	AR
	DYT6	Mixed dystonia	8p	*THAP1* or DYT6	AD
	DYT13	Early-onset primary segmental craniocervical dystonia	1p	-	AD

http://dx.doi.org/10.5772/60765

Clinical category	Designation	Clinical characteristics	Locus	Gene	Inheritance pattern
	DYT17	Idiopathic autosomal recessive primary dystonia	20pq	-	AR
Adult-onset dystonias	DYT7	Adult-onset focal dystonia	18p	-	AD
	DYT21	Late-onset autosomal dominant focal dystonia	2q	-	AD
	DYT23	Adult-onset primary cervical dystonia	9q	*CIZ1*	AD
	DYT24	Autosomal dominant craniocervical dystonia	11p	*ANO3*	AD
	DYT25	Late-onset autosomal dominant primary focal dystonia	18p	*GNAL*	AD
Combined dystonias					
Persistent dystonias					
Dystonias with parkinsonism					
Without any evidence of degeneration	DYT5	Dopa-responsive dystonia or Segawa dystonia	14q/1p	*GCH1 and TH*	AD and AR
	DYT12	Rapid-onset dystonia parkinsonism	19q	*ATP1A3*	AD
	DYT16	Adolescent-onset dystonia parkinsonism	2p	*PRKRA or DYT16*	AR
With evidence of degeneration	DYT3	X-linked dystonia-parkinsonism or lubag	Xq	*TAF1 or DYT3*	XR
Dystonias with myoclonus	DYT11	Myoclonus-dystonia	7q	-	AD
	DYT15	Myoclonus-dystonia	18p	*SGCE*	AD
Dystonias with chorea	DYT4	Dystonia with whispering dysphonia	19p	*TUBB4*	AD
Paroxysmal dystonias					
Paroxysmal dyskinesias	DYT8	Paroxysmal nonkinesigenic dyskinesia 1	2q	*MR-1*	AD

Clinical category	Designation	Clinical characteristics	Locus	Gene	Inheritance pattern
	DYT20	Paroxysmal nonkinesigenic dyskinesia 2	2q	-	AD
	DYT10	Paroxysmal kinesigenic dyskinesia 1	16pq	*PRRT2*	AD
	DYT19	Paroxysmal kinesigenic dyskinesia 2	16q	-	AD
	DYT18	Exercise-induced paroxysmal dyskinesia	1p	*SLC2A1* or GLUT1	AD

*Based on Albanese et al. [3] and Lohmann and Klein [19]

AD – Autosomal dominant, AR – Autosomal recessive, XR – X-linked recessive

Table 1. The hereditary dystonias *

4. Treatment of craniocervical dystonias with BoNT

While BoNT treatment remains the treatment of preference for most focal dystonias, pharmacological and neurosurgical treatments are also important in the treatment algorithm. Treatment with BoNT in properly adjusted doses is known to be effective and safe for cranial and cervical dystonia, but not OMD. In recent years, long-term studies on the efficacy and safety of BoNT-A have been published, a new BoNT-A formulation has been marketed and new studies on BoNT-B have been carried out [30]. Systematic reviews and guidelines recommend that BoNT injections should be offered as a treatment option for CD (for which it has been proven to be effective) and can be offered for blepharospasm, focal upper extremity dystonia and adductor laryngeal dystonia (for which it is probably effective) [30,31].

The first study on the use of BoNT for CD was a single-blind study with 12 patients and used electromyography guidance and a total maximum BoNT-A dose of 200 U (then called Oculinum®) (Smith-Kettlewell Institute, San Francisco, CA, USA). Improvements lasting 4 to 8 weeks were observed in 92 % of the patients, and 25 % reported transient neck weakness [32]. These early results were confirmed by a double-blind, placebo-controlled crossover study of 21 patients using 100 U of BoNT-A which showed an improvement based on investigator ratings and patient assessment of CD severity [33]. Since then some 80 studies have evaluated BoNT in CD. Table 2 shows the main results of some studies. Adverse events included dysphagia and neck weakness [29, 33-38].

While some forms of dystonia are relatively common, such as adult-onset CD, others are less frequent, and not all clinicians have enough clinical experience to guide their practice [39]. OMD is a type of focal dystonia that affects the lower facial, masticatory, labial and lingual musculature. When OMD occurs with blepharospasm, the term cranial dystonia is used.

Meige's syndrome, a variant of OMD, is a combination of upper and lower facial motor dysfunction that includes blepharospasm and OMD [40]. Isolated OMD is relatively rare and represents only 5 % of all dystonias. However, cranial dystonias (OMD, blepharospasm and Meige's syndrome) are the second most frequent dystonias (22 %) [40, 41].

Dystonia is not a stereotyped disorder, and in OMD it has a highly variable presentation. Consequently, treatment must be individualized to accommodate the patients particular requirements and symptoms. OMD dystonia can be classified into the following types: JC, JO, JD, lingual, pharyngeal and mixed [41]. BoNT has become the therapy of choice for OMD, and its use in JO, JC, and JD OMD has been well documented. Although most of the reported literature on OMD consists of open studies, all these have reported improvement with BoNT. In general, JO dystonia is more difficult to treat than JC dystonia [41,42].

	Dose (U)	Motor	Pain improvement
Tsui et al. 1986[33]	100	63 %	87 %
Gelb et al. 1989[34]	50-280	80 %	50 %
Jankovic and Schwartz, 1990[35]	100-300	70.7 %	76.4 %
Greene et al. 1990[36]	30-250	74 %	-
Jankovic et al., 1990[37]	209 (average)	90 %	93 %
Kwan et al. 1998[38]	190	70 %	-
Camargo et al. 2008[29]	100-280 (151.05±52.55)	94.1 %	84.4 %

Table 2. Studies with botulinum toxin A (BOTOX®) for cervical dystonia

5. Diagnosis of dysphagia in dystonias

As it is not easy for patients with CD to notice dysphagia, this condition is very often underdiagnosed [6,29].

Oropharyngeal function is usually investigated with the aid of videofluoroscopy. Clinical and videofluoroscopic evaluations have also indicated a high incidence of swallowing disorders in patients with CD before any treatment such as BoNT injection or rhizotomy [7-9]. In one study, swallowing abnormalities during video fluoroscopic examination were observed in over 50 % of CD patients [7].

In general, videofluoroscopic studies of CD patients show delayed initiation of swallowing and pharyngeal residue [7,10]. CD patients with these signs appear to have "neurogenic dysphagia" [7,43]. In contrast, asymmetric pharyngeal transit of large liquid boluses is consistent with tonic or clonic posturing of the head (and pharynx). Although the postural and neurogenic signs presumably relate to the same underlying neurologic dysfunction and both types might be considered "neurogenic," the authors of some studies suggest that the postural signs were sufficiently selective and specific to warrant a separate classification [7]. Therefore, Riski et al. [7] considered the presence of pharyngeal asymmetry with large boluses to be a sign of "postural dysphagia." Of 43 patients, 16 showed only neurologic signs; three showed only postural signs; and three showed combined postural and neurologic signs. The findings of Riski et al. suggest that swallowing abnormalities in CD are primarily neurogenic but may be solely postural or combined neurogenic and postural in nature. In agreement with this conclusion that CD involves neurogenic dysphagia, similar clinical and electrophysiological findings were reported in patients with OMD and laryngeal dystonia but not CD and in others with CD. Therefore, dysphagia can occur without abnormal head or neck movements [6]. Electrophysiological abnormalities in dystonic muscles are frequent and are all compatible with neurogenic dysphagia [6].

Two-thirds of those who complained of dysphagia showed evidence of swallowing abnormalities, and at least one swallowing abnormality was detected radiographically in half of those who did not complain. This lack of close agreement between subjective reports and videofluoroscopic results may reflect several factors. Firstly, videofluoroscopic examination of swallowing can show dysfunctions; however, as the protocol is standardized, it does not simulate all factors present during meals in the patient's home, e.g., the full range of textures and bolus sizes, the speed of bolus presentation and the presence of external distractions. Secondly, some patients' concerns with the discomfort or cosmetic disability associated with their CD may overshadow the relatively subtle abnormalities in oropharyngeal function. Thirdly, CD patients may have adapted to changes in swallowing function and therefore be asymptomatic [7].

Dysphagia and dysarthria (which account for 10.2 % to 37 % and 0.9 % of complaints, respectively) are the two most common adverse effects of BoNT treatment for OMD [37,42]. Clinical and videofluoroscopic evaluations have also indicated a high incidence of swallowing disorders in CD patients before any treatment such as BoNT injection or rhizotomy [7-9]. In a study by Comella et al., although new radiologic changes occurred in 50 % of CD patients following BoNT treatment, clinically only 33 % of these patients reported new dysphagia symptoms. The severity of new dysphagia symptoms correlated highly with the severity of new radiologic pharyngeal abnormalities. This suggests that rather than being routinely indicated, videofluoroscopic swallowing evaluations should be reserved mainly for patients with the severest clinical symptoms as an objective measure to assess the possibility of aspiration [8].

6. Avoiding dysphagia as an adverse effect of treatment for dystonia

Radiologic findings show that in patients with dysphagia prior to treatment with BoNT-A, the condition did not worsen following treatment [8].

Careful choice of the correct muscle groups with the aid of electromyography before application of BoNT and the use of low dosages may prevent adverse effects [29]. In a study by

Jankovic et al. [37], in which higher average doses of BoNT were used without electromyography guidance, 24 % of CD patients experienced adverse effects, and of these 23 % suffered from dysphagia. In a study by Barbosa et al. [43], who used an average dose of 191 U and did not use electromyography, slightly under half (47 %) of the patients developed dysphagia.

Other factors may have contributed to the low dysphagia indexes found in most studies. For example, the use of a larger number of injection points in each muscle and application in only one sternocleidomastoid (thus reducing diffusion of BoNT-A to the pharynx) can reduce the incidence of dysphagia [29]. Denervation has been shown to occur within a definable area that crosses anatomic barriers, including fascia and bone. Nevertheless, clinical and laboratory data suggest that dysphagia secondary to BoNT therapy is the result of toxin spreading from the sternocleidomastoid injection site to the pharyngeal musculature. Ensuring the injection dose in the sternomastoid does not exceed 100 IU leads to a substantially reduced incidence of this complication [12].

7. Conclusion

Dystonia is an important cause of dysphagia. The main aspects to observe in dystonic patients are:

1. Patients do not normally complain of dysphagia. Comprehensive questioning to confirm this symptom is therefore essential. When indicated, a search for dysphagia in dystonic patients should be performed with videofluoroscopy.

2. Optimization of treatment with BoNT (administration of the lowest possible dose, the use of electromyography and the appropriate choice of muscles) can avoid dysphagia.

Author details

Carlos Henrique Ferreira Camargo[1,2*], Edna Márcia da Silva Abdulmassih[3], Rosane Sampaio Santos[4] and Hélio Afonso Ghizoni Teive[3]

*Address all correspondence to: chcamargo@uol.com.br

1 Department of Medicine, State University of Ponta Grossa, Brazil

2 Hospital Universitário dos Campos Gerais, State University of Ponta Grossa, Brazil

3 Hospital de Clínicas, Federal University of Parana, Brazil

4 Tuiuti University of Parana, Brazil

References

[1] Oppenheim H. Über eine eigenartige Krampfkrankheit des kindlichen und jugendlichen Alters (Dysbasia lordotica progressiva, Dystonia musculorum deformans). NeurolCentrabl. 1911;30: 1090–1107.

[2] Pearce JM. Dystonia. Eur Neurol. 2005;53:151-152.

[3] Albanese A, Bhatia K, Bressman SB, Delong MR, Fahn S, Fung VS, et al. Phenomenology and classification of dystonia: a consensus update. Mov Disord. 2013 Jun 15;28(7):863-873.

[4] Tsui JK. Cervical dystonia. In: Tsui JK, Calne D, eds. Handbook of distonia. New York: Marcel Dekker, Inc; 1995. p. 115–127.

[5] Jankovic J. Etiology and differential diagnosis of blepharospasm and oromandibular dystonia. In: Jankovic J, Tolosa E, eds. In Advances in neurology. Facialdyskinesias. Volume 49 New York, Raven; 1988:103–116.

[6] Ertekin C, Aydogdu I, Seçil Y, Kiylioglu N, Tarlaci S, Ozdemirkiran T. Oropharyngeal swallowing in craniocervical dystonia. J NeurolNeurosurg Psychiatry. 2002 Oct; 73(4):406-411.

[7] Riski JE, Horner J, Nashold BS Jr. Swallowing function in patients with spasmodic torticollis. Neurology.1990;40:1443–1445.

[8] Comella CL, Tanner CM, Defoor-Hill L, et al. Dysphagia after botulinum toxin injections for spasmodic torticollis: clinical and radiological findings. Neurology. 1992;42:1307-1310.

[9] Horner J, Riski JE, Weber BA, et al. Swallowing speech and brainstem auditory evoked potentials in spasmodic torticollis. Dysphagia.1993;8:29–34.

[10] Münchau A, Good CD, McGowan S, et al. Prospective study of swallowing function in patients with cervical dystonia undergoing selective peripheral denervation. J NeurolNeurosurg Psychiatry. 2001;71:67–72.

[11] Whurr R, Bhatia KP, Masarei A, et al. The incidence and nature of dysphagia following botulinum toxin injections for torticollis: a prospective study of 123 patients. J Med Speech Lang Pathol. 1999;7:196–207.

[12] Borodic GE, Joseph M, Fay L, et al. Botulinum A toxin for the treatment of spasmodic torticollis: dysphagia and regional toxin spread. Head Neck. 1990;12:392–398.

[13] Holzer SE, Ludlow CL. The swallowing side effects of botulinum toxin type A injection in spasmodic dysphonia. Laryngoscope.1996;106:86–92.

[14] Ludlow CL, Naunton RF, Sedary SE, et al. Effect of botulinum toxin injections on speech in adductor spasmodic dysphonia. Neurology.1988;38:1220–1225.

[15] Buchholz DW, Neumann S: The swallowing side effects of botulinum toxin type A injection in spasmodic dysphonia. Dysphagia. 1997 Winter;12(1):59-60.

[16] Papapetropoulos S, Singer C. Eating dysfunction associated with oromandibular dystonia: clinical characteristics and treatment considerations. Head Face Med. 2006 Dec 7;2:47.

[17] Bhidayasiri R, Cardoso F, Truong DD. Botulinum toxin in blepharospasm and oromandibular dystonia: comparing different botulinum toxin preparations. Eur J Neurol. 2006 Feb;13Suppl 1:21-29.

[18] .Frucht SJ. The definition of dystonia: Current concepts and controversies. Mov Disord. 2013 Jun 15;28(7):884-888.

[19] Lohmann K, Klein C. Genetics of dystonia: What's known? What's new? What's next? MovDisord. 2013 Jun 15;28(7):899-905.

[20] Defazio G, Berardelli A, Hallett M. Do primary adult-onset focal dystonias share aetiological factors? Brain 2007;130:1183–1193.

[21] Fabbrini G, Defazio G, Colosimo C, et al. Cranial movement disorders: clinical features, pathophysiology, differential diagnosis and treatment. Nat ClinPractNeurol. 2009;5:93–105.

[22] Colosimo C, Suppa A, Fabbrini G, Bologna M, Berardelli A. Craniocervical dystonia: clinical and pathophysiological features. Eur J Neurol. 2010 Jul;17 Suppl 1:15-21.

[23] Cardoso F, Jankovic J. Oromandibular dystonia. In: Tsui JK, Caine DB, eds. Handbook of dystonia. New York:Marcel Dekker 1995: p 181–190.

[24] Meige H. Les convulsions de la face: uneformeclinique de convulsions faciales, bilateraleetmediane. Rev Neurol (Paris). 1910;21:437–443.

[25] Mascia MM, Valls-Sole J, Marti MJ, Sanz S. Chewing pattern in patients with Meige's syndrome. Mov Disord. 2005,20(1):26–33.

[26] Brin MF, Fahn S, Moskowitz C, Friedman A, Shale HM, Greene PE, Blitzer A, List T, Lange D, Lovelace RE, et al. Localized injections of botulinum toxin for the treatment of focal dystonia and hemifacial spasm. Mov Disord. 1987,2(4):237–254.

[27] Papapetropoulos S, Singer C. Primary focal lingual dystonia. MovDisord. 2006;21:429–430.

[28] Schweinfurth JM, Billante M, Courey MS. Risk factors and demographics in patients with spasmodic dysphonia. Laryngoscope. 2002;112:220–223.

[29] Camargo CH, Teive HA, Becker N, Baran MH, Scola RH, Werneck LC. Cervical dystonia: clinical and therapeutic features in 85 patients. Arq Neuropsiquiatr. 2008 Mar; 66(1):15–21.

[30] Albanese A, Asmus F, Bhatia KP, Elia AE, Elibol B, Filippini G, Gasser T, Krauss JK, Nardocci N, Newton A, Valls-Solé J. EFNS guidelines on diagnosis and treatment of primary dystonias. Eur J Neurol. 2011 Jan;18(1):5-18.

[31] Simpson DM, Blitzer A, Brashear A, et al. Assessment: Botulinum neurotoxin for the treatment of movement disorders (an evidence-based review): report of the Therapeutics and Technology Assessment Subcommittee of the American Academy of Neurology. Neurology. 2008;70:1699–1706.

[32] Tsui JK, Eisen A, Mak E, Carruthers J, Scott A, Calne DB. A pilot study on the use of botulinum toxin in spasmodic torticollis. Canadian Journal of Neurological Sciences. 1985;12:314–316.

[33] Tsui JK, Eisen A, Stoessl AJ, Calne S, Calne DB. Double-blind study of botulinum toxin in spasmodic torticollis. Lancet. 1986;2:245–247.

[34] Gelb DJ, Lowenstein DH, Aminoff MJ. Controlled trial of botulinum toxin injections in the treatment of spasmodic torticollis. Neurology. 1989 Jan;39(1):80-84.

[35] Jankovic J, Schwartz K. Botulinum toxin injections for cervical dystonia. Neurology. 1990 Feb;40(2):277–280.

[36] Greene P, Kang U, Fahn S, Brin M, Moskowitz C, Flaster E. Double-blind, placebo-controlled trial of botulinum toxin injections for the treatment of spasmodic torticollis. Neurology. 1990;40:1213–1218.

[37] Jankovic J, Schwartz K, Donovan DT. Botulinum toxin treatment of cranial-cervical dystonia, spasmodic dysphonia, other focal dystonias and hemifacial spasm. J NeurolNeurosurg Psychiatry. 1990 Aug;53(8):633-639.

[38] Kwan MC, Ko KF, Chan TP, Chan YW. Treatment of dystonia with botulinum A toxin: a retrospective study of 170 patients. Hong Kong Med J. 1998 Sep;4(3):279–282.

[39] Gonzalez-Alegre P, Schneider RL, Hoffman H. Clinical, etiological, and therapeutic features of Jaw-opening and Jaw-closing Oromandibular Dystonias: a decade of experience at a single treatment center. Tremor Other HyperkinetMov (NY). 2014 Apr 30;4:231.

[40] Tolosa E, Kulisevsky J, Fahn S. Meige syndrome: primary and secondary forms. Advances in Neurology. 1988;50:509–515.

[41] Tan EK, Jankovic J. Botulinum toxin A in patients with oromandibular dystonia: long-term follow-up. Neurology. 1999 Dec 10;53(9):2102-2107.

[42] Logemann JA. Dysphagia in movement disorders. Adv Neurol.1988;49:307–316.

[43] Barbosa ER, Silva HC, Bittar MS, et al. Tratamento das distoniascervicais com toxinabotulínica: análise de 19 casos. Arq Bras Neurocirurg. 1995;14:135-138.

Chapter 12

Dysphagia in Chronic Obstructive Pulmonary Disease

Livia Scelza, Catiuscia S.S. Greco,
Agnaldo J. Lopes and Pedro Lopes de Melo

Additional information is available at the end of the chapter

1. Introduction

Swallowing is an array of synergistic interdependent movements initiated by complex set of sensory inputs that generate pressures and forces to propel ingested materials through the upper aerodigestive tract and simultaneously protect the upper airway. As seen in Figure 1, the oropharynx is common to both the swallowing and respiratory processes. This functional conflict, therefore, must require fine coordination at the neuronal level to ensure that the peripheral structures produce the intended target behaviour [1].

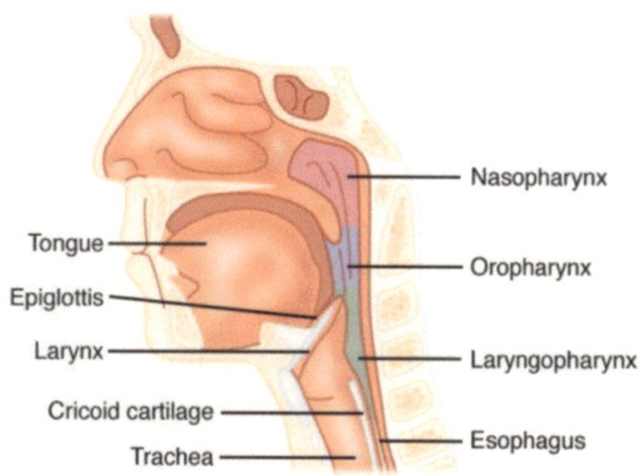

Figure 1. Simplified view of the structures related to swallowing and breathing. Note that the oropharynx is common to both the swallowing and respiratory processes.

Swallowing and breathing are closely related, and synergy of structures is needed for airway protection during the swallowing process to prevent the aspiration of food contents and thus prevent pulmonary complications. The swallowing apnea is described as an important mechanism of airway protection. This may be altered in patients who have lung diseases such as chronic obstructive pulmonary disease (COPD) [2, 3]. COPD is a preventable and treatable disease characterized by progressive limitation of airflow that is usually associated with an abnormal inflammatory response of the lungs to noxious particles and gases [4, 5]. COPD is a major public health problem with high and increasing prevalence [4]. According to World Health Organization (WHO) estimates, 80 million people have moderate to severe COPD [6]. Pulmonary changes can be a detrimental factor to coordination between breathing and swallowing [2, 3, 7, 8]. Swallowing apnea requires a reorganization of the breathing pattern when swallowing. This can be limited by the typical respiratory changes observed in patients with COPD [9].

This chapter discusses the history and current state of our knowledge concerning dysphagia in chronic obstructive pulmonary disease. We also describe the development of instrumentation for the analysis of the swallowing apnea and preliminary results of this analysis in individuals with COPD. The main topics covered by this review will be as follows:

- First we will provide a brief description of dysphagia and the interaction between swallowing and breathing in section 2 and 3, respectively;
- In section 4, we describe the principles of the chronic obstructive pulmonary disease;
- Next, we describe the main results presented in the literature concerning the dysphagia in COPD;
- The development of instrumentation for analysis of swallowing apnea, performed in our laboratory, is presented in section 5;
- Preliminary results of the changes of swallowing apnea in individuals with COPD are described in section 6;
- Finally, we conclude by examining the potential role of the routine analysis of swallowing disorders in COPD in the clinical arena.

2. Dysphagia

Swallowing is a complex sensoriomotor function that depends on the integrity of the mechanoreceptors and chemoreceptors for the sequential stimulation and inhibition of the upper aerodigestive tract; this coordinated process transports foods and liquids through the mouth and pharynx to the esophagus [10] and simultaneously protect the upper airway [1].

Biomechanical events that contribute to secure bolus transport and airway protective mechanisms include: closure of the introitus to the trachea by vocal cord adduction, approximation of the adducted arytenoids to close the laryngeal aditus, epiglottal descent, antero-superior displacement of the larynx away from the path of the bolus, and opening of the upper oesophageal sphincter [11]. During swallowing, the closure of the larynx and the respiratory pause during swallowing are vital protective mechanisms that prevent aspiration [12]. This phenomena is describes schematically in Figure 2.

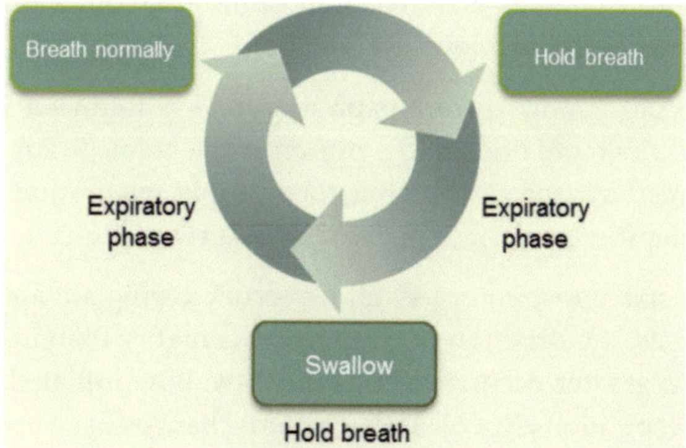

Figure 2. Simplified description of the usual swallowing pattern in healthy adults. Swallowing initiates during the expiratory phase of the breathing cycle. Swallowing interrupts exhalation (swallow apnea), and once the swallow has been completed, breathing resumes with exhalation.

Disordered swallowing, or dysphagia, can develop from lesions in certain areas of the cortex and brainstem that control the swallowing function, or damage to the associated cranial nerves. It is a common problem observed in patients with stroke and head injury [13]. Dysphagia affects at least 12% of patients in acute care hospitals and more than 50% of those in chronic care settings [14]. The presence of dysphagia is associated with aspiration induced chest infections and increases the risk of serious respiratory consequences such as pneumonia. Identification of the patient at risk of aspiration is important from a clinical view point. Due to the risk of aspiration, a significant number of dysphagic patients are fed with a nasogastric tube and /or intravenous fluids [13]. Dysphagia can significantly impact a person's quality of life as well as their health status [15].

3. Coordination of breathing and swallowing

Recent findings have delineated single neurons within medullary networks that demonstrate multifunctionality in the control of both the respiratory and swallowing behaviours [16]. The breathing cycle is not simply repressed during swallowing; it is substituted by a different well-controlled behaviour pattern. Variations in the bolus volume and viscosity characteristics will interfere with the breathing stop time duration [9, 17, 18]. The consistency of these observations has led to speculation that the precise coordination of breathing and swallowing may be an important mechanism to prevent aspiration [19]. The effect of bolus volume influences the swallowed-associated respiratory cycle [9, 20], and this observation notes that these neurological interference engrams may contribute to dyspnoea during meals in some patients with pulmonary disease.

Deglutition apnea is described as an important mechanism of airway protection. It consists of a respiratory pause that occurs involuntarily during each swallow, when the respiratory muscles are centrally inhibited and the airway closes. Breathing ceases just before and during the entire pharyngeal phase of deglutition [3]. The duration of this brief swallow apnea rages between 1 and 2 seconds in liquid swallows in most healthy adults, but there is a variability in the timing depending on the swallow task and bolus viscosity [1, 19, 21, 22].

Deglutition apnea occurs mainly during expiration and is followed by expiration [1, 2, 9, 18-25]. This pattern occurs more often in the presence of a bolus [9, 20]. A different pattern of this coordination of breathing and swallowing, for example, inspiration after swallowing, may increase the risk of aspiration and place patients at an airway protective disadvantage [1].

A modification to the stable respiratory-swallow occurs during advanced ageing. In healthy elderly aged individuals, the duration of deglutition is higher than in young groups [1, 18]. Studies have shown a greater occurrence of liquid swallow initiated and followed by the inspiratory phase of respiration [22, 26]. These pattern changes have not been associated with aspiration, however, they may cause implications on airway protection or bolus clearance in patients with already compromised swallowing function secondary to diseases and other conditions during old age, head and neck cancer, stroke and chronic obstructive pulmonary disease [1].

4. Chronic obstructive pulmonary disease

COPD is a preventable and treatable disease characterized by partially reversible airflow limitation [27, 28]. The limitation is often progressive and is associated with an abnormal inflammatory response of the lungs to noxious particles or gases, especially cigarette smoke [27]. COPD increases mortality in worldwide each year, causing socio-economic damage. The total deaths from COPD are projected to increase by 30% over the next 10 years, unless urgent measures are taken to reduce the risk factors, particularly tobacco use. Estimates indicate that by 2030, COPD may become the third leading cause of death [6].

The COPD is characterized by the presence of chronic bronchitis, obstructive bronchiolitis and emphysema [27, 28]. Chronic bronchitis is inflammation of the airways which deliver air to the lungs. This can lead to an increase in mucus production and consequent narrowing of the bronchi (Figure 3). In emphysema, the tissue that surrounds the smaller airways is damaged and air becomes trapped in the alveoli. These air sacs become overstretched and unable to function correctly causing shortness of breath. The disease process is directly related to an inflammatory response of the lungs, triggering the destruction of the lung parenchyma. Such changes are responsible for airflow limitation and air trapping. [27]. Pathological changes occur in four different regions of the lung: the larger calibre airway, the peripheral airways, the lung parenchyma and the pulmonary vasculature [27-29]. In the larger calibre airways, structural changes occur in the goblet cells and submucosal glands causing mucus hypersecretion and squamous metaplasia, as shown in Figure 3 [27-29].

In the peripheral airways (<2 mm diameter), we observed thickening of the airway wall, peribronchial fibrosis, exudate, narrowing of the airways (obstructive bronchiolitis) and increased inflammatory response. In the lung parenchyma, the structural changes involved destruction of the alveolar wall, apoptosis of epithelial cells and emphysema [27-29]. The main characteristic of COPD is airflow obstruction, which is not fully reversible. Spirometry is the gold standard technique used to assess this obstruction [28, 29].

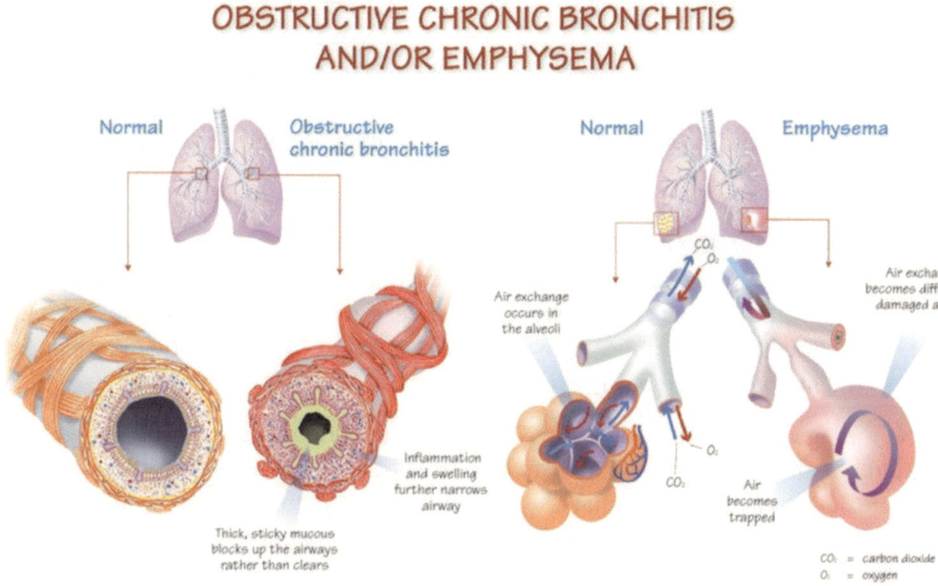

Figure 3. On the left, the effect of chronic bronchitis in which the inflammation of the airways can lead to an increase in mucus production and consequent narrowing of the bronchi. In emphysema (right), the tissue that surrounds the smaller airways is damaged and air becomes trapped in the alveoli. These air sacs become overstretched and unable to function correctly causing shortness of breath. (Source: http://www.livingwellwithcopd.com/en/what-is-copd.html).

The coordination between breathing and swallowing can be severely disrupted in patients with COPD due to their reduced ventilatory capacity. COPD also has the potential to disrupt the coordination of breathing and swallowing because of tachypnoea, an increased tendency to swallow during inspiration, reduced duration of apnea and changes in the mechanics of swallowing. The increase in the elastic and resistive respiratory loads, typical of these patients, is associated with a rapid shallow pattern of breathing that may increase the risk of aspiration [8].

5. Dysphagia in chronic obstructive pulmonary disease

This section focuses on a historically organized review of the main studies presented in the literature. To date, relatively little research has been conducted concerning dysphagia and other swallowing disorders in patients with COPD. The first studies begin in the 1980s, and few studies were conducted until the end of the past millennium. A significant increase was observed in this research area in the 2000s and 2010s.

5.1. The first studies in the 1980s and 1990s

The paper by Coelho [30] is believed to be the first that specifically deals with dysphagia in patients with COPD. The author studied 14 patients with a primary diagnosis of COPD. All of the subjects but one had tracheostomy tubes, and five were ventilator-dependent. Bedside evaluation was performed to assess the oral phase of the swallow and videofluoroscopy was used to examine the pharyngeal phase. Subjects were presented with three consistencies of materials to swallow: liquid, paste and crackers coated with barium. The author observed that ten of the 14 patients demonstrated some degree of dysphagia. The COPD patients tired rapidly and often needed to rest in the midst of chewing foods. Their propensity for fatiguing rapidly is consistent with their performance on other basic activities of daily living. Consistent aspiration was noted in three of these patients and was attributed to a delayed swallowing reflex, decreased pharyngeal peristalsis and cricopharyngeal/oesophageal constriction. Dysfunctional swallowing with no aspiration was observed in 7 of the 14 COPD patients. These patients had difficulties with bolus formation and control, delayed swallowing reflexes and problems with lingual and pharyngeal peristalsis.

In the beginning of the 1990s, Stein et al. [31] performed videofluoroscopy in 25 patients with COPD and identified cricopharyngeal achalasia in 21 of them. In 17 patients, this was judged to be severe, and all were found to have some degree of symptomatic dysphagia. Ten patients had surgical correction and eight had improved pulmonary symptoms. The authors discussed that cricopharyngeal dysfunction may precede airway obstruction and contribute to subsequent progression and exacerbation of airway abnormalities. Alternatively, cricopharyngeal dysfunction may be secondary to COPD because it may increase gastroesophageal reflux by flattening the diaphragm; this reflux leads to cricopharyngeal achalasia, a mechanism that protects the larynx from aspiration of gastric acid.

Shaker et al. [32] used concurrent respirography and submental surface electromyography to study the effects of ageing, tachypnea and bolus volume on the coordination of swallowing in patients with chronic obstructive pulmonary disease. Three groups were studied: 10 young healthy volunteers aged between 18 and 34 years, 11 healthy elderly volunteers aged between 63 and 83 years and 22 patients with COPD aged between 46 and 77 years. Dry and water swallows were observed at rest and during exercise (increased respiratory rate). A total of 2,331 analysable swallows were recorded and analysed for: 1) the respiratory phase in which the swallows occurred; 2) the respiratory phase during which respiration was resumed after swallowing; 3) and the duration of swallow-induced apnea. The author observed that at rest, in the young volunteers the majority of deglutitions were coupled with the expiratory phase of swallowing. The elderly generally initiated swallowing more often in the inspiratory phase compared with the young. Compared with the basal state, the advanced COPD patients swallowed significantly more in the inspiratory phase and resumed their respiration significantly more with inspiration. The reasons for this alteration were not determined; however, the authors noted that derangement in the acid-base balance present in COPD patients may conceivably influence the central coordination of the deglutitive centres. The results of this study indicated that tachypnea, ageing, bolus volume and COPD modify the coordination between deglutition and the phases of continuous respiration.

5.2. Studies performed in the 2000s

One of the first studies published in this decade was performed by Good-Fratturelli et al. [33]. It consisted of a retrospective study that described the swallows of 78 patients with a COPD diagnosis who were seen for videofluoroscopy in 3 years and determined the prevalence of dysphagia in these patients. Patients were given a bolus containing barium in thin and thick liquid, puree, paste and cookie consistencies. Of these patients, 85% were found to have some degree of dysphagia. Bilateral vallecular stasis, bilateral pyriform sinus stasis, oral stasis and delayed pharyngeal swallow response were reported in 60% of the COPD patients. Aspiration was noticed in 42% and laryngeal penetration in 28% of these patients, which were evidenced substantially more with thin and thick liquids compared to semi-solid or solid textures. The authors suggested that the compromised respiratory system, such as the absence of a cough response, or use of quiet but ineffective coughs, may reflect their lack of respiratory strength to clear the airway, and consequently, explains the high prevalence of laryngeal penetration, the inability to expel material from the airway, and aspiration.

Martin-Harris [34] based a study on relevant articles and described the optimal patterns of care and care consideration in patients with COPD and swallowing disorders. The author emphasized that it has been historically reported that the laryngeal cartilage in patients with COPD is often seated more deeply in the neck compared with healthy adults. The lowered basal position of the larynx results in increased distance that the larynx must ascend to achieve maximal closure and facilitate pharyngoesophageal segment (PES) opening. Some patients have oral impairments such as slow bolus preparation and oral bolus transport, and these situations are consistent with their motor behavior in activities of daily living. The labored tongue movement and reduction in oropharyngeal sensation may also contribute to delayed initiation of the pharyngeal swallow. Patients attempting to maintain breathing activity as long as possible before the obligatory apneic pause, and trying to re-establish respiration quickly, while eating semisolids and solids, may present channeling of a bolus to the level of the pyriform sinuses and premature opening of the larynx during the latter stages of swallow. The habitual and sometimes necessary mouth-breathing characteristics of COPD patients, may lead to excessive dryness and adherence of thick and dry materials to the oropharyngeal tissues, with potential post-swallow aspiration.

Oxygen treatments and medications may also confound the problem with xerostomia. The authors suggested an eating and swallowing guideline to reduce the incidence of penetration/aspiration: small and frequent meals; appetite enhancement; environmental control; promotion of relaxation; pacing intake at mealtime; optimizing bolus volume and texture; avoiding sequential swallowing of large volumes of liquid; two swallows per bolus and reflux precautions.

Mokhlesi et al. [35] studied 20 patients with COPD and 20 healthy subjects matched for age and gender. The protocol consisted of swallowing two boluses each of 3 ml and 5 ml of barium liquid, drinking barium liquid from a cup, and swallowing 3 ml barium paste while performing videofluoroscopy. Of these patients, 20% reported dysphagia. The data from the study demonstrate that COPD is associated with abnormal swallowing physiology, including frequent spontaneous and protective manoeuvres and decreased laryngeal elevation during swallowing. A shorter duration of cricopharyngeal opening on three or four bolus types was also observed.

In a later work, Mokhlesi [36] noted that because there is a complex anatomical and functional relationship between the upper gastrointestinal tract and the respiratory tract, it is important to elucidate if this harmonic relationship is disrupted when pulmonary function is compromised, as found in COPD. The aim of the author's article was to review the limited data concerning these important associations and to reinforce the need for additional clinical research in this area. A precise coordination of swallowing and respiration are necessary to avoid dysphagia and aspiration. The mechanisms of coordination between swallowing and airway protective reflexes have precise central and peripheral nervous system integration. COPD may interfere with the precise and complex coordination between swallowing and respiration. The aetiology of the exacerbation of COPD is often unclear. On many occasions, clinicians fail to demonstrate the conditions that are commonly known to cause COPD exacerbation, such as viral or bacterial infections, pulmonary embolism, pneumothorax or myocardial ischaemia. Tracheal aspiration has been suggested to be a cause of exacerbation in some patients with COPD, but there are few data supporting this relationship. In healthy individuals, swallowing interrupts the expiratory phase of respiration and induces an apneic pause of approximately 1 second followed by resumption of respiration with expiration. [21] [19]. However, patients with exacerbations of COPD swallow more often by interrupting the inspiratory phase and resume respiration significantly more with inspiration [32]. In a study of patients with severe COPD who experienced frequent exacerbations, cricopharyngeal dysfunction was diagnosed in 21 or 25 patients (84%). The majority had dysphagia, and eight patients who underwent cricopharyngeal myotomy had significant improvement in swallowing and a decrease in respiratory exacerbations [31]. In a retrospective study of 78 outpatient veterans with COPD referred for a videofluoroscopic swallow examination, the prevalence of dysphagia was 85%. Silent aspiration and laryngeal penetration were noted in 56% of patients. Patients with complaints of dysphagia or unexplained frequent exacerbation of COPD may benefit from detailed swallow evaluations and referral to a speech pathologist. The author (Mokhlesi, [36]) noted that further research was needed to evaluate the role of protective swallowing manoeuvres in stable COPD and their potential failure during acute COPD exacerbation. Additional studies should be performed to determine if occult aspiration is a cause or contributing factor to exacerbation of COPD and, conversely, whether patients with exacerbation are at even greater risk of aspiration.

The study by Kobayashi et al. [37] investigated 2 groups: the first was formed by 25 patients with COPD who had at least one exacerbation during the previous year, and the second group included 25 patients who were stable. They evaluated the swallow reflex by studying the latency of response to the onset of the swallowing action. It was injected 1ml of distilled water into the pharynx through a nasal catheter and the mean latent time of the swallowing reflex was significantly longer in the exacerbation group than in the stable group. Impairment of the swallow reflex was significantly associated with an exacerbation of COPD.

Gross et al. [3] elucidated the relationship between breathing and swallowing in patients with COPD during deglutition. In a prospective study with 25 patients with COPD and 25 healthy control subjects, swallows were analysed simultaneously by surface electromyographic measurements, respiratory inductance plethysmograph and nasal cannula. Patients were given portions of cookies and pudding. The data from that study demonstrated that participants with COPD swallowed the cookie (a bolus that requires mastication) during inhalation significantly more often than normal subjects, and this pattern may increase the frequency of prandial aspiration. Post swallow inhalation occurred significantly more often in the COPD groups with the pudding texture when compared with control subjects. There was no difference in the duration of swallow apnea between the groups for either consistency. However, in the COPD group, the duration of swallow apnea of swallows that occurred during the inhalation phase was significantly longer for both food types. This prolongation could indicate the presence of a compensatory mechanism such as more time for recoil forces to generate higher swallow subglottic pressure or more time for the bolus to traverse the pharynx and enter the oesophagus.

Gross et al. [38] found that patients with stable moderate to severe COPD tend to swallow during inspiration and swallowing is often followed by inspiratory activity. Inspiration just before or just after a swallow increases the risk of inhaling pharyngeal contents. This may be caused because of the negative intrathoracic pressure. Fluoroscopic imaging of swallowing in patients with stable severe COPD and hyperinflation has shown reduced laryngeal elevation and a delayed pharyngeal response. The authors suggested that COPD is a significant risk factor for aspiration among nursing home residents. Alterations in respiratory rate and rhythm during exacerbations of COPD have been associated with an increased tendency for an inspiration-swallow-inspiration sequence when swallowing saliva spontaneously.

Ohta et al. [39] investigated the swallowing function before exacerbation of COPD when it was at a mild stage by performing the simple two-step swallowing provocation test (STS-SPT) and the repetitive saliva swallowing test (RSST). Sixty-four patients with COPD were divided into three groups: mild, moderate and severe. Fifteen healthy subjects were also recruited as a control group. In moderate to severe stages of COPD, the ratio of abnormal to normal swallowing patients estimated by the STS-SPT was higher than in the control group. In contrast, the RSST evaluated the ratio of abnormal to normal swallowing in patients at the mild stage of COPD as being higher than the control; this was also the case in the moderate and severe groups. This study suggest that both STS-SPT and the RSST can be used to evaluate swallowing dysfunction before the exacerbation of COPD occurs. It also suggests that the swallowing dysfunction in COPD may begin in the mild stage and, therefore, aspiration should be monitored from the mild stage in COPD patients. The RSST may be valid to evaluate swallowing at the mild stage.

5.3. Studies performed in the 2010s

Two studies were published in the beginning of this decade. Terada and collaborators [40] evaluated 67 patients with COPD and 19 age-matched controls, and observed that 23 of 86 subjects showed abnormal responses on the STS-SPT test. This behaviour was more frequent among subjects with COPD than controls. The swallowing abnormalities were associated with gastroesophageal reflux disease (GERD) symptoms, the existence of sputum bacteria, and serum C-reactive protein (CRP) levels in patients with COPD at the baseline and were related to an increased risk of frequent exacerbations.

As being part of educational sessions in a Pulmonary Rehabilitation Program, McKinstry et al. [41] discussed with COPD patients about normal swallowing and breathing, symptoms of dysphagia, consequences of aspiration and strategies to improve swallowing. Participants knowledge before and after these sessions was examined by a questionnaire. Of these, 383 patients with COPD underwent basic dysphagia screening and 104 were referred from screening for individual assessment and management of dysphagia. Participants were also asked to complete the standardized dysphagia-specific quality-of-life questionnaire (SWAL-QOL) survey, a dysphagia-specific quality-of-life questionnaire. Statistically significant improvement was found in participant's pre and post questionnaire results on knowledge of dysphagia and COPD. It was found that 27% of participants either exhibited or reported symptoms of dysphagia. Statistically significant improvement was found on 3 subscales of SWAL-QOL 3 months following initiation of treatment. The author concludes that dysphagia management and education of patients in pulmonary rehabilitation programs may contribute towards early identification and self-management of dysphagia and may enhance swallowing-related quality of life.

Cvejic et.al [2] studied 16 patients with COPD and 15 healthy control subjects that underwent videofluoroscopy while swallowing graduated volumes of barium liquid (5, 10 and 20 ml) and 100 ml (continuous cup drinking). Respiratory airflow was assessed using a combination of intranasal pressure measurement and respiratory inductive plethysmography. Electromyography was used to examine swallow timing. Transcutaneous oximetry was used to monitor oxygen saturation. After 36 months, respiratory health status was evaluated by telephone interview. The data of the study demonstrated that scores grading penetration/aspiration were significantly higher in patients with COPD and occurred almost exclusively during the 100 ml liquid swallow. Increased respiratory rates at rest were noted in 3/6 subjects in the COPD group with penetration/aspiration. Transient desaturation was noted after 100 ml liquid swallow in 13 subjects with COPD. The dominant respiratory-swallow pattern associated with smaller barium volumes was expiration-swallow-expiration. Swallowing of 100 ml elicited a different response. In COPD subjects, inspiration-swallow-expiration was observed in 60% compared to 20% of controls. All subjects who experienced penetration/aspiration used this pattern of breathing. The apnea intervals during 100 ml swallows were not different in COPD and controls. Predictive factors linked to impaired swallowing were reduced hyoid elevation and post-swallow pharyngeal residue. All subjects were assessed by telephone interview, and patients with COPD and penetration/aspiration appeared to have more serious adverse outcomes. The authors conclude that normal protective mechanisms during swallowing may be compromised in COPD and that penetration/aspiration may take place when drinking relatively large volumes of fluid.

Singh et al. [8] noted that lung disease including COPD has the potential to disrupt the coordination of breathing and swallowing. The authors suggest that it may happen because of tachypnoea, an increased tendency to swallow during inspiration, a reduced duration of apnoea and changes in the mechanics of swallowing.

The study of Cvejic et al. [2] provided convincing evidence of aspiration during swallowing in patients with stable moderate COPD. In this study, patients with COPD favoured an inspiration-swallow-expiration pattern with larger boluses. Penetration or aspiration was associated with tachypnoea, reduced hyoid elevation, post-swallow pharyngeal residue and a trend towards increased hospitalizations and mortality over 36 months. The Editorial written by Singh [8] pointed out that these findings are important because aspiration may contribute to precipitating or aggravating exacerbations, and increase the morbidity in patient with COPD. Exacerbations of COPD are a major cause of reduced quality of life, reduced activities of daily living and increased health–care costs hospital admission and readmission, and morbidity and mortality [8].

Based on the responses from a self-perception questionnaire, Chaves et al. [7] identified symptoms of dysphagia by comparing 35 patients with COPD and 35 healthy volunteers. There were significant differences between the two groups, and pharyngeal symptoms, airway protection, oesophageal symptoms, history of pneumonia and nutritional symptoms were more common in participants with COPD.

Kobayashi et al. [42] noted that impairment of swallowing and cough reflexes leads to aspiration of oropharyngeal or gastric secretions and their bacteria, resulting in tracheobronchial inflammation and infection. Thus, impairment of these reflexes presents a potential risk factor for COPD exacerbations. The authors suggested that angiotensin-converting enzyme inhibitors can improve the swallowing reflex and protect against aspiration.

Tsuzuki et al. [43] studied sixty-five individuals with COPD during a 1-year follow-up. The repetitive saliva-swallowing test (RSST) and modified water-swallow test (MWST) were performed. The RSST counts the number of dry swallows in 30 seconds while sitting; fewer than three dry swallows was determined to be abnormal. Patients with abnormal RSST results had a significantly greater prevalence of exacerbations during the 1-year follow-up. Cold water (3ml) is placed on the floor of the mouth in the MWST. The MWST result was determined to be abnormal if the individual was unable to swallow, or experiences dyspnea, coughing, or wet-hoarse dysphonia after swallowing in either of two trials. The MWST results were not associated with exacerbations in participants with COPD. The small number of participants with abnormal results suggests that the MWST is not suitable for detecting dysphagia associated with COPD exacerbations. A cough peak flow (CPF) <270L/min was also associated with a higher frequency of exacerbations. The CPF results showed that the participants with dysphagia and a low CPF cannot eject residue in the pharynx or penetrated or aspirated boluses. The RSST is useful to detect dysphagia associated with exacerbations in individuals with COPD. The authors recommended that individuals with abnormal RSST results undergo videofluoroscopy or videoendoscopy to check their swallowing functions.

Clayton et al. [44] noted that relatively little research has been conducted on the prevalence of dysphagia and other swallowing disorders in patients with COPD until 2012. The authors suggested that COPD may weaken the strength of swallow and increase the prevalence of aspiration. The impaired ability to use expired air to clear the larynx and protect the airway, combined to weakening of swallow, may contribute to an increased risk for aspiration of pharyngeal contents and aspiration pneumonia. The authors suggested that one hypothesis is that a laryngopharyngeal sensory deficit exists. Thus, the primary goals of this study were to identify the prevalence of laryngopharyngeal sensory impairment as determined by the laryngeal adductor reflex (LAR) threshold in patients with proven COPD and to characterize the relationship between laryngopharyngeal sensory impairment and the severity of COPD. The laryngopharyngeal sensory discrimination test (LPSDT) was performed. The study included 20 COPD patients and a control group with 11 volunteers. The study revealed that patients with COPD have a significantly worse level of laryngopharyngeal sensory impairment as defined by the LAR threshold. No relationship was identified between the severity of laryngopharyngeal sensory impairment and the severity of COPD (as defined by the FEV_1 testing). The diagnosis of COPD was strongly related to laryngopharyngeal sensory impairment, but the severity of COPD did not correlate with deterioration in laryngopharyngeal sensitivity. The presence of COPD itself is enough to predict impairment of laryngopharyngeal sensitivity.

In a recent study, Terzi et al. [45] evaluated fifteen consecutive chronic obstructive pulmonary disease patients with exacerbations requiring ICU admission and non-invasive ventilation (NIV). The objectives of this study were to evaluate swallowing during NIV in COPD patients with acute respiratory failure and, if appropriate and based on the results, to develop and evaluate a simple alteration in the ventilator design to eliminate ventilator insufflations during swallowing. Swallowing and breathing interactions were investigated noninvasively by chin electromyography, cervical piezoelectric sensor, and inductive respiratory plethysmography. Two water volumes (5 and 10 ml) were tested in random order. The results indicated that swallowing during NIV is feasible in patients with COPD experiencing acute exacerbations, swallowing efficiency and the breathing-swallowing pattern improve with NIV compared with spontaneous breathing and dyspnea decreases during swallowing when using NIV.

The work recently published by Chaves et al. [46] emphasizes that previous studies have indicated consistent aspiration in COPD patients. It is believed that this phenomenon was mainly related to delayed swallowing reflex and problems with lingual and pharyngeal peristalsis as a result of bilateral weakness and incoordination of the related muscles. When combined with an impaired ability to use expired air to clear the larynx and protect the airway, a weak swallow may contribute to an increased risk for aspiration of pharyngeal contents and may consequently lead to aspiration pneumonia. This work discuss that although the cause of impaired laryngopharyngeal sensitivity remains unclear, a few hypotheses have been introduced: (1) the use of inhaled corticosteroids and anticholinergics may have an effect on the sensory mucosa of the laryngopharynx; (2) laryngeal edema caused by smoking and the presence of chronic cough commonly reported in COPD patients may contribute to reduced sensation. The purpose of the study by Chaves et al. [46] was to evaluate swallowing transit times and valleculae residue characteristics of stable COPD patients who have no swallowing complaints. The population included 20 patients with COPD and 20 healthy controls. Swallows were assessed through videofluoroscopy. The protocol included swallows of 3, 5 and 10 ml of liquid consistency; swallows of 7 ml of paste consistency, and swallows of a solid biscuit. The data of the study indicated that stable COPD patients and healthy controls did not present any signs of penetration-aspiration for any tested consistency. Patients with COPD presented longer pharyngeal transit time (PTT) during the ingestion of 10 ml of the liquid consistency and during the ingestion of the paste consistency. In cases of exacerbation, patients are more likely to have difficulties in prolonging swallowing events, so this manoeuvre might be difficult to execute. Regarding the duration of the tongue base contact (TBC) with the posterior pharyngeal wall, COPD patients also presented longer durations for liquid and paste consistencies. The authors concluded that the risk for aspiration in the COPD population is not limited to the presence of valleculae residue, and this cannot be seen as an isolated factor in an attempt to explain swallowing alterations in this population. Stable COPD may present physiological adaptations as a protective swallowing manoeuvre to avoid aspiration/penetration of pharyngeal contents.

Table 1 summarizes the studies conducted on the prevalence of dysphagia and other swallowing disorders in patients with COPD to date.

Reference	Subjects	Reference test	Oral impairment	Pharyngeal impairment	Presence of aspiration	Coordination of breathing and swallowing
Coelho (1987)	14 COPD patients	Videofluoroscopy and bedside evaluation	Difficulties with bolus formation and control	Delayed swallowing reflex, decreased pharyngeal peristalsis and cricopharyngeal and esophageal constriction	3 of 14 patients (21%)	Not tested
Stein et al. (1990)	25 COPD patients with cricopharyn geal dysfunction	Videofluoroscopy	Not tested	Cricopharyngeal achalasia	Not tested	Not tested
Shaker et al. (1992)	21 healthy subjects and 22 COPD patients	Electromyography and respirography	Not tested	Not tested	Not tested	Swallowing occurred during inspiration in exacerbation of COPD
Good-Fraturelli et al. (2000)	78 COPD patients	Videofluoroscopy	Oral stasis	Bilateral vallecular and pyriform sinus stasis, delayed pharyngeal swallow response.	42% of patients evidenced aspiration with thin and thick liquid, more than with semi-solid or	Not tested

Reference	Subjects	Reference test	Oral impairment	Pharyngeal impairment	Presence of aspiration	Coordination of breathing and swallowing
					solid textures.	
Martin-Harris et al.(2000)	Review of literature, no subjects were tested	Review of literature and care guidelines based on clinical deductions from experience in the evaluation and treatment of patient with COPD and dysphagia	Altered oropharyngeal sensation, slow lingual motility, slow and effortful chewing and bolus preparation, oropharyngeal xerostomia	Delayed laryngeal closure, prolonged laryngeal ascent and descent, premature laryngeal opening, pharyngeal residue, channeling of food to pyriform sinuses	Post-swallow aspiration may occur with thick and dry materials	Not described
Mokhlesi et al.(2002)	20 COPD patients and 20 healthy subjects	Videofluoroscopy	Reduced tongue control, reduced antero-posterior tongue movement, reduced tongue stabilization, reduced tongue strength, and reduced tongue base retraction.	Frequent spontaneous and protective maneuvers, delayed pharyngeal swallow, decreased laryngeal elevation, shorter duration of cricopharyngeal opening	Not observed	Not tested
Kobayashi et al.(2007)	25 stable COPD patients, and 25 that had one exacerbation during the previous year	Injection of 1 ml distilled water into pharynx	Not tested	Mean latent time of swallowing reflex was longer in exacerbation group of COPD	Not tested	Not tested
Gross et al. (2009)	25 COPD patients and 25 control subjects	Electromyography, nasal cannula and respiratory inductance plethysmography	Not tested	Not tested	Not tested	Swallowing during inhalation, and post swallow inhalation were observed more often in COPD

Reference	Subjects	Reference test	Oral impairment	Pharyngeal impairment	Presence of aspiration	Coordination of breathing and swallowing
						than in normal subjects
Ohta (2009)	64 COPD patients	STS-SPT and RSST	Not tested	Impairment of triggering of the swallowing response and the frequency of saliva swallowing, may begin in the mild stage of COPD	Not tested	Not tested
Terada et al. (2010)	67 COPD patients and 19 healthy subjects	Simple Two-Step Swallowing Provocation Test (STS-SPT)	Not tested	Impairment of triggering of the swallowing response was more frequent in COPD than in normal subjects	Not tested	Not tested
McKinstry et al. (2010)	55 COPD patients	Dysphagia screening and Swal-QOL	Not tested	Not tested	Not tested	Not tested
Cvejic et al. (2011)	16 COPD patients and 15 control subjects	Videofluoroscopy, eletromyography, and respiratory inductive plethysmography	Not tested	Reduced hyoid elevation and post-swallow pharyngeal residue	4 of 16 patients(2 5%) in 100ml liquid barium	Inspiration-swallow-expiration pattern was observed more often in COPD than in control subjects
Kobayashi et al. (2011)	25 stable COPD patients, and 25 that had one exacerbation during the previous year	Simple Two-Step Swallowing Provocation Test (STS-SPT)	Not tested	Not tested	Not tested	Angiotensin-converting enzyme inhibitors protect against aspiration tracheobronchitis and exacerbations of COPD.
Chaves et al. (2011)	35 COPD patients and 35 healthy subjects	Self perception questionnaire	Not tested	Airway protection and pharyngeal symptoms were common in	Not tested	Not tested

Reference	Subjects	Reference test	Oral impairment	Pharyngeal impairment	Presence of aspiration	Coordination of breathing and swallowing
				participants with COPD		
Tsuzuki et al. (2012)	65 COPD patients	Repetitive Saliva Swallowing Test (RSST) and Modified Water-Swallow Test (MWST)	Not tested	Reduced number of swallows in RSST, and dyspnea, coughing or wet-hoarse dysphonia after swallowing in MWS in patients with COPD	Not tested	Not tested
Clayton et al. (2012)	20 COPD patients and 11 healthy subjects	Laryngeal sensory discrimination test (LPSD)	Not tested	COPD patients have a worse level of laryngopharyngeal sensory impairment	Not tested	Not tested
Terzi et al. (2014)	15 COPD patients	Electromyography and respiratory inductive plethysmography during noninvasive ventilation	Not tested	Not tested	Not tested	Swallowing efficiency and the breathing-swallowing pattern improve with NIV compared with spontaneous breathing
Chaves et al. (2014)	20 COPD patients and 20 healthy controls	Videofluoroscopy	Longer duration of the tongue base contact with the posterior pharyngeal wall	Longer pharyngeal transit time	Not observed	Not tested

Table 1. Summary of the studies that evaluated the prevalence of dysphagia and other swallowing disorders on patients with COPD.

6. Development of instrumentation for the analysis of the coordination between respiration and swallowing in COPD patients

This section briefly describes the development of a configurable system that may be used for ambulatory and/or home analysis of swallowing using telemedicine and internet data exchange developed in our laboratory [24]. The general architecture of the instrument is described in Figure 4.

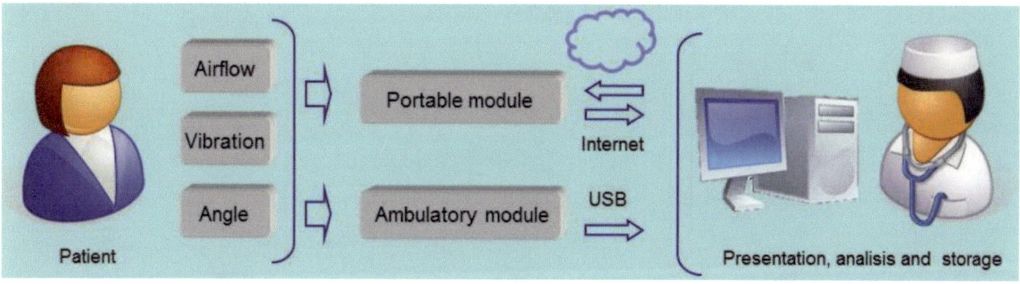

Figure 4. Simplified block diagram of the configurable instrument for the analysis of swallowing disorders.

The instrument allows an unobtrusive monitoring of respiration during feeding using a nasal airflow measurement system based on a nasal cannula attached to a sensitive pressure transducer (176PC; Honeywell Inc., New York, U.S.A.) through a long and flexible connection tube (100 cm length, 4 mm, i.d.). Intranasal air pressure recordings yield minimally intrusive and accurate information about the direction of airflow in real time.

Also included in the basic instrument is a system used to monitor the elevation of the larynx. This movement prevents the entering of the material in the tracheal airway and gives rise to a characteristic vibration pattern that can be used to detect the pharyngeal phase of the swallowing mechanism [47]. This mechanical vibration was measured using an electret microphone (CZN-15E; Ningbo Yuelong Electronics Co., Zhejiang, China) which was placed on the throat at the level of the thyroid cartilage by an apparatus similar to a collar.

The angle of the glass used to drive water was used to non-invasively monitor the beginning of water entering the mouth of the volunteer. To this end, inclinometry data have been obtained from a dual axis accelerometer (ADXL213, Analog Devices Inc., Norwood, MA, U.S.A.). The resulting analogue output value is then used in conjunction with a lookup table to determine the corresponding glass angle relative to the line of gravity.

The module dedicated to telemonitoring applications is battery operated. This subsystem also includes a Palmtop iPAQ HP hx2490 with 520 MHz, 64 Mb of RAM and 192 Mb of ROM, with operational system Microsoft® Windows Mobile® 5.0. For ambulatory application, a data acquisition system was developed using an 18F4550 microcontroller (Microchip, Arizona, USA).

Regardless of the method used for data acquisition (ambulatory or telemonitoring), the final analysis of the airflow, mechanical vibration and glass angle signals is performed by a dedicated software (Figure 5). It allows the user to automatically calculate the time in the course of the swallowing apnea (s) and the phase in which the swallowing apnea started and stopped in the respiratory cycle (inspiration or expiration).

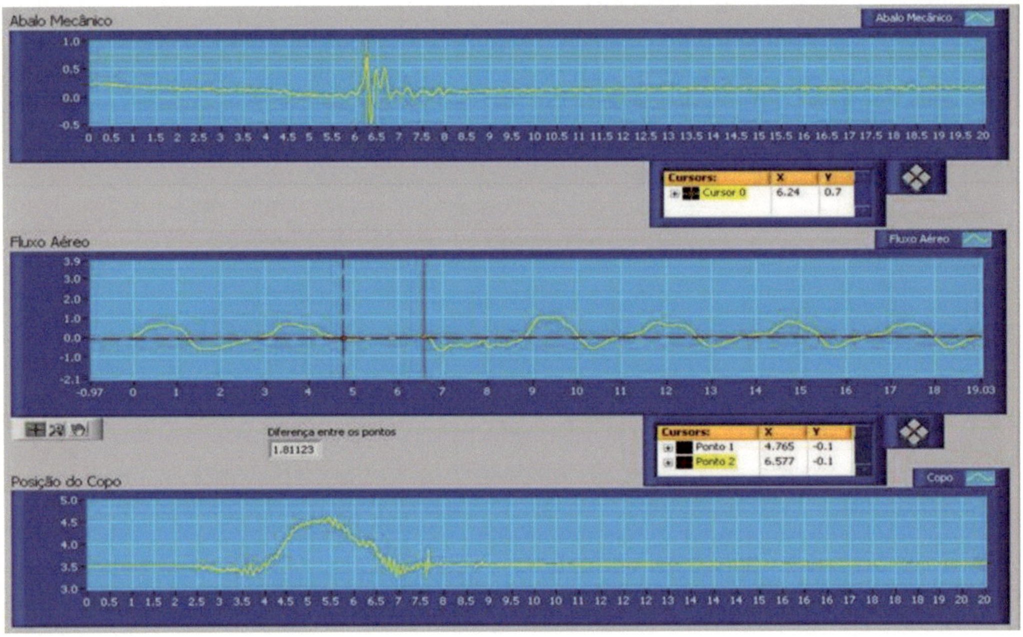

Figure 5. Front panel of the program used to automatically calculate the time in the course of the swallowing apnea (s) and the phase in which the swallowing apnea started and stopped in the respiratory cycle (inspiration or expiration).

Representative examples of the typical morphology of the nasal airflow, mechanical vibration and glass angle signals obtained during a swallowing of 20 mL of water in a normal subject and a dysphagic patient are presented in Figure 6.

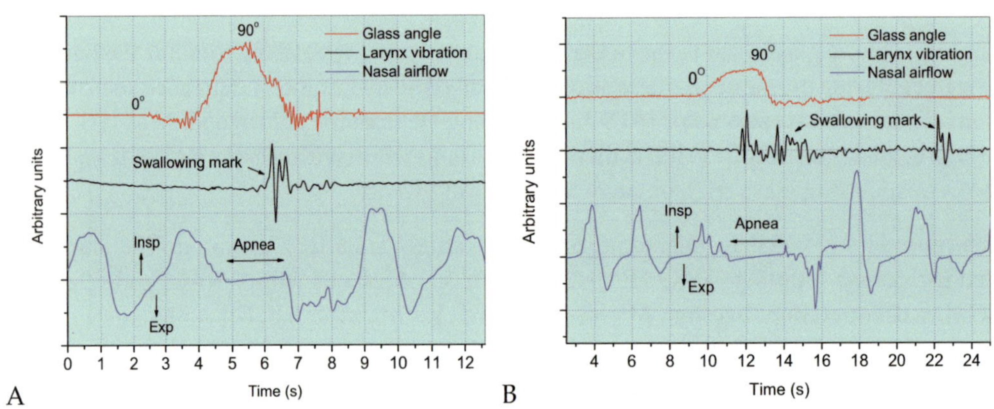

Figure 6. Typical glass angle, larynx mechanical vibration and nasal airflow normal signal morphology during swallowing of 20 mL of water in a normal (A) and a dysphagic patient (B).

As seen in Figure 6A, the movement necessary to drive water into the mouth of the volunteer is described by the increase in the glass angle. When the angle is near 90^0 and water is beginning to enter the mouth of the volunteer, the swallowing apnea begins. The absence of airflow, which can be observed in the end of the inspiration cycle, demarks the beginning of the deglutition process (near 4.8 s). After the beginning of this event, Figure 6A shows the presence of the mechanical vibration signal indicating the action of protective mechanisms including the movement of the larynx-hyoid complex. Note a small delay between water entering the mouth (glass angle = 90^0) and the movement of the larynx-hyoid complex. After a period of approximately 1.5 s, the apnea reaches its end, and an expiration phase is initiated. Meanwhile, the returning of the glass to the initial position is described by a correspondent gradual reduction of the associated signal to zero.

A representative recording in a patient with dysphagia is shown in Figure 3B. Water entering the mouth of the patient (near 11 s) is accompanied by a first swallowing mark (larynx vibration signal) which lasted approximately 4 s. The corresponding apnea period also lasted approximately 4 s. Note that these periods were higher than that presented by the normal volunteer. An important characteristic of this patient is the constant presence of coughing during liquid swallowing. This is related to a clinical history of three cerebral vascular accidents (CVA). This behaviour is in conformity with the hypothesis of an adaptation mechanism in which the patient increases swallowing times to protect itself from aspiration. While similar to the normal subject, the apnea was followed by expiration and a transitory hyperventilation. Figure 3B also shows a second swallowing mark and a second apnea event (≅22s), which was preceded by an expiratory event. This occurs because the patient was not able to swallow all of the 20 mL of water in the first swallowing, therefore, a second swallowing event was necessary. The detailed description presented in Figure 3B confirms the potential of the proposed instrument in the analysis of abnormal swallowing events.

7. Preliminary results of the analysis of swallowing apnea in individuals with chronic obstructive pulmonary disease

This section presents new results concerning the evaluation of swallowing apnea in patients with COPD. This analysis was performed using the instrument described in the previous section. The primary hypothesis is that swallowing apnea in COPD patients is altered during liquid swallowing compared with age-matched healthy subjects.

7.1. Patients and methods

The study included a control group formed by eleven healthy subjects and twelve outpatients with COPD. The volunteers initially were analysed using spirometry and plethysmography [48]. This study was approved by the Ethics Committee of the State University of Rio de Janeiro. Informed consent was obtained from all volunteers before inclusion in the study.

The variables studied were: forced expiratory volume in the first second (FEV1), forced vital capacity (FVC), the ratio of forced expiratory volume to forced vital capacity (FEV1 / FVC), forced expiratory flow between 25 and 75% of the FVC curve (FEF 25-75%), total lung capacity (TLC), functional residual capacity (FRC), residual volume (RV) and the ratio of residual volume and total lung capacity (RV / TLC). The exams were performed by swallowing saliva and water at volumes of 5, 10 and 20 mL. Patients were instructed to swallow each volume three times. Twelve swallows of each patient were studied (276 total swallows).

7.2. Results

Table 2 shows the biometric, spirometric and plethysmographic characteristics of these volunteers. Volunteers in the two groups were comparable considering age, weight and height, showing no statistically significant differences. In general, the pulmonary function parameters were highest in normal subjects and lower in patients.

	Control n=11	COPD n=12	p-value
Age (years)	69.8 ± 6.8	71.3± 6.1	ns
Weight (kg)	69.98 ± 10.3	61.4 ± 17.4	ns
Height (cm)	160.8 ± 9.9	156.9 ± 9.0	ns
IMC (kg/m²)	24.7 ± 5.5	27.0 ± 2.8	ns
FEV_1 (%)	106.8 ± 12.7	69.9 ± 29.7	0.001
FVC (%)	103.9 ± 13.0	95.0 ± 24.1	ns
FEV_1/CVF	81.2 ± 4.00	56.1 ± 16.1	<0.0001
FEF25-75(%)	117.0 ± 24.5	34.3 ± 24.9	<0.0001
TLC (%)	100.7 ± 6.5	114.0 ± 9.4	<0.0001
FRC (%)	86.3 ± 14.1	112.7 ± 2.2	0.003
RV (%)	98.9 ± 14.1	148.5 ± 38.6	<0.0001
RV/TLC	39.9 ± 6.40	52.9 ± 10.8	0.0003

Table 2. Biometric and pulmonary function characteristics of the investigated subjects. Ns: non-significant.

Figure 7 shows that, in contrast with the control subjects (p=ns), the increase of the offered volume resulted in a longer duration of swallowing apnea in patients with COPD (p<0.05).

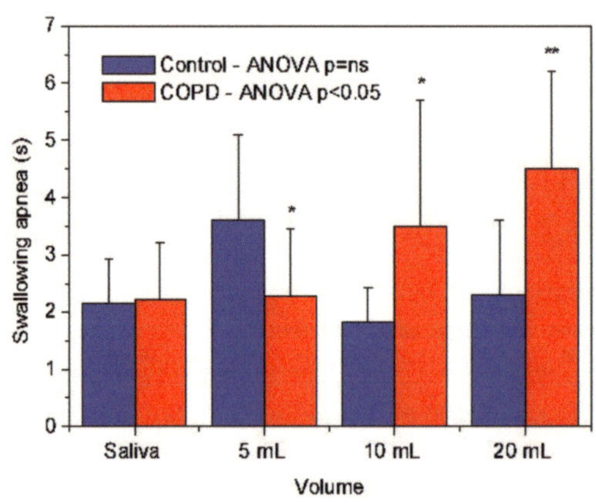

Figure 7. Time interval of swallowing apnea in healthy subjects and patients with COPD for different volumes of water. * p < 0.02; ** p < 0.002 in comparison with the control group.

The COPD patients had longer swallowing apnea with volumes of 10 mL ($p<0.02$) and 20 mL ($p<0.002$). A higher number of swallows in the pattern of inspiration-apnea-inspiration was observed in the COPD group, especially in the volumes of 10 and 20 mL (Figure 8).

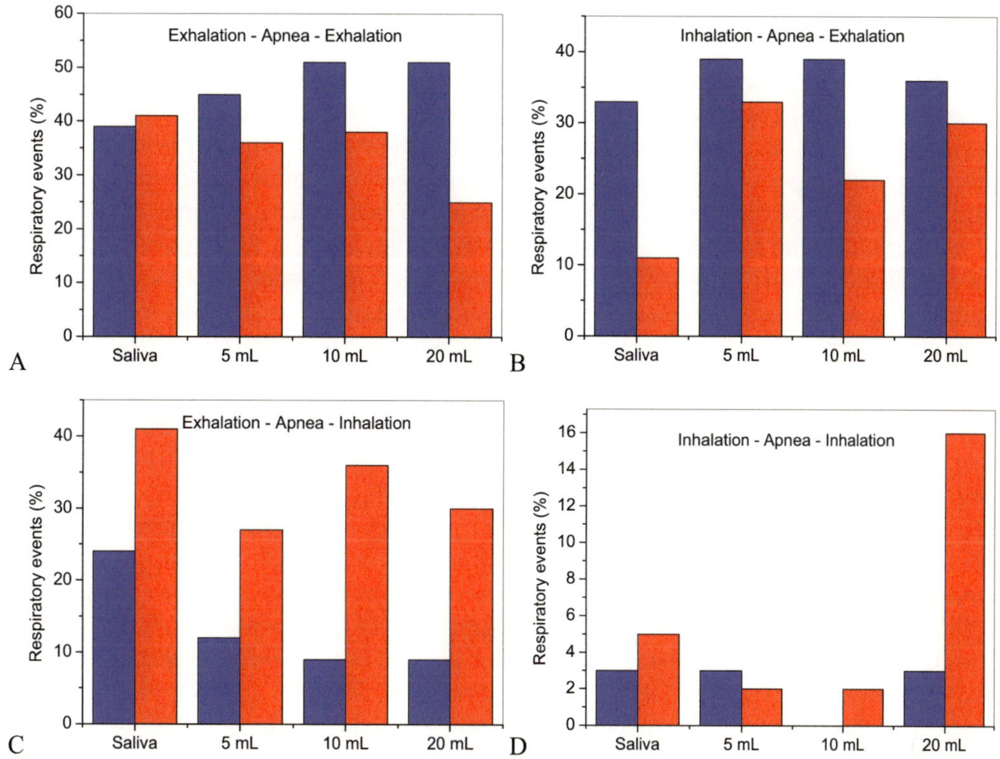

Figure 8. Percentage of exhalation-apnea-exhalation (A), inhalation-apnea-exhalation (B), exhalation-apnea-inhalation (C) and inhalation-apnea-inhalation (D) events in healthy (blue) and COPD patients (red) for different water volumes. 276 swallows were studied.

7.3. Discussion

Leslie et al. [49] suggested that the apnea time significantly increases with volume in normal elderly subjects. In contrast, Esteves and colleagues [24] found no increase in apnea time and swallowing with volume in normal young subjects. In the results described in Figure 7, the increase in volume did not result in increased swallowing apnea time in elderly individuals. Note that, in the volume of 5 ml, individuals of the control group had significantly longer apnea times than that observed in the swallowing of saliva, 10 and 20 mL of water ($p<0.02$). This result may be related to the relatively small number of individuals analysed.

In contrast with that observed in normal volunteers, the presence of COPD resulted in increased apnea time with the bolus volume (Figure 7). We can also observe that patients with COPD had apnea times significantly higher during conditions of higher volume (10 mL and

20 mL). These findings disagree with those described in the study by Gross [38], which observed no difference in apnea time between the COPD and control group. These authors note, however, that in the swallows of COPD patients in which apnea occurred in inspiration time, the apnea interval was longer. Physiologically, the presence of longer periods of apnea in COPD could indicate a compensatory mechanism for airway protection against aspiration of food residuals.

The control group presented an increased number of swallows in the standard-expiration apnea-expiration (EE) pattern in all studied volumes (Figure 8). This is in close agreement with previous studies [9, 20, 22, 50]. This finding supports the theory that swallowing during the expiratory phase represents less risk of aspiration and therefore may be considered a protective mechanism of the airways. Swallowing during the inspiratory phase may facilitate the entry of food and saliva into the airways during and after swallowing [22]. Other patterns were also observed in this group. In order of increasing frequency: inspiration-apnea-expiration (IE), expiration-apnea-inspiration (EI), and inspiration-apnea-inspiration (II). This result is consistent with that reported by Martin-Harris [22]. The pattern II presented the smallest frequency in all volumes, which agrees with previous results [9, 20, 22].

COPD patients more frequently showed the EE and EI patterns (Figure 8). Similar findings were reported in the study conducted by Cjevic [2]. The pattern II occurred less frequently compared with other patterns. Comparing the swallowing of COPD patients with control subjects, it can be observed that the pattern EI (Figure 8C) occurs more frequently in COPD patients compared to control subjects. This phenomenon was observed in all studied volumes. Considering the pattern II (Figure 8D), we observe that this also occurs more frequently in COPD, particularly in exams using 20 mL. In agreement with the present work, the study by Gross [38] describes that patients with COPD had pre and post inspiration swallowing apnea more often than the control subjects. These results are consistent with the observation that the inspiration after swallowing facilitates aspiration of food and saliva.

8. Conclusions

This chapter initially provided a brief overview of dysphagia, coordination of breathing and swallowing, and COPD. This was followed by a historical review that described the research through the decades on swallowing in COPD. In addition to these previous studies, new results were presented. This analysis provides evidence that (1) the apnea interval increases with the swallowed volume in COPD; (2) COPD patients had higher swallowing apnea time compared to controls in larger volumes; (3) the occurrence of inspiratory patterns after swallowing increases in COPD, which may facilitate the occurrence of aspiration in these patients, and (4) the prototype that was described in section 6 is suitable for clinical studies.

Routine clinical evaluation of swallowing disorders in COPD has yet to gain full acceptance, but the evidence of the importance of these analyses is growing fast. The results of the present study, together with the results described in the historical review, provide additional evidence that patients with COPD might present modifications in deglutition and a specialized evaluation is necessary for safe deglutition, especially in case of acute exacerbation.

Acknowledgements

The authors would like to thank the Brazilian Council of Research and Development (CNPq), the Rio de Janeiro State Foundation for Research (FAPERJ), and the Rio de Janeiro State University – PROCIÊNCIA Program for research grants.

Author details

Livia Scelza[1,2], Catiuscia S.S. Greco[1,2], Agnaldo J. Lopes[3] and Pedro Lopes de Melo[1,4*]

*Address all correspondence to: plopeslib@gmail.com

1 Biomedical Instrumentation Laboratory, Institute of Biology and Faculty of Engineering, Rio de Janeiro/RJ, Brazil

2 State University of Rio de Janeiro, Brazil

3 Pulmonary Function Laboratory, Pedro Ernesto University Hospital, Rio de Janeiro/RJ, Brazil

4 Clinical and Experimental Research Laboratory in Vascular Biology, Institute of Biology, State University of Rio de Janeiro, Pavilhão Haroldo Lisboa da Cunha, Sala 104, Maracanã, Rio de Janeiro/RJ, Brazil

References

[1] B. Martin-Harris, "Clinical implications of respiratory-swallowing interactions," *Curr Opin Otolaryngol Head Neck Surg,* vol. 16, pp. 194-9, Jun 2008.

[2] L. Cvejic, R. Harding, T. Churchward, A. Turton, P. Finlay, D. Massey, *et al.*, "Laryngeal penetration and aspiration in individuals with stable COPD," *Respirology,* vol. 16, pp. 269-75, Feb 2011.

[3] R. D. Gross, C. W. Atwood, Jr., S. B. Ross, J. W. Olszewski, and K. A. Eichhorn, "The coordination of breathing and swallowing in chronic obstructive pulmonary disease," *Am J Respir Crit Care Med,* vol. 179, pp. 559-65, Apr 1 2009.

[4] Gold, "Global Strategy for The Diagnosis, Management, And Prevention of Chronic Obstructive Pulmonary Disease (Revised 2013)," *Global Initiative for Chronic Obstrutive Lung Disease,* 2013.

[5] C. D. Mathers and D. Loncar, "Projections of global mortality and burden of disease from 2002 to 2030," *PLoS Med,* vol. 3, p. e442, Nov 2006.

[6] W. H. O.-. WHO, "Burden of COPD. Available form: <http:// http://www.who.int/respiratory/copd/burden/en/>," 2012.

[7] D. Chaves Rde, C. R. Carvalho, A. Cukier, R. Stelmach, and C. R. Andrade, "Symptoms of dysphagia in patients with COPD," *J Bras Pneumol,* vol. 37, pp. 176-83, Mar-Apr 2011.

[8] B. Singh, "Impaired swallow in COPD," *Respirology,* vol. 16, pp. 185-6, Feb 2011.

[9] H. G. Preiksaitis, S. Mayrand, K. Robins, and N. E. Diamant, "Coordination of respiration and swallowing: effect of bolus volume in normal adults," *Am J Physiol,* vol. 263, pp. R624-30, Sep 1992.

[10] C. Ertekin and I. Aydogdu, "Neurophysiology of swallowing," *Clin Neurophysiol,* vol. 114, pp. 2226-44, Dec 2003.

[11] B. K. Medda, M. Kern, J. Ren, P. Xie, S. O. Ulualp, I. M. Lang, *et al.*, "Relative contribution of various airway protective mechanisms to prevention of aspiration during swallowing," *Am J Physiol Gastrointest Liver Physiol,* vol. 284, pp. G933-9, Jun 2003.

[12] J. A. Logemann, P. J. Kahrilas, J. Cheng, B. R. Pauloski, P. J. Gibbons, A. W. Rademaker, *et al.*, "Closure mechanisms of laryngeal vestibule during swallow," *Am J Physiol,* vol. 262, pp. G338-44, Feb 1992.

[13] N. P. Reddy, R. Thomas, E. P. Canilang, and J. Casterline, "Toward classification of dysphagic patients using biomechanical measurements," *J Rehabil Res Dev,* vol. 31, pp. 335-44, Nov 1994.

[14] T. S. Dozier, M. B. Brodsky, Y. Michel, B. C. Walters, Jr., and B. Martin-Harris, "Coordination of swallowing and respiration in normal sequential cup swallows," *Laryngoscope,* vol. 116, pp. 1489-93, Aug 2006.

[15] S. M. Molfenter and C. M. Steele, "Physiological variability in the deglutition literature: hyoid and laryngeal kinematics," *Dysphagia,* vol. 26, pp. 67-74, Mar 2011.

[16] A. Jean, "Brain stem control of swallowing: neuronal network and cellular mechanisms," *Physiol Rev,* vol. 81, pp. 929-69, Apr 2001.

[17] M. M. Costa and E. M. Lemme, "Coordination of respiration and swallowing: functional pattern and relevance of vocal folds closure," *Arq Gastroenterol,* vol. 47, pp. 42-8, Jan-Mar 2010.

[18] W. G. Selley, F. C. Flack, R. E. Ellis, and W. A. Brooks, "Respiratory patterns associated with swallowing: Part 1. The normal adult pattern and changes with age," *Age Ageing,* vol. 18, pp. 168-72, May 1989.

[19] H. G. Preiksaitis and C. A. Mills, "Coordination of breathing and swallowing: effects of bolus consistency and presentation in normal adults," *J Appl Physiol (1985),* vol. 81, pp. 1707-14, Oct 1996.

[20] J. Smith, N. Wolkove, A. Colacone, and H. Kreisman, "Coordination of eating, drinking and breathing in adults," *Chest,* vol. 96, pp. 578-82, Sep 1989.

[21] B. J. Martin, J. A. Logemann, R. Shaker, and W. J. Dodds, "Coordination between respiration and swallowing: respiratory phase relationships and temporal integration," *J Appl Physiol (1985),* vol. 76, pp. 714-23, Feb 1994.

[22] B. Martin-Harris, M. B. Brodsky, Y. Michel, C. L. Ford, B. Walters, and J. Heffner, "Breathing and swallowing dynamics across the adult lifespan," *Arch Otolaryngol Head Neck Surg,* vol. 131, pp. 762-70, Sep 2005.

[23] M. S. Klahn and A. L. Perlman, "Temporal and durational patterns associating respiration and swallowing," *Dysphagia,* vol. 14, pp. 131-8, Summer 1999.

[24] G. P. Esteves, E. P. Silva Junior, L. G. Nunes, C. S. Greco, and P. L. Melo, "Configurable portable/ambulatory instrument for the analysis of the coordination between respiration and swallowing," *Conf Proc IEEE Eng Med Biol Soc,* vol. 2010, pp. 90-3, 2010.

[25] A. I. Hardemark Cedborg, K. Boden, H. Witt Hedstrom, R. Kuylenstierna, O. Ekberg, L. I. Eriksson, *et al.*, "Breathing and swallowing in normal man--effects of changes in body position, bolus types, and respiratory drive," *Neurogastroenterol Motil,* vol. 22, pp. 1201-8, e316, Nov 2010.

[26] L. J. Hirst, G. A. Ford, G. J. Gibson, and J. A. Wilson, "Swallow-induced alterations in breathing in normal older people," *Dysphagia,* vol. 17, pp. 152-61, Spring 2002.

[27] J. Vestbo, S. S. Hurd, A. G. Agusti, P. W. Jones, C. Vogelmeier, A. Anzueto, *et al.*, "Global strategy for the diagnosis, management, and prevention of chronic obstructive pulmonary disease: GOLD executive summary," *Am J Respir Crit Care Med,* vol. 187, pp. 347-65, Feb 15 2013.

[28] E. W. Russi, W. Karrer, M. Brutsche, C. Eich, J. W. Fitting, M. Frey, *et al.*, "Diagnosis and management of chronic obstructive pulmonary disease: the Swiss guidelines. Official guidelines of the Swiss Respiratory Society," *Respiration,* vol. 85, pp. 160-74, 2013.

[29] ATS/ERS. (2004, 10-09-2014). American Thoracic Society/European Respiratory Society Standards for diagnosis and management of patients with COPD.

[30] C. A. Coelho, "Preliminary findings on the nature of dysphagia in patients with chronic obstructive pulmonary disease," *Dysphagia,* vol. 2, pp. 28-31, 1987.

[31] M. Stein, A. J. Williams, F. Grossman, A. S. Weinberg, and L. Zuckerbraun, "Cricopharyngeal dysfunction in chronic obstructive pulmonary disease," *Chest,* vol. 97, pp. 347-52, Feb 1990.

[32] R. Shaker, Q. Li, J. Ren, W. F. Townsend, W. J. Dodds, B. J. Martin, *et al.*, "Coordination of deglutition and phases of respiration: effect of aging, tachypnea, bolus vol-

ume, and chronic obstructive pulmonary disease," *Am J Physiol,* vol. 263, pp. G750-5, Nov 1992.

[33] M. D. Good-Fratturelli, R. F. Curlee, and J. L. Holle, "Prevalence and nature of dysphagia in VA patients with COPD referred for videofluoroscopic swallow examination," *J Commun Disord,* vol. 33, pp. 93-110, Mar-Apr 2000.

[34] B. Martin-Harris, "Optimal patterns of care in patients with chronic obstructive pulmonary disease," *Semin Speech Lang,* vol. 21, pp. 311-21; quiz 320-1, 2000.

[35] B. Mokhlesi, J. A. Logemann, A. W. Rademaker, C. A. Stangl, and T. C. Corbridge, "Oropharyngeal deglutition in stable COPD," *Chest,* vol. 121, pp. 361-9, Feb 2002.

[36] B. Mokhlesi, "Clinical implications of gastroesophageal reflux disease and swallowing dysfunction in COPD," *Am J Respir Med,* vol. 2, pp. 117-21, 2003.

[37] S. Kobayashi, H. Kubo, and M. Yanai, "Impairment of the swallowing reflex in exacerbations of COPD," *Thorax,* vol. 62, p. 1017, Nov 2007.

[38] R. D. Gross, C. W. Atwood, S. B. Ross, J. W. Olszewski, and K. A. Eichhorn, "The Coordination of Breathing and Swallowing in Chronic Obstructive Pulmonary Disease," *American Journal of Respiratory and Critical Care Medicine,* vol. 179, pp. 559-565, Apr 1 2009.

[39] K. Ohta, K. Murata, T. Takahashi, S. Minatani, S. Sako, and Y. Kanada, "Evaluation of swallowing function by two screening tests in primary COPD," *Eur Respir J,* vol. 34, pp. 280-1, Jul 2009.

[40] K. Terada, S. Muro, T. Ohara, M. Kudo, E. Ogawa, Y. Hoshino, *et al.*, "Abnormal swallowing reflex and COPD exacerbations," *Chest,* vol. 137, pp. 326-32, Feb 2010.

[41] A. McKinstry, M. Tranter, and J. Sweeney, "Outcomes of dysphagia intervention in a pulmonary rehabilitation program," *Dysphagia,* vol. 25, pp. 104-11, Jun 2010.

[42] S. Kobayashi, M. Hanagama, M. Yanai, and H. Kubo, "Prevention of chronic obstructive pulmonary disease exacerbation by angiotensin-converting enzyme inhibitors in individuals with impaired swallowing," *J Am Geriatr Soc,* vol. 59, pp. 1967-8, Oct 2011.

[43] A. Tsuzuki, H. Kagaya, H. Takahashi, T. Watanabe, T. Shioya, H. Sakakibara, *et al.*, "Dysphagia causes exacerbations in individuals with chronic obstructive pulmonary disease," *J Am Geriatr Soc,* vol. 60, pp. 1580-2, Aug 2012.

[44] N. A. Clayton, G. D. Carnaby-Mann, M. J. Peters, and A. J. Ing, "The effect of chronic obstructive pulmonary disease on laryngopharyngeal sensitivity," *Ear Nose Throat J,* vol. 91, pp. 370, 372, 374 passim, Sep 2012.

[45] N. Terzi, H. Normand, E. Dumanowski, M. Ramakers, A. Seguin, C. Daubin, *et al.*, "Noninvasive ventilation and breathing-swallowing interplay in chronic obstructive pulmonary disease*," *Crit Care Med,* vol. 42, pp. 565-73, Mar 2014.

[46] R. de Deus Chaves, F. Chiarion Sassi, L. Davison Mangilli, S. K. Jayanthi, A. Cukier, B. Zilberstein, *et al.*, "Swallowing transit times and valleculae residue in stable chronic obstructive pulmonary disease," *BMC Pulm Med,* vol. 14, p. 62, 2014.

[47] C. S. Souza, J. A. Junior, and P. L. Melo, "A novel system using the Forced Oscillations Technique for the biomechanical analysis of swallowing," *Technol Health Care,* vol. 16, pp. 331-41, 2008.

[48] SBPT, "Diretrizes para Testes de Função Pulmonar," *J Bras Pneumol,* vol. 28, 2002.

[49] P. Leslie, M. J. Drinnan, G. A. Ford, and J. A. Wilson, "Swallow respiratory patterns and aging: presbyphagia or dysphagia?," *J Gerontol A Biol Sci Med Sci,* vol. 60, pp. 391-5, Mar 2005.

[50] A. I. H. Cedborg, K. Boden, H. W. Hedstrom, R. Kuylenstierna, O. Ekberg, L. I. Eriksson, *et al.*, "Breathing and swallowing in normal man - effects of changes in body position, bolus types, and respiratory drive," Neurogastroenterology and Motility, vol. 22, pp. 1201-+, Nov 2010.

Chapter 13

Histopathological Change of Esophagus Related to Dysphagia in Mixed Connective Tissue Disease

Akihisa Kamataki, Miwa Uzuki and Takashi Sawai

Additional information is available at the end of the chapter

http://dx.doi.org/10.5772/60509

1. Introduction

Dysphagia is one of the symptoms in patients with connective tissue diseases (CTDs), although it is not directly fatal and is a frequent complication. The frequency of esophageal dysmotility is 46-92%, 30-88%, 21-72%, and 50% in patients with systemic sclerosis (SSc), mixed connective tissue disease (MCTD), systemic lupus erythematosis (SLE), and polymyositis/dermatomyositis (PM/DM), respectively [1-8]. While the cause of esophageal dysfunction in patients with CTDs has been unclear, there are some reports that suggest the accumulation of extracellular matrix, neuropathy, and autoantibody as the cause of esophageal dysfunction in patients with SSc [9-11]. On the other hand, there are few reports relating to the cause of esophageal dysfunction in MCTD patients, despite its frequency. Therefore, we examined the histopathological characteristics of esophageal lesions in MCTD patients using 27 autopsy cases in Japan [12].

2. Histopathological analysis of esophagus in MCTD patients

2.1. Comparison between changes in the upper, middle, and lower portion of the esophagus.

To date, there have been studies demonstrating a high frequency of esophageal symptoms in patients with MCTD [1-7,13] (Table 1). In our study, evidence of histological changes was found in 25 of the 27 cases examined (91%). The differences may be due to differences in the method of measurement. Esophageal dysmotility in MCTD patients is sometimes associated with the dilatation of the distal esophagus (Figure 1). The main sites of esophageal change were generally different between CTDs [8]. In patients with SSc and MCTD, the lower portion of the esophagus changes histologically. Therefore, we examined 3 different regions of the esophagus, which we defined as follows: 1) upper, at the height of the ring around the cartilage of the trachea; 2) middle, at the height of the bifurcation of the trachea; and 3) lower, just above the esophago-cardiac junction. We compared histological changes for each portion. Of 12 cases examined, 9 showed slight to severe changes in the lower portion, 3 showed slight to severe changes in the middle portion, and none showed histopathological changes in the upper portion. According to these results, the lower portion was involved in many cases of MCTD.

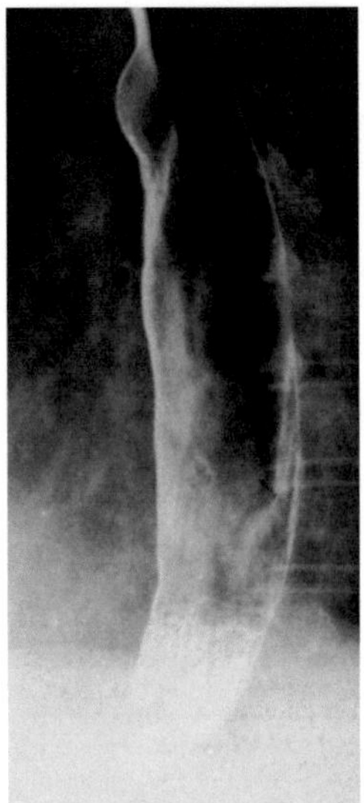

Figure 1. X-ray photograph of esophagus in MCTD patients.

Symptoms and dysmotility	Actual number (Frequency)	Reference
Abnormal esophageal motility	8/17 (47.1%)	Bennett (1980) [1]
Esophageal symptoms	11/17 (64.7 %)	Gutierrez (1982) [2]
• Heartburn	10/17 (58.8%)	
• Regurgitation	6/17 (35.3%)	
• Dysphagia	1/17 (5.9%)	
Abnormal esophageal motility	14/17 (82.4%)	
Esophageal symptoms		Dantas (1985) [3]
• Dysphagia	6/12 (50%)	
Abnormal esophageal motility	6/12 (50%)	
Esophageal symptoms		Marshall (1990) [4]
• Heartburn or regurgitation	29/61 (47.5%)	
• Dysphagia	23/61 (37.7%)	
Abnormal esophageal motility	21/35 (60.0%)	
Esophageal symptoms	14/21 (66.6%)	Doria (1991) [5]
• Heartburn	5/21 (23.8%)	

Symptoms and dysmotility	Actual number (Frequency)	Reference
• Regurgitation	5/21 (23.8%)	
• Dysphagia	4/21(19.0%)	
Abnormal esophageal motility	15/21 (71.4%)	
Abnormal esophageal motility	15/17 (88.2%)	Lapadula (1994) [6]
Abnormal esophageal motility	10/18 (55.6%)	Rayes (2002) [7]
Esophageal symptoms		Calerio (2006) [15]
• Heartburn	9/24 (37.5%)	
• Dysphagia	18/24 (75%)	
Abnormal esophageal motility (cine-esophogram)	23/24 (95.8%)	

Table 1. The frequency of esophageal involvement in patients with mixed connective tissue disease.

2.2. Comparison between changes in the inner circular muscular layer and outer longitudinal muscular layer of the esophagus

As regards histological changes in the muscular layers, the inner circular muscular layer (IM) exhibited more severe changes than the outer longitudinal muscular layer (OM) in 17 of 27 cases (63%). Eight cases (30%) showed similar changes. Two cases (7%) showed no pathological changes in either IM or OM, and no cases (0%) showed more severe involvement of OM than IM. Muscular dynamisms of IM and OM in esophageal motility are different. The IM is fairly active and subject to greater stress than the OM [14]. Furthermore, esophageal regurgitation often occurs and exerts direct effects on the IM, particularly in the lower esophagus. Thus the IM in the lower portion may carry a larger physical stress than the OM. Therefore, more severe histological changes may occur in the IM of the lower portion than in the OM.

2.3. Cellular and tissue change

In our study, the most striking change of the esophagus in MCTD was severe atrophy and occasional disappearance of muscular fibers followed by fibrosis in muscular layer (Figure 2). In contrast to smooth muscle, however, striated muscle of the upper esophageal portion exhibited no marked changes. Similar histopathological changes occur in SSc [15,16]. In SSc patients, histological features are also characterized by degeneration and disappearance of smooth muscle cells with fibrosis, especially in the IM of the lower portion [17]. In our study, ganglionic cells had not decreased in number and were not particularly atrophic except in severely fibrotic areas. Vascular changes were also not overly severe in non-fibrotic regions, although slight intimal thickening of small vessels was sporadically found in the fibrotic area. The vein wall was injured and smooth muscle cell disruption and inflammatory cell invasion were observed (Figure 3).

2.4. Pathogenesis of esophageal lesions

The factors that seem to be associated with esophageal dysfunction have been reported in some studies, and include extracellular matrix degradation, disorder of blood circulation, and

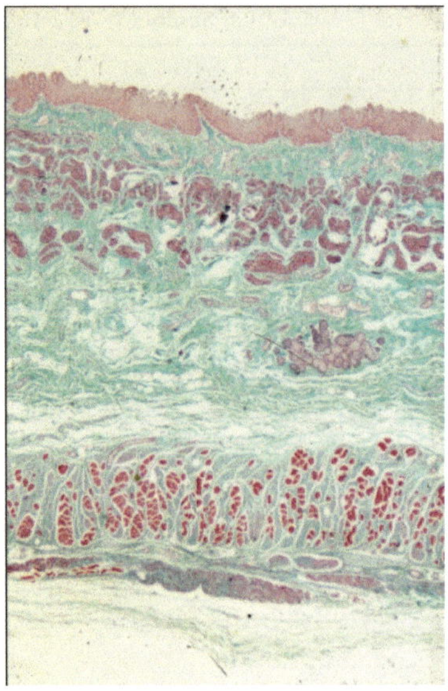

Figure 2. Esophageal muscle degeneration and fibrosis in MCTD patients.

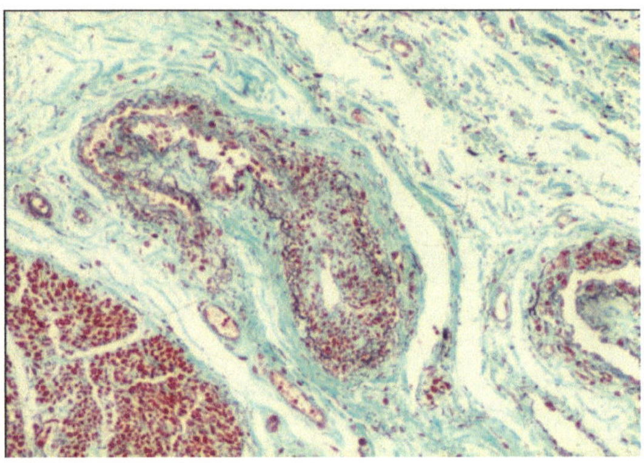

Figure 3. Vascular changes in the esophagus of MCTD patients.

autoantibodies [10,18-20]. Our hypothesis was that autoantibodies are associated with the pathogenesis of esophageal lesions. In immunohistochemical studies, anti-human IgG and anti-C3 antibodies reacted positively with muscle tissues showing a myolytic appearance accompanied by edema and inflammatory cell infiltration in MCTD autopsy case (Figures 4). No IgM deposition was found (Figure 4). The reactivity of IgG extracted from sera of MCTD patients against normal esophageal tissues was then assessed. Esophageal tissues used here were non-cancerous parts taken intraoperatively from esophageal cancer patients without specific immunological disorder. The IgG reacted with smooth muscle cells in the muscularis mucosa, muscular layer and venous wall, the ganglion cells in Auerbach's plexus, and squamous epithelium of the esophagus (Figure 5), but did not react with striated muscle in upper portion (Figure 5 A,B). IgG from MCTD patients also reacted with primary-cultured smooth muscle cells prepared from surgical specimens of esophagus (unpublished data) (Figure 6). These results suggested that antibodies in the serum of patients with MCTD attack smooth muscle tissues as well as other tissues of the esophagus.

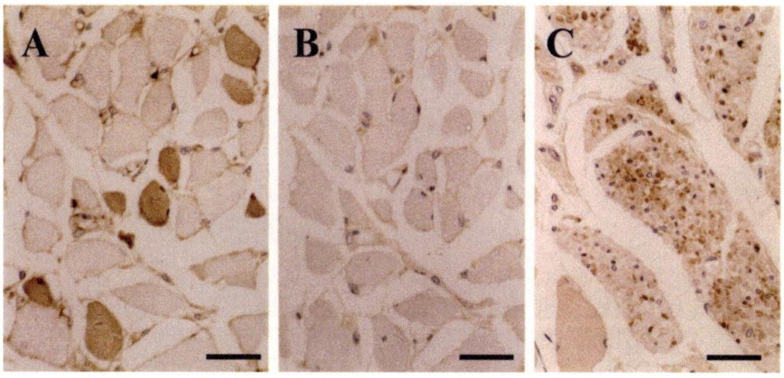

Figure 4. Immunoglobulin and complement deposition in the muscular layer of the esophagus from MCTD patients. Deposition of IgG (A), IgM (B), and complement C3 (C).

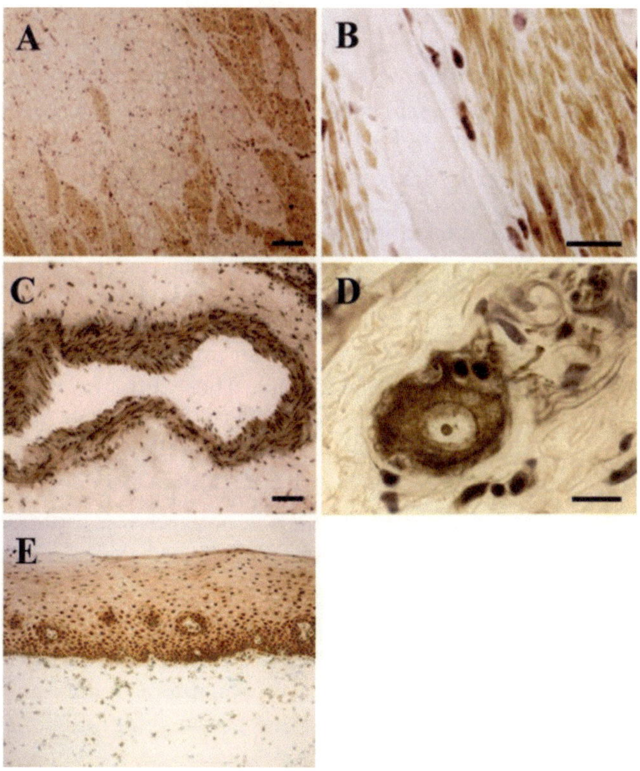

Figure 5. Reaction of IgG from MCTD patients with smooth muscles and other cells composing the esophagus. (A) Esophageal smooth muscle tissue, (B) Higher magnification of esophageal smooth muscle tissue, (C) Medial smooth muscle of the venous wall, (D) Ganglionic cell in Auerbach's plexus, (E) Squamous epithelium of esophagus

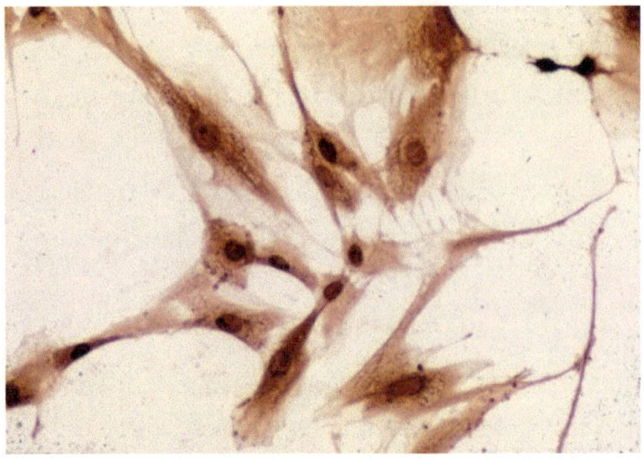

Figure 6. Reaction of IgG from MCTD patients with primary-cultured smooth muscle cells from esophagus.

3. Discussion

Histopathological features of the esophagus in SSc and MCTD patients are similar, but muscular change in SSc is more progressive than in MCTD patients in our study. It has been suggested that there is no association between manometric abnormality and cutaneous symptoms in MCTD patients, and the characteristics of SSc are not always linked to esophageal dysfunction [5]. The pathological mechanism of esophageal dysfunction in MCTD may be similar but not always identical to that in SSc.

In patients with CTDs, autoimmune inflammation occurs in systemic organs such as kidney, lung, skin and blood vessels, and so on. The gastrointestinal tract is also involved though the histological features and grades are different from disease to disease even in the same CTD.

In CTDs, many kinds of autoantibodies may play an important role in causing the various symptoms and diseases, whether they are fatal or not. These differ from disease to disease and from tissue to tissue. We showed that IgG from MCTD patients reacts to various tissues such as kidney and lung (unpublished data) (Figure 7). It is well known that pulmonary hypertension is the fatal cause of MCTD. Anti-endothelial cell antibody (AECA) was identified in the serum of MCTD patients, and was especially high in patients with pulmonary hypertension [21]. We now examine the antigen of AECA in endothelial cells of small pulmonary vascular vessels [22]. As for the autoantibody of MCTD against esophagus, our study revealed that IgG extracted from MCTD patients showed a positive immunohistochemical reaction not only for the smooth muscle cells of esophagus, but also for the ganglion cells in Auerbach's plexus, the vascular walls in esophageal muscular tissues, and squamous epithelium of the esophagus. Dysphagia in MCTD and SSc patients may be one of the symptoms often occurring as an autoimmune reaction.

The reason why the inner layer of the lower portion incurs more severe damage than other portions has not been clarified. Esophageal manometry shows that this portion sustains more intense mechanical stress in peristalsis than the outer layer or upper portions. Thus autoantibodies, mechanical stress and regurgitation may induce the severe dysphagia in MCTD and other CTDs.

Motility dysfunction is not a direct cause of death, but a strong association between esophageal dysmotility and interstitial lung disease in patients with MCTD is indicated [23]. Therefore, care must be taken with diagnosis.

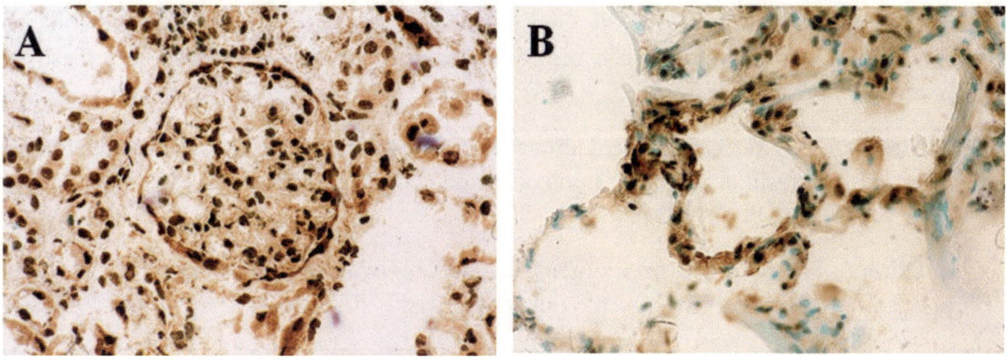

Figure 7. Reaction of IgG from MCTD patients with various tissues. (A) kidney, (B) lung

Acknowledgements

This research was partly supported by a Grant-in-Aid for Scientific Research from the Ministry of Health, Labour and Welfare of Japan.

Author details

Akihisa Kamataki[1], Miwa Uzuki[2] and Takashi Sawai[3,4*]

*Address all correspondence to: sawai@wonder.ocn.ne.jp

1 Department of Pathology, Iwate Medical University, Shiwa, Japan

2 Department of Nursing, Tohoku Bunka Gakuen University, Sendai, Japan

3 Department of Pathology, Tohoku University, Sendai, Japan

4 Department of Pathology, Sendai Open Hospital, Sendai, Japan

References

[1] Bennett RM, O'Connell DJ. Mixed connective tissue disease: a clinicopathologic study of 20 cases. Semin Arthritis Rheum. 1980;10(1):25-51.

[2] Gutierrez F, Valenzuela JE, Ehresmann GR, Quismorio FP, Kitridou RC. Esophageal dysfunction in patients with mixed connective tissue diseases and systemic lupus erythematosus. Dig Dis Sci. 1982;27(7):592-7.

[3] Dantas RO, Villanova MG, de Godoy RA. Esophageal dysfunction in patients with progressive systemic sclerosis and mixed connective tissue diseases. Arq Gastroenterol. 1985;22(3):122-6.

[4] Marshall JB, Kretschmar JM, Gerhardt DC, Winship DH, Winn D, Treadwell EL, et al. Gastrointestinal manifestations of mixed connective tissue disease. Gastroenterology. 1990;98(5 Pt 1):1232-8.

[5] Doria A, Bonavina L, Anselmino M, Ruffatti A, Favaretto M, Gambari P, et al. Esophageal involvement in mixed connective tissue disease. J Rheumatol. 1991;18(5): 685-90.

[6] Lapadula G, Muolo P, Semeraro F, Covelli M, Brindicci D, Cuccorese G, et al. Esophageal motility disorders in the rheumatic diseases: a review of 150 patients. Clin Exp Rheumatol. 1994 Sep-Oct;12(5):515-21.

[7] Rayes HA, Al-Sheikh A, Al Dalaan A, Al Saleh S. Mixed connective tissue disease: the King Faisal Specialist Hospital experience. Ann Saudi Med. 2002;22(1-2):43-6.

[8] Sheehan NJ. Dysphagia and other manifestations of oesophageal involvement in the musculoskeletal diseases. Rheumatology (Oxford). 2008;47(6):746-52.

[9] Hendel L, Ammitzbøll T, Dirksen K, Petri M. Collagen in the esophageal mucosa of patients with progressive systemic sclerosis (PSS). Acta Derm Venereol. 1984;64(6): 480-4.

[10] Stacher G, Merio R, Budka C, Schneider C, Smolen J, Tappeiner G. Cardiovascular autonomic function, autoantibodies, and esophageal motor activity in patients with systemic sclerosis and mixed connective tissue disease. J Rheumatol. 2000 Mar;27(3): 692-7.

[11] Zuber-Jerger I, Müller A, Kullmann F, Gelbmann CM, Endlicher E, Müller-Ladner U, et al. Gastrointestinal manifestation of systemic sclerosis--thickening of the upper gastrointestinal wall detected by endoscopic ultrasound is a valid sign. Rheumatology (Oxford). 2010;49(2):368-72.

[12] Uzuki M, Kamataki A, Watanabe M, Sasaki N, Miura Y, Sawai T. Histological analysis of esophageal muscular layers from 27 autopsy cases with mixed connective tissue disease (MCTD). Pathol Res Pract. 2011;207(6):383-90.

[13] Caleiro MT, Lage LV, Navarro-Rodriguez T, Bresser A, da Costa PA, Yoshinari NH. Radionuclide imaging for the assessment of esophageal motility disorders in mixed connective tissue disease patients: relation to pulmonary impairment. Dis Esophagus. 2006;19(5):394-400.

[14] Bansal A, Kahrilas PJ. Has high-resolution manometry changed the approach to esophageal motility disorders? Curr Opin Gastroenterol. 2010;26(4):344-51.

[15] Reynolds TB, Denison EK, Frankl HD, Lieberman FL, Peters RL. Primary biliary cirrhosis with scleroderma, Raynaud's phenomenon and telangiectasia. New syndrome. Am J Med. 1971;50(3):302-12.

[16] Rohrmann CA Jr, Ricci MT, Krishnamurthy S, Schuffler MD. Radiologic and histologic differentiation of neuromuscular disorders of the gastrointestinal tract: visceral myopathies, visceral neuropathies, and progressive systemic sclerosis. AJR Am J Roentgenol. 1984;143(5):933-41.

[17] Schneider HA, Yonker RA, Longley S, Katz P, Mathias J, Panush RS. Scleroderma esophagus: a nonspecific entity. Ann Intern Med. 1984;100(6):848-50.

[18] Jinnin M, Ihn H, Yamane K, Asano Y, Yazawa N, Tamaki K. Serum levels of tissue inhibitor of metalloproteinases in patients with mixed connective tissue disease. Clin Exp Rheumatol. 2002;20(4):539-42.

[19] Flick JA, Boyle JT, Tuchman DN, Athreya BH, Doughty RA. Esophageal motor abnormalities in children and adolescents with scleroderma and mixed connective tissue disease. Pediatrics. 1988;82(1):107-11

[20] Takeda Y, Wang GS, Wang RJ, Anderson SK, Pettersson I, Amaki S, et al. Enzyme-linked immunosorbent assay using isolated (U) small nuclear ribonucleoprotein polypeptides as antigens to investigate the clinical significance of autoantibodies to these polypeptides. Clin Immunol Immunopathol. 1989;50(2):213-30.

[21] Sasaki N, Kurose A, Inoue H, Sawai T. A possible role of anti-endothelial cell antibody in the sera of MCTD patients on pulmonary vascular damage relating to pulmonary hypertension. Ryumachi. 2002;42(6):885-94.

[22] Kamataki A, Sasaki N, Hatakeyama A, Sawai T. Analysis of the serum reactivity against possible target proteins for anti-endotheial cell antibodies from sera of mixed connective tissue disease patients with pulmonary hypertension. Arth Rheum. 2007;56(9): S643

[23] Fagundes MN, Caleiro MT, Navarro-Rodriguez T, Baldi BG, Kavakama J, Salge JM, et al. Esophageal involvement and interstitial lung disease in mixed connective tissue disease. Respir Med. 2009;103(6):854-60.